Recovery from Brain Damage
RESEARCH AND THEORY

Recovery from Brain Damage
RESEARCH AND THEORY

Edited by
STANLEY FINGER
Washington University
St. Louis, Missouri

PLENUM PRESS • NEW YORK AND LONDON

Library of Congress Cataloging in Publication Data

Main entry under title:

Recovery from brain damage.

   Includes bibliographies and index.
   1. Brain damage. 2. Neuropsychology. 3. Diseases—Animal models. I.
Finger, Stanley.
RC386.2.R4   616.8   77-27585
ISBN 0-306-31107-0

© 1978 Plenum Press, New York
A Division of Plenum Publishing Corporation
227 West 17th Street, New York, N.Y. 10011

Printed in the United States of America

Contributors

C. Robert Almli
Department of Psychology
Ohio University
Athens, Ohio 45701

Arthur Benton
Departments of Neurology and
    Psychology
University of Iowa
Iowa City, Iowa 52242

J. Jay Braun
Department of Psychology
Arizona State University
Tempe, Arizona 85281

George E. Corrick
Department of Psychology
Indiana University
Bloomington, Indiana 47401

Stanley Finger
Department of Psychology
Washington University
St. Louis, Missouri 63130

Gabriel P. Frommer
Department of Psychology
Indiana University
Bloomington, Indiana 47401

Michael S. Gazzaniga
Department of Psychology
State University of New York
Stony Brook, New York 11794
                    and
Department of Neurology
Cornell Medical College
New York, New York 10021

Robert B. Glassman
Department of Psychology
Lake Forest College
Lake Forest, Illinois 60045

Stanley D. Glick
Department of Pharmacology
Mount Sinai School of Medicine
City University of New York
5th Ave. and 100th St.
New York, New York 10029

David Johnson
Department of Psychology
Ohio University
Athens, Ohio 45701

Bryan Kolb
Department of Psychology
University of Lethbridge
Lethbridge, Alberta, Canada

Scott Laurence
Department of Psychology
Clark University
Worcester, Massachusetts 01610

Barry S. Layton
Departments of Neurology and
    Psychology
St. Louis University
St. Louis, Missouri 63104

Ulf Norrsell
Department of Physiology
University of Göteborg
Göteborg, Sweden

Donald G. Stein
Department of Psychology
Clark University
Worcester, Massachusetts 01610

Edward M. Stricker
Department of Psychology
University of Pittsburgh
Pittsburgh, Pennsylvania 15260

Arthur W. Toga
Departments of Neurology and
    Psychology
St. Louis University
St. Louis, Missouri 63104

J. M. Warren
Department of Psychology
The Pennsylvania State University
University Park, Pennsylvania,
    16802

George Wolf
Division of Natural Sciences
State University of New York
Purchase, New York 10577

Thomas A. Woolsey
Departments of Anatomy and
    Neurobiology
Washington University
    School of Medicine
St. Louis, Missouri 63110

Michael J. Zigmond
Department of Biology
University of Pittsburgh
Pittsburgh, Pennsylvania 15260

Betty Zimmerberg
Department of Pharmacology
Mount Sinai School of Medicine
City University of New York
5th Ave. and 100th St.
New York, New York 10029

Preface

It has long been recognized that damage to the mammalian central nervous system may be followed by behavioral recovery, but only recently has close attention been directed to specific factors which may enhance or retard restitution. This is evident in the rapidly growing number of journal articles and scientific paper sessions dealing with "recovery of function," as well as in the publicity given by the popular press to some of the findings in this field.

The present text seeks to examine the foundations of brain lesion research, to review recent material on a number of factors which appear to contribute to recovery after brain damage, and to present models which have been proposed to account for these effects. In order to best accomplish these goals, a number of key workers in these areas were asked to examine and describe research literatures dealing with specific problems or methodological manipulations associated with brain damage and behavior, using their own experiments and those of others to illustrate important points. In addition, significant interpretive and theoretical issues were to be evaluated in each chapter.

An attempt to summarize the issues and findings in this field has not been undertaken in the past, although there is one edited publication on recovery phenomena which presents in detail the research programs of several scientists.* It was hoped that the broader, more general approach of the current volume would appeal to a larger population of readers, particularly to those involved in brain lesion research, and those wishing to survey particular effects relating to brain damage, behavior, and recovery of function for clinical or educational reasons.

*Stein, D. G., Rosen, J. J., and Butters, N. (Eds.), *Plasticity and recovery of function in the central nervous system.* New York: Academic Press, 1974.

The present volume begins by discussing the logic and role of the lesion experiment in the neural sciences. This is followed by two chapters (Part II) which evaluate the generality of lesion data across laboratory species, and the possible application of some of these findings to man. The third part of the book examines both the proximal and distal anatomical effects of brain damage and the difficulties inherent in correlating anatomical data with performance.

The chapters in Part IV review the status of some of the factors which have been associated with recovery after brain damage. These variables include age at the time of insult, duration of the postoperative recovery period, speed of growth of the lesion, and the role of spared fragments of target tissue in mediating behavior. Other factors, including the use of pharmacological agents, enriched environments, and specific testing procedures, also are examined in this part of the book.

The concluding chapters (Part V) look at theories of recovery and at the doctrine of localization of function in the light of recent findings. This section compares and analyzes some of the models which have been proposed to account for sparing and recovery after brain damage. Here, special attention is devoted to the ever-present possibility that at least some goal-directed acts may reflect less than truly "recovered" abilities upon closer analysis.

While principally aimed at providing specific information about brain injury and behavior, it is hoped that the present volume will have a number of general effects. One is to convey a feeling for the complexities and difficulties involved in interpreting the results of brain lesion research. Another is to help clarify and resolve some of the important interpretive and theoretical issues in this area so as to pave the way for new conceptual advances. Most of all, it is hoped that this book, with its emphasis on recovery phenomena, will be able to stimulate new research in a rapidly developing field whose important questions are only beginning to be answered.

Stanley Finger

St. Louis, Missouri

Contents

Chapter 3

The Interplay of Experimental and Clinical Approaches in Brain Lesion Research

ARTHUR BENTON

PART III: ANATOMICAL RESPONSE TO CNS INJURY

Chapter 4

Lesion Experiments: Some Anatomical Considerations

THOMAS A. WOOLSEY

Chapter 5

Brain Lesions: Induction, Analysis, and the Problem of Recovery of Function

GEORGE WOLF, EDWARD M. STRICKER, and
MICHAEL J. ZIGMOND

PART IV: EXPERIMENTAL MANIPULATIONS AND BEHAVIORAL RECOVERY

Chapter 6

Age, Brain Damage, and Performance

DAVID JOHNSON and C. ROBERT ALMLI

Chapter 9

Testing Procedures and the Interpretation of Behavioral Data

ULF NORRSELL

Chapter 10

Subtotal Lesions: Implications for Coding and Recovery of Function

GABRIEL P. FROMMER

Chapter 13

Sensory Restriction and Recovery of Function
BARRY S. LAYTON, GEORGE E. CORRICK,
and ARTHUR W. TOGA

PART V: ACCOUNTING FOR SPARING AND RESTITUTION

Chapter 14

Recovery after Brain Damage and the Concept of Localization of Function
SCOTT LAURENCE and DONALD G. STEIN

Chapter 15

Is Seeing Believing: Notes on Clinical Recovery
MICHAEL S. GAZZANIGA

PART I

THE DOMAIN OF BRAIN-LESION RESEARCH

The Logic of the Lesion Experiment and Its Role in the Neural Sciences

ROBERT B. GLASSMAN

(1) Since the logic of the lesion method is similar to that of other methods, it should not be singled out in regard to the inadequacy of our concepts of brain function and the possible localization of functions. In fact, molar studies of the effects of lesions on behavior may yield reductionistic formulations which cannot be achieved in any other way. Those who devise such formulations must be aware of their metaphorical foundations. (2) The possibility of ever disentangling the variables that constitute systems even less complex than the brain has been questioned, when prior knowledge of the plan of construction is unavailable. However, certain evolutionary considerations suggest that the brain may be very amenable to study by the lesion method. (3) Because science is concerned with relatively inaccessible mechanisms, it is easy to lose sight of the fact that scientific method rests on the same foundation as do the much more rapid evaluations involved in everyday perception. Everyday perception involves the integration of multiple cues with past experience. In science, *single* cues take much effort to obtain. In this way, it can be seen that the double-dissociation criterion for lesion studies is really a special case of the search for converging information. It is proposed that certain procedures more general than double dissociation be used in planning and evaluating experiments on the brain. That is, we should seek (a) not merely double dissociations but multiple dissociations and (b) not merely dissociations but *associations*, or

ROBERT B. GLASSMAN • Department of Psychology, Lake Forest College, Lake Forest, Illinois 60045

overlaps, in the neural substrates of behaviors. Only this more general procedure, involving multiple lesions and observations of many behaviors, can provide bases for making inferences about the properties of the neural substrates and for integration of such inferences with data obtained from anatomy and physiology. (4) Since brain scientists are dealing with a system of immense complexity, they must face the necessity of relaxing parsimony while elaborating multiple, alternative, complex theories. More time and resources must be devoted to these attempts to integrate theoretically the broad range of available clues about brain and mind.

1. INTRODUCTION

A characteristic of the human mind is that it can do only so many things in a given interval of time, or in a lifetime. Although in retrospect well-developed ideas may seem clear and easy to learn, progress would not be possible if the commitment of effort required to recognize and learn them were not many times less than the time it takes to work them out. As a consequence we have research specialties, but also the possibility of communication among specialties.

Metascientific philosophies which might help scientific specialists by giving them a more objective view of their own behavior take a long time to develop and require their own specialists, each of whom must limit his subject matter. But our need for philosophy is immediate; we must therefore borrow some time from research to do our own amateur philosophizing. When we do so, it becomes clear that there are trends within specialties with regard to the types of questions asked, models built, and methods used. As examples, computer-type models and terminology have been popular in neuroscience for some years now and biochemical and pharmacological techniques now seem to be increasingly common. The reasons for these and other trends must be examined to see whether they are due in part to fortuitous factors or whether it is clear that these paths, more than any other conceivable ones, provide the best routes to a basic understanding of mind and brain.

If scientific progress were impossible unless all scientists were philosophers, very little progress would be made. Once grounded in such basics as the need for careful observation, systematic taking of data, and control experiments, our intuitive handling of problems and raising of questions is often effective. Nevertheless, scientists are subject to the same social influences as are other human beings, for example, tendencies to adopt traditions and to fall into patterns of behavior similar to those around us. On occasion, scientists' intelligence may not help them to avoid these tendencies so much as to do well at rationalizing poor decisions. With regard to the problem at hand, careful examination of reasons sometimes given for using or not using the lesion method may help us to see whether these decisions are being made for the right reasons. Since logic is not autochthonous with each substantive field, the following arguments are relevant to more than the lesion method alone.

2. CONCEPTUAL AND METHODOLOGICAL PROBLEMS: WHAT IS A "FUNCTION"?

We sometimes first identify as a methodological problem what turns out to be a much broader, conceptual one. Although almost all scientists would agree that science involves analysis, to some people the conceptual foundation of the lesion method is the more specific, reductionistic idea that the activities of an organism can be derived from functions which can be localized. The most important question one can ask about this assumption is whether a given conceptual decomposition into functional units is unequivocal or whether we are faced, as is physical science, with the problem of complementarity (Turner, 1971; Markowitz, 1973), i.e., alternative ways of analyzing a phenomenon, some of which may be equally useful for their respective purposes but which do not correspond to each other clearly. This issue of complementarity is related to the question of the quality of the concept of a function (Meyer, 1958), or the "what" question, which is at least as important as the "where" (Teuber, 1955). Although this issue applies to any scientific problem, it has tended to arise frequently with specific regard to the lesion method. This is because with the lesion method it is easy to commit the excess of reifying a discovered relation between independent and dependent variables as a controlling "part."

In the absence of well-worked-out ideas about what sorts of relations are being sought, the "where" question often emerges too strongly, leading to explicit or implicit interpretations of results in terms of "centers." It has been pointed out that discovery of a lesion-induced deficit does not imply that the area in question is a "center" for the "function" suggested by the deficit (Gregory, 1961, p. 324). Even if the problem of complementarity is set aside for the moment, and the definition of function is assumed to be unequivocal, it is possible that a particular deficit occurred because only one of many important lines of communication was cut, either because the target structure was really a link in a functional chain or because inadvertent damage was done to passing fibers. This is a criticism cast in methodological and anatomical terms. A related psychological and conceptual criticism involves noting that functions, however they are defined, have many aspects. Impairment of any one aspect could have a surprisingly large or small effect on the function. Lashley's studies of a phenomenon as complex as maze learning appear to have been particularly susceptible to this criticism (Zangwill, 1961), and Lashley himself noted the possibility that an apparent mass-action effect could be due to certain other factors, e.g., summated sensory deficits with the larger lesions (Beach, Hebb, Morgan, and Nissen, 1960). In this way, the "search for the engram" can be seen as a simplistic way of posing a question. Similarly, some current descriptions of split-brain phenomena imply a grander localization than the data warrant—e.g., localization of consciousness—in view of the possibility that an alteration of only one of many aspects of a function might cause a profound alteration of certain measures.

Other methodological points that temper any interpretation in terms of local centers are as follows. The possibility of indirect effects among interconnected areas has been noted (Jones and Powell, 1973, p. 601; Schoenfeld and Hamilton, 1977), e.g., changes in concentration of neurotransmitters may occur at various places remote from the localized lesions (Thompson, 1971, p. 152). The idea of diaschisis (von Monakow, 1914) raises this point in a more general way. Side effects may occur following lesions including possible irritative effects of electrolytic damage (Thompson, 1967, p. 47) or scarring from thermocautery (Milner, 1970, p. 40). Such accidents can yield experimental effects due to stimulation of adjacent tissue rather than to loss of the area in question. What appears to be mass action of one region may really result from inadvertent, progressive invasion of a neighboring one (Lashley, in Beach et al., 1960), i.e., this may represent mass action of the neighboring regions.

In addition to such "extraneous side effects," some authors have viewed as problems with the lesion method various phenomena that might also be seen as providing interesting conceptual issues, i.e., effects of lesion size, recovery time, age, experience (Thompson, 1971; see also other chapters of this volume), release effects generally and those which yield recovery when a second lesion is made, the serial-lesion effect, and the possibility of functioning of small remnants (Chow, 1967, p. 711; Zangwill, 1961, p. 69). These are methodological problems only so long as the researcher is unaware of them. Once discovered, they demand methodological refinements but remain important conceptual problems which challenge our notion of the functions studied. The most difficult methodological–conceptual problem may be the question of what is a significant finding. On some occasions statistical significance may be obtained with a very "small phenomenon." Yet in some such cases, the finding of any indication whatsoever that an area participates somehow in a particular behavior may be extremely important.

The study of the brain involves the same sorts of objective thinking that would be applied to any other complex physical system. A general consideration of the meaning of "function" may therefore give more perspective on the study of the brain. In his provocative essay "The Brain as an Engineering Problem," Gregory (1961) described similarities in the difficulties and heuristics involved in studying the brain compared with those of studying a machine. People who work with machines may sometimes have an advantage over those who study the brain, in that the functions of many machines are known, limited, and well-defined. Populations of machines have identical parts, each of which seems to be defined by both its function and its physical boundary. One problem with the lesion method is that our starting point for delimiting the boundaries of parts is less obvious. Gall, viewing the work of Flourens through the walls of a glass house, criticized the attempt to localize functions by the lesion method, in part on the basis of lack of knowledge of boundaries (Young, 1970). Though anatomical and physiological progress has presented us with better *prima facie* definitions of functional regions, the doubt about the best way to dissect the system conceptually remains. Nevertheless, it is easy to overstate the contrast between the study of machines and the study of organisms. Although someone who is troubleshooting a machine can often find the difficulty merely by replacing parts step by step, machines are "modular" in geometry only according to certain conceptual decompositions. Some functional relations among and within modules may not be easily bounded. Moreover, a repair technician may not understand his modules in the same sense as does the designer of the machine.

A scientist trying to learn about an unknown machine is in much the same position as one who studies the brain, even if the machine's function as a whole is known (Gregory, 1961). Arbib (1972, pp. 11–12) gives an illustration of this fact in describing the failure of a group of sophisticated users of computers to figure out how to operate a new computer before the manual arrived, though it was a variant of models with which they were familiar. Perhaps part of the reason why machines are hard to figure out is that technological artifacts undergo a certain degree of evolutionary progress by trial and error in much the same way as do other parts and products of living systems. A part originally present to serve one function may turn out to be able to serve others simultaneously and will be modified to improve these abilities. Refinements are made which may be comprehensible only to someone who has observed the drawbacks of earlier models. However, in contrast to the pessimistic point made by Gregory and Arbib, it will be suggested later that evolution may nevertheless yield living systems that are eminently amenable to study by the lesion method.

A related example of confusion about functional localization with brain lesions is the "holist criticism." This says that brain lesions do not show you what the region in question does, but rather what the rest of the whole complex brain system does *without* the part in question. A methodological response to this criticism involves preparation of simplified organisms by ablation (Chow, 1967, p. 708) or transection (Thompson, 1967, pp. 424–427) procedures. With such preparations, one observes the variety of behaviors that remain rather than concentrating on the few that have been lost, as is more typical of ablation studies. However, it would be dangerous to take too seriously the holist criticism, which smacks of naive realism as much as do interpretations in terms of centers. The holist criticism is an overreaction to the overinterpretation of lesion data, which leads to talk of centers. Above all, it must be recognized that similar holist criticisms apply to most methods, e.g., (1) electrical stimulation does not tell you what the stimulated region does normally, it tells you how the system as a whole responds to abnormal conditions at that point; (2) infusion of a putative neurotransmitter at a particular locus does not tell you about the responsiveness of that region, it tells you how the whole system reacts to an unusual amount of the substance at that point; (3) a single-unit recording tells you, not about properties of that unit, but about the entire system to which it is connected. All of these criticisms have a certain validity as cautions regarding methodological care and overinterpretation, but it is incorrect to go so far as to use them to justify the elimination of a method.

In vitro studies and histological techniques may be less open to holist criticism; however, it is not obvious that such techniques alone will lead to understanding of the nervous system. Naturalistic observations of the behavior of whole organisms can supplement these more molecular studies and naturalistic techniques obviously cannot be criticized as dealing with abnormalities. However, while our ultimate goal is an understanding of the whole organism, science proceeds by isolating causal factors. Since naturalistic research does not attempt this by actual manipulation, it must do so by selective attention and comparison of situations. The naturalistic method may then also be susceptible to a holist-type criticism: the isolated independent variable may be more of a determinant of the particular dependent measure than other variables, but how does one know whether or not this is true only in the particular context in which measurements were taken? Furthermore, it is not obvious that naturalistic methods would supplement anatomical and physiological methods adequately to answer all questions about how a nervous system works. The point is that no single procedure allows us a direct apprehension of reality; rather, observations are no more than cues or indicators which must be worked into a conceptual scheme. Though this is a truism that all scientists appreciate in the general case, the aforementioned confusions do occur.

A simple, concrete case will help to show the degree of overstatement involved in the holist criticism of the lesion method. As Milner (1970, p. 40) points out, the ancient Greeks already knew about the functions of peripheral nerves, based on instances in which the nerves had been injured. It seems evident that the Greeks must have had to do some reasoning to separate out, say, effects of sectioning nerves from those of sectioning blood vessels and other tissue, and it is even possible that subsequent research might have proven them wrong. However, the reasonableness of a conclusion about peripheral nerve function based on instances of severing cannot be doubted. Of course, what we are actually seeing in such a case is the behavior of the remainder of the system which lacks a segment of peripheral nerve, but the inference from that behavior is hardly problematical.

3. REDUCTIONISM AND METAPHOR IN PHYSIOLOGICAL PSYCHOLOGY

The susceptibility of biobehavioral techniques to confusion about their significance, particularly in regard to localization of function, will be more understandable if we go so far here as to try to consider more carefully the general issue of the nature of explanation. In particular, we should be aware that there are certain inadequacies in the casually reductionistic notion that understanding something involves a description in terms of the "parts." Instead it is suggested here that expression of all new observations and ideas should be viewed as an *ad hoc* contrivance, using metaphors from past experience to label similarities. When dealing with ideas there is always a danger that irrelevant aspects of metaphors, sometimes derived from more "concrete" or familiar modes of expression, may take over. Thus, when conceptually dissecting a system into "parts," there is a danger of thinking that we are talking about concrete parts when we are really referring to patterns. The difference is that real parts are bounded on spatial dimensions whereas metaphorical parts, or patterns, are distinguished along other qualitative dimensions. Even when a geometrically bounded part does correspond to a functional part, not all functions and interrelations will be obvious on brief gross inspection. One learns this the hard way when trying to repair an instrument so simple that it is constructed of visible components that act in a purely mechanical manner, such as a typewriter.

For an example closer to physiological psychology, while learning appears to lead to new *connections* among *stimuli* and *responses* and while learning is undoubtedly embodied in the brain, it takes a leap of faith to expect to see local neural representations of stimuli and responses and of connections between them. This leap has sometimes been taken with little reflection. Perhaps such components will someday be found, but it is also possible to begin to imagine alternative, complex systems which can learn but which do not localize these conceptual "parts" in spatial compartments. For instance, though sensory receiving areas are partly separated from motor regions, it is conceivable that an integrated representation of the proper response to a recognized stimulus pattern lies within a single small brain region.

In this vein, Gregory (1961) has warned that the terms used in describing the output of a system will generally be inadequate for describing the internal goings on; for example, we do not see the spark of the engine represented in the output of a car, but rather we see the wheels turning. Horel (personal communication), in a similar manner, has recommended that a careful distinction be made between behavioral functions and brain functions. He notes that von Monakow recommended distinguishing between localization of symptoms and localization of function. These distinctions are important and are consistent with a more general message, most often heard during arguments in support of basic research; that is, that scientific sophistication consists in part in a willingness to solve problems indirectly rather than by seizing on their most immediate associations. Though there is nothing advantageous about indirectness *per se*, a willingness to use indirect methods allows integration of a greater amount of relevant information in solving a problem. The confusion between brain function and psychological function can occur only before this sophistication is fully attained. Although it has been pointed out that there are a number of aspects of Gall's work that should be appreciated, e.g., his attempt to be systematic and empirical (Young, 1970), phrenology is an excellent example of naiveté in regard to this failure to be indirect and to differentiate between brain function and psychological function. In phrenology, the source of ideas about parts into which the system could be decomposed was the vocabulary of common language, and the application of this vocabulary was very direct. Modern attempts to understand the brain in terms of interactions among areas concerned primarily with "emotion," "motivation," "sensation," and "movement" also use our common vocabulary. This vocabulary has, of course, evolved to serve us in describing psychological functions, and will not necessarily be well suited for describing brain functions.

Attempts to be more scientific have sometimes not involved efforts to broaden our repertoire of alternative concepts and terms; rather they have merely expurgated certain common terms from the vocabulary of a faction of researchers and have replaced others with technical ones having more limited reference than their common counterparts. Thus, like phrenologists, we still look for centers of "sensation" but not of "will." But narrowed vision is not the way to solve the problem of brain function. While current knowledge and vocabulary may not always suggest the right path to take in an investigation, these provide the only places from which to begin. Awareness of some of the preconceptions implicit in our terms can make their meanings more susceptible to felicitous modifications. For example, though gross neuroanatomical structures were originally named after familiar things such as seahorses and feet, modern anatomy and physiology are not impaired by the survival of these names. Perhaps the Latinization served a real function, in this regard, as a warning that the common term was used with reservation.

Some would argue that anatomical and physiological descriptions are precisely what is required in describing brain function, as distinct from and as underlying psychological function. The trouble is that anatomy and physiology alone do not seem to provide the questions that must be asked about behavior. Without these questions we may be doomed to endless cataloguing of findings, without much integration. To say this is most definitely not to contradict the reductionistic foundations of science, especially as similar arguments can be made about all levels of natural phenomena. For example, we have learned about many properties of atoms not so much via direct observations in particle physics as by means of inferences from more molar studies in chemistry. In fact, it is important to realize that even particle physicists do not observe their entities directly but by means of a complicated structure of inferences from the actual observations of larger entities. In this respect, brain research is particularly vulnerable to the possibility of a naive kind of reductionism. Histological techniques do allow us actually to see cells and certain obvious aggregations of cells. This may sometimes distract us from seeking alternative functional units.

4. THE SURPRISING SOURCE OF METAPHORS USED IN STUDYING THE BRAIN

Common experience, as reflected in our vocabulary, has been one source of metaphors for behavior and technology has been another fruitful source. For Aristotle the imprint left by a stylus in clay was analogous to human memory (Milner, 1970, p. 425), and Descartes was inspired in the concept of the reflex by certain hydraulic phenomena (Herrnstein and Boring, 1966). While the modern age has given us the computer and hologram metaphors, applications of these remain very speculative. On the other hand, the servo system and the idea of coding are modern technological metaphors which have proven invaluable to all aspects of brain research.

Reductionism is often thought of as involving an explanation in terms of parts that are more basic. However, it is difficult to give a general definition of the quality of being basic. Chemical elements are obviously simpler than compounds. But in mathematics the idea that axioms are elemental absolute truths has been discarded. It would perhaps be better to say only that we try to reduce complexities to terms that appear nonproblematical or at least more familiar. The idea of servo systems and of coding have passed about as stringent a test of nonvagueness as humans have been able to devise, i.e., machinery has been built which embodies these ideas. Yet a nagging question remains: Technology has given neuroscientists these ideas by some stroke of fortune, but isn't this a peculiar position for a scientist to find himself in—having to wait for developments in other areas for ideas about what to look for in his own? Will there be no more fundamental advances in the understanding of brain function if no other technological ideas turn out to be useful? The answer to this question is ironic and requires that we take a second look at the ideas of the servo system and of coding. It is evident that technologists are not more creative than other people after all; the original source of the ideas of servo systems ("regulatory," "seeking," "hunting") and coding is in fact the observation of living systems and of human behavior!

Fortunately, this realization need not bring us full circle. Though the starting point for the embryogenesis of new ideas is in metaphors with familiar things, these ideas can come to be used in explanatory ways that are not naively direct. Recognizing that this is a feature of scientific thought opens the way to using this method more self-consciously. In other words, one should range broadly in the search for ideas from familiar things about metaphorical parts useful in the conceptual decomposition of a complex system. However, further questions about whether these parts are nonproblematical and about other, alternative decompositions should be shelved only temporarily. To give a concrete example (using a rather extreme suggestion), in explaining a complex system such as the human brain, it would be reasonable to hypothesize a part that had all of the properties of a human mind, except for having a personality that in some defined way was simpler than that of the whole human. For example we might "experiment" theoretically with the idea of a single-minded actor interested only in feeding, who devises various strategies in competing with inner homunculi having other motivations. Such metaphors might constitute a useful system description at an explanatory level intermediate in complexity between the whole human and a collection of single-variable reflex arcs or servo systems. If a plausible explanation of much of behavior could be given using such molar concepts, then additional questions would next have to be faced about how the parts of these parts functioned together, and also questions about whether alternative reductions were possible. Luria has expressed the view that an adequate modern approach to brain function involves neither strict localization nor antilocalization theorizing but rather consideration of systems in which there are complex interactions of jointly functioning parts. Nevertheless, a conceptual gap remains between this exhortation and a clear statement of possible hypothetical neural entities which could explain his behavioral findings from frontally damaged patients (Luria, 1973). This gap could be closed if more ideas about possible mechanisms were tried out.

5. ARE BRAINS MORE OR LESS EASY TO ANALYZE THAN MACHINES?

With the brain we are apparently faced with a system of such enormous complexity, possibly basically different from any other familiar system, that we must wonder whether in the final analysis all metaphors and analyses that we can think of will be hopelessly inadequate and ambiguous. Arbib's anecdote about the manual-less computer suggests that this may be true even of machines, as does Gregory's analogy in which he notes how unlikely it would be that an ablation or stimulation of part of a television set would tell us much about how the set works. Even people experienced in electronics do much better with a circuit diagram in front of them and with preexisting knowledge of the functions of aggregates of components. Against the threat of such despair, we can cling first to the copious empirical evidence that specific changes in behavior are seen when ablations or stimulations are carried out on the brain and, second, to the faith that some of the ideas that these changes suggest are indeed approximations to the truth. This faith may actually be valid for two possible reasons. The first is that our analogy with machines may be overly pessimistic and our heuristics used in studying either machines or living systems may really be more powerful in action than we can appreciate in retrospect. Since there do seem to be some system similarities across many levels of complexity (Miller, 1971), our metaphors have a chance of success; however, there are also real differences among systems. Nevertheless, scientists in other areas have been able to perform the bootstrap operation of describing the unique aspects of systems using newly evolved concepts. The issue of conceptual novelty will be considered again further below (Section 11).

The second possible reason that localization studies in physiological psychology might be giving us valid ideas is that there may be something special about organisms that lends them to this. Gregory (1961, pp. 321–322) notes that the problem of discovering functional localization is especially difficult in systems such as televisions in which an output event is the outcome of a series of several causally necessary prior events. He points out that a piano, on the other hand, consists of a number of rather independent machines (the 88 sets of keys, hammers, and strings) in one package, and the function of these might be isolated easily by a lesion. In comparing human brains with computers, a number of authors have pointed to the more "parallel" as opposed to "serial-processing" nature of the former (Arbib, 1972). It should be recognized, parenthetically, that if it happened to be the function of each individual piano key that was of interest we would again be in trouble due to the causal chain problem, i.e., breaking a link any place between the ivory and the strings would give the same output deficit.

Earlier it was said that living systems and machines in general may be decomposed conceptually in a variety of ways, only some of which were reasonably "modular" in concrete, geometric terms. Is there any *a priori* reason for expecting the brain to be particularly modular in this respect as we move away from the microscopic level of cells toward the more molar matter–energy patterns that must be important in determining behavior? This question is closely related to the question of parallel elements versus causal chain. An affirmative answer is implied in the work of Ashby (1960), who argues that any system that gains organization by an evolutionary process of natural selection must be composed of subsystems that are sufficiently independent of each other that a random perturbation in one part does not destroy the entire existing organization. On much the same basis, Simon (1969) has argued that any complex organized system must involve sets of subassemblies contained within other subassemblies, in a manner defined as hierarchical. Though some of these functional systems will not be geometrically modular, these considerations suggest that in working with living systems we might expect a lesion experiment to successfully isolate a functional unit more frequently than if we were dealing with machines.

Another implication of natural selection also turns out to yield a fortunate state of affairs for the lesion method. This is the fact that the only plausible way in which a natural selection process can work is for the evolutionary route from one form to another (and, in particular, from lower to more highly organized forms) to involve tiny steps. Each

for justification, psychology has many more journals devoted primarily to empiricism than to theory, whereas theoretical physics is an established area. An example of the tendency to try first for the simplest solutions is the assumption sometimes made that if stimulation of some area has one effect, then ablation should have the opposite effect. If taken more seriously than as one of several alternative hypotheses, this is a variant of the "centers" fallacy.

An obvious extension of the foregoing comments on the need for a more generalized form of the double dissociation criterion in lesion studies is that multiple independent and dependent variables should be the rule in any study. To say this alone does not give guidance about where to seek those variables nor what to do with the findings. This will obviously depend on various aspects of the particular investigation. However, it must be emphasized that current research and editorial practice is highly inadequate in this regard. It should be every experimenter's duty not to be exceedingly parsimonious in his discussion sections. Rather, having first related his data to other findings of most obvious relevance, the author should then proceed to construct as many elaborate fantasies as he can which seem to tie his work into the broader context of the problem of how the mind works. This should be done because while science properly emphasizes observation, it is inherently interpretive (Campbell, 1974). Observation does not yield understanding automatically. It is better to be conscious of alternative interpretations than to have an unconscious one partially determining one's description of data. Such an unconscious interpretation will be arbitrary and often simplistic. Theoretical fantasies should be elaborated even if it is feasible to present only some of them in a detailed, published discussion.

As indicated earlier, our use of language in our individual prescientific ontogenies is a metaphorical backdrop for current descriptive statements. While pure objectivity is impossible for mortals, we can approximate it by using the perspective of time to step back and look repeatedly at previous theoretical efforts. In so doing we can try to understand what pertinent and extraneous factors contributed to these efforts and can try to adjust them accordingly. Whether a theory or explanation is pertinent can be determined by examining alternative explanations. These help to reveal whether the initial explanation has excessive, irrelevant, or superstitious assumptions—or whether it contains too few!

The principle of multiple alternative theories goes hand in hand with the principle that multiple measures should be carried out. To speak of "refined" observational techniques by themselves begs the question of what is being sought. On closer examination it will often turn out to be the case that the term "additional" techniques would be more appropriate. This is true to a much lesser extent in anatomy and physiology, where the theoretical foundations appear less problematical. That is, it is quite reasonable to speak of intracellular microelectrodes or histochemical techniques as refinements because the unit we are homing in on is, unequivocally, the neuron or its contents or parts. In the case of behavioral investigations, one can speak of refinements only on the basis of a theoretical assumption about what is being sought, e.g., if it is assumed that an area is sensory, then one can design more accurate instruments for presenting stimuli. But, insofar as we are not sure of how to analyze the brain, it is variety that should be sought. This includes varieties of behavioral techniques for a given lesion and a variety of lesions for a given behavior, as well as histological and physiological studies of areas. To some extent, this is simply to court serendipity, but to do so having consciously come prepared with alternative theories which not only lean on what is known, but which attempt to recognize frankly and to fill in the large gaps of what is not known.

To compound this suggestion, it is further suggested that scientists should permit each other a certain amount of vagueness in public communications, so long as a serious attempt is made to identify these parts of a theory for the reader. This may provide a way in which many minds can make use of a potentially fruitful idea. In other words, we ought to reexamine the principle that all theory should yield unequivocal predictions immediately. Again, explicit theories that are incompletely formulated seem preferable to unconscious ones or to mere cataloguing of data.

The broad use of theory proposed here involves the difficult intellectual effort of thinking of many things at once, but if this is not done we may be condemning ourselves to a meandering dialectic of hypotheses and deductions. Each of these may seem reasonable to us at each point in time, but this will be for reasons which are largely fortuitous and which lead us in a random walk. An unfortunate property of ideas is that they seem obvious, once they find their way into the social group. But like hair styles, today's paradigm may seem quaint tomorrow. This can happen not because of a thorough exploration of alternatives, but because of arbitrary attention to a few together with ignorance of others.

Occam's razor (Lowry, 1971), or strict parsimony, is not merely inappropriate when dealing with a system that is known to be complex, it is a downright self-indulgence and an inexcusable concession to the limited capacity of the researcher's mind. The game of science as now played usually requires that empirical findings be marshalled by a researcher after he makes his predictions. Yet it is often true that, with some effort, numerous other theoretical explanations can be seen to be equally unifying of the data in question. We tend to look askance at *post hoc* reinterpretations because it seems too easy to generate too many. To allow such reinterpretation would seem to throw things too wide open, making us vulnerable to a new scholasticism of endless cheap talk. But the unfortunate effect of having little public outlet for theoretical debate is that the one public theoretical explanation of a body of data is licensed by the happenstance that it is simple and that it comes from the experimenter's mouth. Such an explanation is arbitrarily selected and must bear only an accidental relation to the truth.

8. PERCEIVING COMPLEX SYSTEMS

An example of the fallacy of "refined methods" is the claim, sometimes encountered, that a certain biochemical technique, by virtue of its special selectivity, provides a more accurate localization of function than would a comparable lesion study of behavior. While local implantation of a chemical may help to isolate structures, in some cases the new technique may carry with it new possibilities for artifacts. The tendency for liquid intracranial injections to ride up the outside of the cannula is an example. More important, use of the single behavioral method alone, in the context of a biochemical procedure or any other manipulation, leaves the researcher with a mere variant of the idea that functions are things that are to be understood by localizing them. The word "system" has sometimes been abused by researchers who have found that a particular outcome results from electrically or chemically stimulating the brain at a number of specified points. In the same sense, if a lesion in any of a set of widely dispersed structures yields the same behavioral result, the set could be called a "system." Although such experimentation and interpretation is partially consistent with the above exhortation to use multiple methods, it does not go far enough.

The most simple-minded interpretation of an ablation study of a single area involves a conclusion about "spot localization" of a "center." But studies of how a single behavior is affected by manipulations in multiple areas can lead to a hardly less trivial concept of "protuberant localization." Even additional, converging information, say about localization of a particular transmitter substance in the "protuberant field," may not be of much help. A related problem arises when pharmacologists speak of the "receptor" for some psychoactive substance. This is a reification, in terms of a hypothetical neural entity, quite analogous to that of the "center." The same problems are present with either local or distributed "centers" as discussed above. That is, we need information about both similarities and differences in a spectrum of behavioral effects obtained on manipulating these structures. This must include information about the varying degrees to which different behaviors overlap anatomical regions. Otherwise, there is no way that we have of making inferences about how information is processed.

The exhortation to think of elaborate fantasies and to use multiple methods in science is an extrapolation from what human beings appear to do normally in perceiving the world. Much of modern psychology views perception as an active process; our perceptions depend on past experience and on the hypotheses with which we enter a situation, as well as on the stimuli arising in the situation (e.g., Gregory, 1970). When encountering a new source of cues, it is common practice to view it from many angles, touch it, manipulate it, listen to it, etc.; that is, one performs a variety of tests that enable him to relate the new source to past experience. All of science can be seen as an extension of this sort of common sense—what other source could there possibly be for the logic of scientific method? Animals have some of the same capability; there is a classroom film about perception in which E. G. Boring, discussing the ability of animals and people to achieve object constancy, went so far as to declare with tongue only partly in cheek that "the chicken is a scientist." The need to use elegant methodologies and instruments to extend this commonsense process arises in science when cues are not easy to come by. On different occasions this may occur when the source of cues is very small or at a great distance, if it is concealed by a barrier (such as the skull), or if its activity consists of forms of energy to which our receptors are not sensitive. These circumstances introduce no fundamentally new contingencies that are not already coped with by our commonsense methods, except to strain our memories and our patience while formulating the perception.

Sometimes more complicated factors are involved, e.g., it is difficult to get a clear view of a process that takes a long time, or one which involves many jointly acting variables. But these are also merely practical problems requiring ingenuity in taking data but not necessarily requiring innovation in interpretive methods. The trick is to display the data in a way convenient for our perceptual systems. We should acknowledge that science is an extension of the commonsense process of perceiving because it will help us to avoid fallacies analogous to ones we would never be in danger of making in everyday life. In the well-known fable about the blind men and the elephant, each blind man came up with a different conception depending on the part that he touched; for example, the one who felt a leg concluded that "an elephant is very much like a tree!" It is clear even to a child that each blind man was also a fool for extrapolating so far and so simplistically from a single observation. If the blind men had been prepared with multiple, alternative hypotheses, they would have felt compelled to make additional observations. Yet a similar error is very easy for an intelligent person to commit when he follows a long and painstaking (yet single variable) investigation with a conclusion about neural centers.

An argument against Occam's razor has been presented above, i.e., it is obvious that excessively parsimonious explanations will fail when there are ample indications that a phenomenon is complex. More importantly, if hypotheses are well constructed, it should turn out to be the case that the greater the variety of findings that can be considered at once, the *fewer* the alternative explanations that will appear possible. In this view, the scientist is analogous to the hero of a detective story; only the acute mind of Sherlock Holmes is capable of scanning boldly over a wide range of alternatives to find the one that fits all the clues, while Watson looks on but does not *observe*. More generally, science is a form of problem solving in which, like any other, clues are integrated and alternative hypotheses tested. Under all conditions of problem solving, the unsuccessful onlooker is bewildered because the clues themselves did not shout out the answer.

Scientific problem solving may be considered to involve both implicit (Polanyi, 1966) and explicit processes. Before well-formulated hypotheses arising from one clue are ever explicitly checked against others, many are eliminated or not even thought of because they are absurd, i.e., inconsistent with accepted knowledge and heuristics. This implicit factor is a necessary one because there is not enough time to think of everything, but it can be responsible for failures to solve certain difficult problems, as when an apparently outlandish idea turns out to be valid. The related issue of "functional fixedness" has been studied by experimental psychologists (Wason and Johnson-Laird, 1968).

By assuming that certain ideas are improper, the specialist takes a gamble that the limited range of phenomena he studies and ideas he considers will ultimately fall together in such a way as to explain others. This can be an arbitrary position and it would be better if attempts such as that of Pribram (1971) to integrate a broad range of data into brain theory, even including evidence from subjective experience, were to become more common. As with lesion data and other kinds of experimental results, such information is to be taken not at face value but as a clue. The source of relevant ideas may sometimes turn out to be surprising and to involve extensive reasoning. The use earlier in this paper of ideas about evolutionary processes is another example of an attempt to range further afield than the usual empirical sources in search of ideas which can both augment our conception of brain function and limit possible alternative interpretations.

There is a kind of economics involved in the decision about which of many possible multiple measures to concentrate on. Some time ago, Meyer (1958) argued that anatomical verification might sometimes be insufficiently relevant to justify the effort involved. That is, for a "molar analysis" of behavior we might simply be happy to find that there exists a lesion which differentially affects several behaviors. Not only may anatomical correlates sometimes have little relevance, but they may actually interfere with conceptualization if allowed to dominate the interpretation of a certain experiment. It has sometimes been found that lesion or stimulation in a particular anatomical structure gives rise to the same behavioral phenomenon in many cases—but not in all cases (e.g., Valenstein, 1973). This is not necessarily a cause for shame, to be covered up by averaging of data. On only some of these occasions will it be adequate to say that there must have been some inaccuracy of electrode placements or that anatomical regions simply do not correspond precisely to functional ones.

To see this, recall first Gregory's warning that output function may not correspond in any obvious way to internal functional units, and recall that however simple a behavioral measure is, such a measure is dependent on the activity of a complex system of interacting parts. Consider the possibility that the goal-directed character of organisms' behavior is such as to enable them to invoke strategies beyond those which involve alternative usage of peripheral sensory and motor organs when confronted by some obstacle. Conceivably, organisms also have some range of options as to which sets of neural structures to use in performing tasks. The initial tendency of one particular individual to use one or the other option might be determined by past experience or by very slight innate differences, say, in the number of cells in a nucleus. Repeated use of particular options would exaggerate individual differences, through learning.

9. HOW TO PAMPER YOUR PERCEPTUAL SYSTEM

Restating some of the comments of the previous section in the language of popular social science, we could say that the scientist is inherently alienated from the reality which is his source of data. While we obtain quick answers in everyday perception, in science it takes so long to learn a small fact that we easily lose perspective on the relative importance of findings. Insofar as an individual scientist is capable of keeping his attention focused on his goal, he must suffer continuing tension and frustration during his prolonged effort. Because physiological phenomena generally take place on a more rapid time scale than behavioral ones, physiology is inherently a more satisfying enterprise. For a similar reason, among those who study behavior, psychopharmacology is a lively area of research. You give a drug and, bingo, you see an effect; try a different drug in the same animal and promptly see a different effect. Contrast this with the long time it takes to pin down a finding by means of lesion experiments. One kind of personal solution to this problem for the researcher interested in questions requiring the lesion method is to cherish the artistry of a well-conducted experiment. One does the work for its own sake. We all must adopt this attitude to a degree; however, as necessary as it is, it succeeds in reducing our alienation from the reality we seek only by the defense mechanism of denial. This attitude leaves us open to the danger of stagnation, i.e., of doing beautiful but arbitrary and ultimately useless research. The broad perspective must always be borne in mind, difficult though this is. This perspective comprises alternative theories and a constant searching for ideas about how to answer big questions as quickly as possible.

There is no one simple formula which translates this general advice into specific methods for all types of lesion experiment. In studying somatosensory and motor functions, which are highly (though not completely) lateralized, the present author has kept his "alienation from reality" at a tolerable level by using retention techniques in doing single-organism studies (e.g., Glassman, 1970; Glassman, Forgus, Goodman, and Glassman, 1975; Glassman and Glassman, 1977). In studying sensory and motor function, the animal can be used as its own control not only in the sense of preoperative baseline versus postoperative measures, but also in the sense of comparing the two sides of the body before and after unilateral lesions. In addition, I have gone so far as to use the method of serial enlargement of lesions—in spite of the possibilities of (a) confounding by the serial lesion effect, (b) confounding by synergetic effects, and (c) distortion of the anatomical results of the first lesion—to use the animal further as its own control in comparing different sizes and placements of lesion. The uncertainties introduced during these procedures seem to me to have been less important for the time being than the opportunity to grasp a phenomenon in individual cases.

In most of this research, some simple and quickly administered neurological tests (modified from those used by Sprague, 1966) have proven to be just as sensitive as a test of learned discrimination. The quantification of these neurological tests according to defined criteria, on a four-point scale, appears to be just as meaningful quantitatively as the more variable, day-to-day percent-correct score in discrimination learning. The rapidity of these tests has facilitated testing of individual animals in several measures. As in everyday perception, such a procedure allows separating figure from ground (Hochberg, 1972), i.e., it allows an appreciation not only of what the effect is but also of what it is not.

10. THE QUALITATIVE NATURE OF INVESTIGATION

The extent to which scientific endeavor is an extrapolation of our common ability to perceive, understand, and solve problems is often missed because we are distracted by the quantitative aspect of scientific endeavor. Although quantification is a prominent characteristic of science, the role which it plays is often overstated. Except possibly in some special cases, quantification is useful not for its own sake but because it contributes to decisions about which alternative qualitative descriptions are best or because it modifies and refines a qualitative description. The qualitative description is the real locus of understanding.

A number of authors have argued that human understanding is an outgrowth of the sort of distal, multidimensional perception which is characteristic of vision (Campbell, 1974; Gregory, 1970), and Lorenz (1959) has argued, similarly, that what the scientist strives for is a Gestalt perception of multiple interrelations. Although one might disagree with Lorenz's position on the basis that it is used largely to justify a naturalistic methodology, notoriously susceptible to confounding of variables, there is no question that a scientist must develop a perspective about the role of his selected variables in the reality he is trying to perceive. The writings of these authors should be read carefully.

It is possible to find evidence for the importance of "Gestalt perception" closer to physiological psychology. Consider the richness of information present in a stained section of neural tissue, in comparison with the poverty of results of an ablation study in which some single behavioral measure is affected by a lesion. The latter result, though taking much longer to arrive at than an anatomical preparation, is more heavily dependent on an interpretive framework and on interrelations with other studies, as argued earlier. To carry the histological example further, consider the additional richness of information given for us to apprehend in one fell swoop by a scanning electron micrograph, as opposed to what we would see in a section of the same material. This is not to say that the former gives all of the information that would be seen in the section but that for certain purposes, when a three-dimensional surface is of interest, it gives more information and demands less painstaking inference.

As another example, consider how present methodology constrains us so that we can observe electrical activity of only a few points at a time in the brain. Bearing in mind the facility with which we can apprehend the rich spatial array of a histological preparation, we would certainly be in an excellent position if we could somehow focus in on distributions of electrical and chemical activity in a similar manner in living preparations and if we could slow these down on "instant replay." Instead, the preparations that we are capable of constructing are used in a painstaking manner to build up to a conception, but not to an immediate perception of the distribution of activity. Multiple-channel recording attempts to surmount this problem but, again reflecting on the richness inherent in a histological preparation, this method is still only a poor approximation to the ideal.

Among lesion studies the most interesting are not those which measure differences of a single variable but those in which an entire syndrome is described, e.g., the Klüver–Bucy (1939) syndrome. Because behavioral phenomena extend over long periods of time with respect to a human observer's life, and because they take up a relatively large amount of room, we are in a position with regard to them analogous to what we would be up against if we had to view histological preparations only one point at a time and if only a few points on a given slide could be observed. We would then have to fall back on an inferential method and on quantitative, statistical measurements of optical density distributions in order to arrive at a conception of what a section looked like. Under conditions such as these our facility for language appears to be invaluable in taking us from point to point among data and ideas, and in seeking out inconsistencies that might be immediately obvious if we could only see it all at once.

There is only one way in which it might be claimed that we have a kind of scientific advantage in studying the more difficult problems of behavior, in comparison with pure anatomy. Recalling that all observation and description has theoretical underpinnings, the very ambiguity of the behavioral enterprise makes it difficult to agree prematurely on units of analysis. In this manner it might be claimed that it is unfortunate that the histologist can hardly help seeing his units in the cells and other structural formations. The laws of Gestalt perception (Hochberg, 1972) weld these together for him in his eye–brain system before he ever has a chance to bring judgment to bear. For example, it is hard for an observer to conceive of a structure delimited by a closed contour as anything but a unit; similarly, symmetrical patterns are automatically imbued with significance, etc. It is difficult to take this too seriously as a criticism of anatomical method because it throws things too wide open; if you cannot start by assuming that a cell is a cell, where can you start? Nevertheless, this criticism may have some validity in that it alerts us to look for aspects of functional organization which are not reflected in the most obvious aspects of structure.

Behavioral researchers often look to physics for guidance about how to be good scientists, but in physics too one can see the same subordination of quantification to qualitative description, e.g., of an atomic model. The solar system model of the atom could not possibly have been arrived at by direct visualization. It represents a structured set of inferences from measurements. Though in modern physics one is careful not to take such models too literally—for example, one speaks not of the position of an electron but of a probability distribution—the physicist still uses terms to describe networks of relations, e.g., emission, particle, velocity, that are reminiscent of common experience.

11. EMERGENCE

An explanation is most satisfying when it is "elegant." Such an explanation gives us a simple concept which enables us efficiently to answer a broad variety of new questions. As noted at several earlier points, explanations involve explicit analogies and analogies implicit in descriptive terms, relating present problems to earlier ones. If description and explanation were not possible, we would not be discussing the issue; nevertheless, the possibility is amazing, as Einstein recognized in his often quoted remark that the most incomprehensible thing about the universe is its comprehensibility.

New phenomena can always be related to past experience, at least in the primitive sense of being describable using our old vocabulary. Description could be considered a kind of unconscious reduction which by itself is suggestive of new ideas and experimental observations. Somewhat less frequently, it is possible to arrive at an explicit, self-conscious reductionistic formulation. All such formulations might be said to involve a heavy contribution of hindsight. What is obvious after the fact is often not obvious before; therefore to a lesser degree formulations yield foresight or predictability. Occasionally, persistent failures to arrive at a reductionistic formulation lead researchers to speculate that an "emergent property" has been encountered, one that cannot be explained in terms of prior knowledge. It is not yet clear whether this is an ontological issue or an epistemological one but there is some hope that the problem will eventually be solvable by philosophers of science, by general systems theorists (Laszlo, 1973), or by amateur philosophers who spend their professional time in laboratories.

The philosophical subfield of evolutionary epistemology (Campbell, 1974) should be attractive to physiological psychologists because it views knowledge as a biological phenomenon. Like other biological phenomena, the evolution of knowledge is seen as being ultimately dependent on an evolutionary process of trial and error. If this is so, then some form of the concept of emergence would be inescapable, and pure reasoning techniques, no matter how powerful, would not be able to predict everything that there is to be known. Nevertheless, it is in the nature of scientific reductionism to go as far as it can in perceiving similarities among systems, that is, similarities of those observed now or in the future to those observed before. Sometimes, alternative, valid explanations differ in efficiency or elegance. In this regard, Boulding has wondered whether Copernicus would have been unnecessary if Ptolemy had had computers available, which he could have used for simulation techniques (Kuhn, 1974).

Some multiple-variable problems, which in principle seem as if they ought to be comprehensible, are extremely refractory to exact analysis; Bertalanffy (1962) gives as an example the three-body problem in physics. Though the situation with three interacting masses appears simple, it is impossible to analyze into "one-way [relations] between cause and effect." The brain of course has many more than three elements and more possibilities for complex interactions involving feedback loops. Loci of cause and effect are not easily or unequivocally defined. We should probably hold off, for the time being, on judging to what extent studies of the brain are hopelessly doomed to cataloguing "emergent facts" as opposed to what extent efficient formulations can be created that will make us feel that we have discovered important, underlying truths. Though the results of lesion studies are likely to contribute significantly to such formulations, it is ironic that, due to the great wisdom of hindsight, they may also contribute to the impression that such molar techniques were never really necessary to a healthy, reductionistic science!

12. REFERENCES

Arbib, M. A. *The metaphorical brain.* New York: Wiley, 1972.

Ashby, W. R. *Design for a brain.* New York: Wiley, 1960.

Beach, F. A., Hebb, D. O., Morgan, C. T., and Nissen, H. W. *The neuropsychology of Lashley.* New York: McGraw-Hill, 1960, pp. 432–434.

Bertalanffy, L. von. General system theory—a critical review. 1962. Reprinted in W. Buckley (Ed.), *Modern systems research for the behavioral scientist*. Chicago: Aldine, 1968, pp. 11–30.

Campbell, D. T. Natural selection as an epistemological model. In R. Naroll and R. Cohen (Eds.), *A handbook of method in cultural anthropology*. Garden City, N.Y.: The Natural History Press, 1970, pp. 51–85.

Campbell, D. T. Evolutionary epistemology. In P. A. Schilpp (Ed.), *The philosophy of Karl Popper*. Vol. 14, I and II. *The library of living philosophers*. LaSalle, Ill.: Open Court Publishing Co., 1974, pp. 413–463.

Chow, K. L. Effects of ablation. In G. C. Quarton, T. Melnechuk, and F. O. Schmitt (Eds.), *The neurosciences*. New York: Rockefeller University Press, 1967, pp. 705–713.

Darwin, C. *The origin of species*. New York: Washington Square Press, 1963 (reprinted).

Glassman, R. B. Cutaneous discrimination and motor control following somatosensory cortical ablations. *Physiology and Behavior*, 1970, *5*, 1009–1019.

Glassman, R. B. Similar effects of infant and adult sensorimotor cortical lesions on cats' posture. *Brain Research*, 1973, *63*, 103–110.

Glassman, R. B., Forgus, M. W., Goodman, J. E., and Glassman, H. N. Somesthetic effects of damage to cats' ventrobasal complex, medial lemniscus or posterior group. *Experimental Neurology*, 1975, *48*, 460–492.

Glassman, R. B., and Glassman, H. N. Distribution of somatosensory and motor behavioral function in cat's frontal cortex. *Physiology and Behavior*, 1977, *18*, 1127–1152.

Gregory, R. L. The brain as an engineering problem. In W. H. Thorpe and O. L. Zangwill (Eds.), *Current problems in animal behavior*. Cambridge: University Press, 1961, pp. 307–330.

Gregory, R. L. *The intelligent eye*. New York: McGraw-Hill, 1970.

Hebb, D. O. Drives and the CNS (conceptual nervous system). *Psychological Review*, 1955, *62*, 243–254.

Herrnstein, R. J., and Boring, E. G. *A source book in the history of psychology*. Cambridge: Harvard University Press, 1966, pp. 266–272.

Hochberg, J. Perception, I. color and shape. In J. W. Kling and L. A. Riggs (Eds.) *Woodworth and Schlosberg's experimental psychology*. Third edition, Vol. I, *Sensation and perception*. New York: Holt, Rinehart and Winston, 1972, pp. 395–474.

Jones, E. G. and Powell, T. P. S. Anatomical organization of the somatosensory cortex. In A. Iggo (Ed.), *Handbook of sensory physiology, Vol. II: Somatosensory system*. New York: Springer–Verlag, 1973, pp. 579–620.

Klüver, H., and Bucy, P. C. Preliminary analysis of functions of the temporal lobes in monkeys. *Archives of Neurology and Psychiatry*, 1939, *42*, 979–1000. Reprinted in R. L. Isaacson (Ed.), *Basic readings in neuropsychology*. New York: Harper and Row, 1964, pp. 60–86.

Krantz, D. L. Toward a role for historical analysis: the case of psychology and physiology. *Journal of the History of the Behavioral Sciences*, 1965, *1*, 278–283.

Kuhn, A. *The logic of social systems*. San Francisco: Jossey-Bass, 1974, p. 478.

Laszlo, E. *Introduction to systems philosophy*. New York: Harper Torchbooks, 1973.

Lorenz, K. Z. Gestalt perception as a source of scientific knowledge. *Zeitschrift für experimentelle und angewandte Psychologie*, 1959. Reprinted in K. Z. Lorenz, *Studies in animal and human behaviour*, Vol. II. Cambridge: Harvard University Press, 1971, pp. 281–322.

Lowry, R. *The evolution of psychological theory*. Chicago: Aldine-Atherton, 1971, p. 121.

Luria, A. R. *The working brain*. New York: Basic Books, 1973, pp. 27–34.

Markowitz, D. Generalized complementarity re-entered. *Journal of Theoretical Biology*, 1973, *40*, 399–402.

Marshall, J. F., Turner, B. H., and Teitelbaum, P. Sensory neglect produced by lateral hypothalamic damage. *Science,* 1971, *174,* 523–525.

Meyer, D. R. Some psychological determinants of sparing and loss following damage to the brain. In H. F. Harlow and C. N. Woolsey (Eds.), *Biological and biochemical bases of behavior.* Madison: University of Wisconsin Press, 1958, pp. 173–192.

Miller, J. G. The nature of living systems. *Behavioral Science,* 1971, *16,* 277–301.

Milner, P. M. *Physiological psychology.* New York: Holt, Rinehart and Winston, 1970.

Polanyi, M. *The tacit dimension.* Garden City, N.Y.: Doubleday, 1966.

Pribram, K. H. *Languages of the brain.* Englewood Cliffs, N.J.: Prentice-Hall, 1971.

Schoenfeld, T. A. and Hamilton, L. W. Secondary brain changes following lesions: a new paradigm for lesion experimentation. *Physiology and Behavior,* 1977, *18,* 951–967.

Simon, H. A. *The sciences of the artificial.* Cambridge: MIT Press, 1969.

Skinner, B. F. *Science and human behavior.* New York: Macmillan, 1953.

Sprague, J. M. Visual, acoustic, and somesthetic deficits in the cat after cortical and midbrain lesions. In D. P. Purpura and M. Yahr (Eds.), *The thalamus.* New York: Columbia University Press, 1966, pp. 391–417.

Teitelbaum, P. Levels of integration of the operant. In W. K. Honig and J. E. R. Staddon (Eds.), *Handbook of operant behavior.* Englewood Cliffs, N.J.: Prentice-Hall, 1977, pp. 7–27.

Teuber, H-L. Physiological psychology. *Annual Review of Psychology,* 1955, *6,* 267–296.

Teuber, H-L. Perception. In J. Field, H. W. Magoun, and V. E. Hall (Eds.), *Handbook of physiology, Section 1: Neurophysiology,* Vol. III. Washington, D.C.: American Physiological Society, 1960, pp. 1595–1668.

Thompson, R. Introducing subcortical lesions by electrolytic methods. In R. D. Myers (Ed.), *Methods in psychobiology.* New York: Academic Press, 1971, pp. 131–154.

Thompson, R. F. *Foundations of physiological psychology.* New York: Harper and Row, 1967.

Turner, M. B. *Realism and the explanation of behavior.* New York: Appleton-Century-Crofts, 1971, pp. 228–229.

Valenstein, E. S. *Brain control, a critical examination of brain stimulation and psychosurgery.* New York: Wiley, 1973.

von Monakow, C. Diaschisis. In *Die Lokalisation im Grosshirn und der abbau der Funktion durch kortikale Herde.* Wiesbaden: J. F. Bergmann, 1914, pp. 26–34. Reprinted in K. H. Pribram (Ed.), *Brain and behaviour 1, mood states and mind.* Baltimore: Penguin, 1969.

Waddington, C. H. Discussion. In P. S. Moorhead and M. M. Kaplan (Eds.), *Mathematical challenges to the neo-Darwinian interpretation of evolution.* Philadelphia: Wistar Institute Press, 1967, p. 70.

Wason, P. C., and Johnson-Laird, P. N. *Thinking and reasoning.* Baltimore: Penguin, 1968.

Weiskrantz, L. Treatments, inferences, and brain functions. In L. Weiskrantz (Ed.), *Analysis of behavioral change.* New York: Harper and Row, 1968, pp. 400–414. (*a*)

Weiskrantz, L. Some traps and pontifications. In L. Weiskrantz (Ed.), *Analysis of behavioral change.* New York: Harper and Row, 1968, pp. 415–429. (*b*)

Young, R. M. *Mind, brain and adaptation in the nineteenth century.* Oxford: Clarendon Press, 1970.

Zangwill, O. L. Lashley's concept of cerebral mass action. In W. H. Thorpe and O. L. Zangwill (Eds.), *Current problems in animal behavior.* Cambridge: University Press, 1961, pp. 59–86.

PART II

SPECIES VARIABLES

2

Generalizations in Neuropsychology

J. M. WARREN and BRYAN KOLB

Although rats are obviously not little men in white fur suits, physiological psychologists use rats as research subjects far more frequently than any other species. Few psychologists who work with rats affect a strong interest in rats for the sake of rats, however. They believe that rats are typical mammals, and that therefore brain–behavior relations found in rats apply to mammals generally. Students of primate biopsychology, however, reject the idea that experiments with rats only can provide a satisfactory neurology of mammalian behavior (e.g., Wilson, 1976).

The disagreement over the traditional emphasis on rats in physiological psychology is a special case of the concern of this chapter: When can one reasonably generalize results from neurobehavioral studies on one species to other species of mammals?

Questions about the existence and meaning of similarities between taxa are critical in many other fields in biology. Taxonomists, for example, have dealt with such problems since long before the birth of physiological psychology. Their experience suggests both the difficulties encountered in interpreting comparative material and ways to overcome them.

J. M. WARREN • Department of Psychology, The Pennsylvania State University, University Park, Pennsylvania   **BRYAN KOLB** • Department of Psychology, University of Lethbridge, Lethbridge, Alberta, Canada   This paper deals only with mammals. Most biopsychological work is done with mammals, and the authors' experience with nonmammalian taxa is severely limited.

The establishment of homology is never absolutely one hundred percent certain, but to insist on that fact as a deficiency of evolutionary taxonomy would tend to negate the value of any and all scientific endeavor. Some homologies, for instance between the humeri of men and apes, are as nearly certain as that the sun will rise tomorrow. Others have lower degrees of probability. Some that seemed nearly certain when inadequately studied have turned out to be almost certainly not homology but homoplasy, as in the example of the litopterns and horses. The same example shows that gathering more data and applying more numerous and precise criteria can be sufficiently definitive even in such difficult cases (Simpson, 1961).

The situation is much the same in comparative neuropsychology. Conclusions once held as almost certain are contradicted and revised as more adequate experimental data are obtained. Several recent revisions of traditional views in neuropsychology, however, collectively form a coherent pattern and suggest the following model for predicting some agreements and disagreements among species in the behavioral effects of brain dysfunction.

1. CLASS-COMMON BEHAVIOR

Wild animals are adapted to survive and reproduce in a characteristic ecological niche by means of a unique, species-specific set of motor patterns and sensitivities to sign stimuli, correlated with events and situations that are significant for survival and reproduction. An ethogram is a comprehensive description of the behavior patterns of a species; every species has a distinctive ethogram that differs from that of every other species. By now the idea that each species has its own inventory of motor patterns and sign stimuli and its own overall pattern of behavioral organization is generally accepted in the study of animal behavior (Alcock, 1975; Brown, 1975; Eibl-Eibesfeldt, 1970; Hinde, 1970; Warren, 1972, 1973).

Evolutionary theory tells us that this must be the case. No two species can long survive in precisely the same niche, so no two species have been exposed to exactly the same selection pressures. It is consequently most improbable that any two species could ever evolve identically organized behavioral repertoires.

In the recent literature one gains the impression that some behavioral psychologists have learned the lesson of species-specificity in behavior too well. They write as if the behavior of each species developed in complete independence, or perhaps as a result of special creation. This view is of course a counsel of despair regarding the possibility of generalization in neuropsychology. It is also wrong. More broadly trained biologists have long recognized that many species may share common structural and behavioral traits.

> From the point of view of usefulness taxonomic characters range between
> two extremes: those that are so invariable in a large taxonomic group that
> they are useless for classification, like the two eyes of vertebrates, and those
> that are either so variable or so easily affected by the environment that they
> do not even permit discrimination between closely related taxa, like size or
> color in some animals. Between these extremes are those characters which
> are constant within a given taxonomic group (species, genus, family) but
> vary between it and another taxonomic group. There are many behavior
> characters that fall into this category (Mayr, 1958, pp. 344–345).

Lorenz also saw that many species may have the same behavioral
character in common. "But is it not possible that beneath all the variations in individual behavior there lies an inner structure of inherited
behavior which characterizes all members of a given species, genus or
larger taxonomic group—just as the skeleton of a primordial ancestor
characterizes the form and structure of all animals today?" (Lorenz,
1958). The answer is yes; the taxonomic group that shares a common
behavior pattern may sometimes be large indeed.

> Anyone who has watched a dog scratch its jaw or a bird preen its head
> feathers can attest to the fact that they do it in the same way. The dog props
> itself on the tripod formed by its haunches and two forelegs and reaches a
> hindleg forward in front of its shoulder. Now the odd fact is that most birds
> (as well as virtually all mammals and reptiles) scratch with precisely the same
> motion. A bird also scratches with a hindlimb (that is, its claw), and in doing
> so it lowers its wing and reaches its claw forward in front of its shoulder.
> One might think that it would be simpler for the bird to move its claw di-
> rectly to its head without moving its wing, which lies folded out of the way
> on its back. I do not see how to explain this clumsy action unless we admit
> that it is inborn. Before the bird can scratch, it must reconstruct the old spa-
> tial relationship of the limbs of the four-legged common ancestor which it
> shares with mammals (Lorenz, 1958).

In general, it appears that each mammalian species has a unique
behavioral repertory, and, at the same time, shares similar behavioral
traits and capacities with other mammals. For example, all mammalian
mothers provide milk and maternal care to their young, and all mammals tested learn operant behavior under complex schedules of reinforcement and master tasks that seem beyond the capacity of "lower"
vertebrates (Warren, 1977).

Behaviors and behavioral capacities demonstrable in all mammals
will be designated *class-common behaviors*. The term *class-common* may be
useful as a reminder that many discrete behaviors are not species-
specific and also to define a reference point on the continuum of interspecific specificity–generality in behavior, near the opposite end of
the scale from species-specific.

Ethologists have drawn essentially the same distinction between class-common and species-specific in studies of the constancy of individual behavior patterns in mammals. Some behavior patterns like grooming are conservative, showing relatively little change across species. Other patterns like courtship and copulation are phylogenetically labile, with marked differences occurring among closely related species as a result of strong selection for sexual isolation (Dewsbury, 1975).

2. CLASS-COMMON NEURAL MECHANISMS

Class-common behaviors permit mammals to cope successfully with problems of adaptation that confront all mammalian species. It is reasonable to hypothesize that the basic neural mechanisms responsible for class-common behaviors are also class-common. Class-commonality in respect to behavior and underlying neural mechanisms implies that observations on one species may be validly generalized to other species of mammals.

A consideration of the problems every mammal must solve if it is to long endure suggests the behaviors most likely to be mediated by common neural substrates. All mammals must detect and interpret sensory stimuli, relate this information to past experience, and act appropriately. The behavioral evidence indicates that these functions are carried out in qualitatively similar ways when animals are observed under neutral conditions, i.e., in the absence of sign stimuli significant for the species. It seems unlikely that the basic sensory, associative, and motor functions of the brain have changed drastically in the evolution of the mammals. Stimulation and evoked-potential studies reveal a similar topography in the motor, somatosensory, visual, and auditory cortices of the mammals. There are no gross qualitative discontinuities in the organization of the sensory and motor fields between placental mammals and marsupials or monotremes.

The phyletic stability of the organization of the motor and sensory areas in the brains of mammals implies strong and persistent selection for efficient function, a view supported by the convergent evolution of similar systems in nonmammalian species. The barn owl, for example, has independently evolved visual receptor cells in the Wulst that are very similar to those in the striate cortex of cats and monkeys (Pettigrew and Konishi, 1976).

Class-common behaviors are largely those necessary for mammals to construct a valid model of their environment from present and past experience. Species-specific behaviors have been selected to promote survival in a unique niche and way of life. The distinction and the interaction of the two sorts of behavior is apparent in the response of monkeys and cats to a brief noise from an invisible speaker. A monkey is frightened and tries to get away from the sound source, while a cat is fascinated by the sound and tries to get as close to the source as she can. These are species-specific reactions, eminently appropriate for the cat as predator, and the monkey as potential prey. However, cats, monkeys, and every other species of mammal observed to date are very well endowed with the forms of sensitivity to acoustic stimuli needed to localize accurately sources of sound (Masterton, Heffner, and Ravizza, 1969). All mammals must localize sounds accurately and have evolved neural circuits to mediate sound localization; this is class-common behavior. How an animal responds to a sound is determined by whether it is a predator or a possible prey and by other characteristics of its species; this is species-specific behavior.

3. SOME EVIDENCE FOR CLASS-COMMON NEURAL MECHANISMS

We have argued that there is no basic qualitative difference in the neural bases for such class-common behaviors as sensory, associative, and motor functions in mammals. The perceptive and erudite reader will recognize this position as a direct contradiction of the literature on the encephalization and encorticalization of function in mammals. These notions were based on inadequate evidence and have been discredited; the best evidence for class-common effects of lesions on behavior comes from the experiments which disconfirmed the encephalization concept.

3.1. The Phylogeny of Mammalian Vision

> It has long been recognized, especially by comparative anatomists, that the central nervous system exhibits an orderly development in phylogeny characterized by the shifting of function from lower towards higher centers ("encephalization"), and nowhere is the growth of dominance in higher centers more strikingly illustrated [than] in the evolution of visual function (Fulton, 1949, pp. 349–350).

Fulton's view was based on the following evidence. Rats deprived of the visual cortex lose pattern vision but can discriminate brightness, avoid obstacles, and recognize food by sight. Dogs after occipital lobectomy act as if blind, move cautiously and slowly in unfamiliar surroundings, exploring carefully with the paws. Operated dogs can discriminate brightness, but show no sign of object vision. The picture is much the same in cats without the visual cortex. Klüver's (1941) monkeys could discriminate total luminous flux, but neither visual size nor brightness. The occipital monkey "appears to have no serviceable vision" (Fulton, 1949, p. 351).

The classical picture of a steady phyletic progression from rats to monkeys in the severity of the syndrome resulting from destruction of the visual cortex is untenable today. Helen, Humphrey's (1974) chronic monkey with almost no striate cortex, avoided obstacles and found currents with great efficiency. Monkeys with no striate cortex also learned both shape and color discriminations (Schilder, Pasik, and Pasik, 1972), and pattern-discrimination learning has been demonstrated by striatectomized cats (Doty, 1971) and rats (Weiskrantz, 1974).

There is thus no basis for postulating any major disparity among mammals in regard to the visual functions that are lost or remain after removal of the striate cortex.

The chief reasons for the more severe symptoms reported by early researchers on the visual cortex compared to those seen by contemporary investigators are two. First, the early lesions were bigger; occipital lobectomies destroy, in addition to the striate cortex, much of the extrastriate visual cortex, which contributes importantly to the visual guidance of behavior (Weiskrantz, 1974). In recent years, students of visual cortical functions have been at pains to confine their ablations to striate or nonstriate visual cortex only, unless they plan deliberately to invade both areas.

Second, behavioral assessment techniques have improved. The most dramatic example is the close and warm relationship Humphrey developed with Helen over a period of years which permitted him unequivocally to show Helen's ability to avoid obstacles in the real world outside the laboratory without the striate cortex. There have also been very significant advances in the development of displays to elicit the best visual performance from striatectomized mammals (Schilder *et al.*, 1972; Weiskrantz, 1974).

3.2. Ablation of Auditory Cortex

Research on the effects of decorticating the auditory projection cortex in mammals is characterized by a high level of agreement in the findings obtained from different species of mammals (Ravizza and Belmore, in press). Monkeys with ablations of the auditory cortex are severely impaired in their ability to approach the site of a brief sound, but they can respond differentially to sounds presented at different loci in space if the response is lever pressing, not movement through space

(H. Heffner and Masterton, 1975). Like monkeys, hedgehogs, bush-babies, and cats are grossly impaired when required to approach the site of a brief sound signal in localization tests (Neff, Arnott, and Fisher, 1950; Ravizza and Diamond, 1974). Like monkeys, opossums are not impaired in localizing sounds when tested on a conditioned suppression task that did not entail approaching the sound source (Ravizza and Masterton, 1972). Thus, all of the species sampled reacted the same way in the same circumstances, being impaired when obliged to use sound localization cues to guide a directed approach, but not impaired when the location of a sound in space was the discriminative stimulus for a response that did not demand directed movement. To the limited extent that the number of species permits, the data suggest transspecific generality in the effect of response requirement on performance and give a different kind of support for the position that the basic functions of the auditory cortex are similar in mammals. If the functions are common, they should be affected in the same way by the same variations in experimental parameters, as is true in this illustration.

3.3. Encephalization of Motor Functions

A generation ago it was widely held that the effects of motor as well as visual decortication become progressively more serious as one goes from rats to cats and dogs to primates. Lassek (1954), for example, contrasted the effects of injuries to motor cortex in monkeys and carnivores in the following terms. Decortication of Brodmann's area 4 in primates causes "an enduring paralysis of isolated movements especially in the digits. A flaccid type of paralysis occurs in the proximal joints whereas the wrists and fingers pass through a period of moderate spasticity" (Lassek, 1954, pp. 65–66). On the other hand, "the motor cortex appears to be largely dispensable in mammals ranking below primates. Ablation of area 4 in the cat or dog is attended by only negligible and transitory deficits" (Lassek, 1954, p. 67).

Note that this comparison is not based upon comparable response measures. The most profound defects in monkeys were in manual activities, while only posture and locomotion were observed in experimental cats and dogs. And it is well known that the action of proximal effectors is less severely disturbed by motor lesions than distal effectors in the same species.

The view that the motor cortex is largely dispensable in carnivores is not sustained by more recent work. Large lesions in the motor cortex produce a severe and permanent impairment in the ability of cats to manipulate objects and especially to make controlled extension responses with the forepaw; these deficits persist throughout postoperative observation periods as long as six months (Forward, Warren, and Hara, 1962; Warren, Cornwell, Webster, and Pubols, 1972).

These experiments indicate that the motor cortex makes a significant contribution to the normal behavior of intact cats and cast doubt upon the notion of an abrupt discontinuity, a quantal jump, in cortical motor functions between cats and monkeys. The defect in manipulation seen in cats is all the more cogent an argument against the presumed uniqueness of the primate motor cortex when one considers that cats have only a very modestly developed corticospinal system (R. Heffner and Masterton, 1975). It seems likely that species of carnivores like racoons, with more precise control of the hand and digits, would show an even more monkey-like set of changes in manual responses after motor cortex lesions than cats.

3.4. The Frontal Cortex and Learning by Rats

For years it was believed that the mediodorsal thalamic nucleus (MD) projected to the frontal pole in rats. Lesions in the frontal polar region were generally unsuccessful in producing behavioral symptoms of the sort found in carnivores and primates (Warren and Akert, 1964), suggesting a major difference in rodents versus carnivores and primates.

The resolution of this paradox, indicative of a qualitative disjunction in the role of the frontal cortex in learning by rats and other mammals, followed quickly upon Leonard's (1969) discovery that MD in rats projects to a medial region anterior to the genu of the corpus callosum and to a lateral suprahinal strip (sulcal cortex), but not to the frontal pole.

Divac (1971) showed that lesions in the medial frontal field significantly impaired spatial reversal performance in rats, but frontal polar lesions did not; defective performance in reversal learning is one of the most dependable symptoms of frontal injuries in different species of mammals. Disruption of reversal learning after medial frontal lesions and sparing after frontal pole lesions indicates that only the former is similar to the frontal system in other mammals.

A more complete answer to the question of the similarity between the functions of the frontal cortex and learning in rats and other mammals was obtained by Kolb, Nonneman, and Singh (1974). On the basis of thalamocortical connections, the rat's medial frontal cortex is like the dorsolateral cortex in monkeys, and the sulcal cortex of rats like the orbital cortex in monkeys. The possibility that the anatomically similar areas mediate similar learned behavior in the two species was examined by testing rats with medial and sulcal frontal lesions on tasks known to be differentially affected by dorsolateral and orbital frontal lesions in monkeys. Rats with medial frontal lesions were severely impaired on delayed response and spatial reversal learning. Rats with lesions in the sulcal cortex showed greatly exaggerated perseveration on a DRL 20 schedule and in extinction. The defects in the two groups of rats correspond very closely to those seen in monkeys with frontal lesions restricted to the dorsolateral and orbital cortex. Thus there is a virtually identical division of labor between the subfields of frontal cortex that receive projections from the parvo- and magno-cellular portions of MD in rats and monkeys. It is clear that the initial appearance of a difference in frontal lobe functions between rats and other mammals resulted from improper identification of the frontal cortex in rats.

3.5. Cerebral Asymmetry in Monkeys

Most neuroscientists are of the opinion that the functions of the cerebral hemispheres are differentiated only in humans (Levy, 1977; Warren, 1976). A large number of experiments with monkeys subjected to unilateral ablation and split brain procedures and tested on visual learning tasks confirm this view (Hamilton, 1977a,b; Warren and Nonneman, 1976).

Our faith in the dogma that cerebral asymmetry is associated with language and therefore present only in humans is shaken, although not yet definitively destroyed, by Dewson's (1977, in press) suggestive findings on hemispheric asymmetry in monkeys tested on delayed matching to sample with auditory signals. The monkeys are rewarded for choosing green on trials when noise is presented, and red on trials with a tone. Ablation of the left superior temporal gyrus permanently impairs delayed matching performance; lesions in the right superior temporal gyrus and auditory projection cortex do not.

Dewson's sample is small and his task is complex and somewhat difficult to interpret unambiguously. Yet his findings fit well into the argument that species-unique adaptations in sensory, associative, and cognitive functions are rather rare among mammals.

Similar behavioral changes result from comparable brain lesions in several species of mammals. This finding is compatible with the notion that class-common behaviors are based upon class-common neural mechanisms. If this is so, why do some mammals have larger and more elaborately differentiated cerebral cortexes than others?

Perhaps mammals with more highly developed cortex have additional sensory and associative capacities beyond those which are mediated by class-common mechanisms, these extra capabilities being the functional correlates of the advances in cerebral complexity. No one knows. The behaviors studied in ablation and stimulation experiments are typically close to the lowest common denominator of mammalian capacity, about equally appropriate for opossums, rats, and monkeys.

With more adequate behavior testing, integrative behaviors and neural mechanisms may be found that are not common to all mammals. It is likely, however, that such advanced neural mechanisms will be functionally superimposed upon, and supplement rather than replace, the class-common mechanisms characteristic of all mammals. This speculation is based partially on observations of intact mammals. Chimpanzees are not conspicuously more adept than most other mammals on classical conditioning or learning set tasks, which require class-common abilities, but differ from nonanthropoid mammals in their acquisition of paralinguistic behaviors like sign language (Warren, 1977).

4. SPECIES-SPECIFIC NEURAL MECHANISMS

The sensible place to look for species-specific neural mechanisms to control species-specific behaviors is in the limbic system and hypothalamus, where lesions usually disrupt species-specific behavior. Yet the experimental literature yields no convincing suggestions of genuinely species-unique neural circuits in this part of the brain. The evidence indicates instead that the functional organization of the limbic system is class-common, not species-specific. The basic structural plan of the limbic system is the same in all mammals. Lesions in the same limbic structure produce similar sorts of changes in the behavior of diverse species (Isaacson, 1974).

The class-common organization of the hypothalamus is more obvious. Mammals with lesions in the ventromedial nucleus are fat and aggressive, no matter what their species-specific pattern of feeding and agonistic behaviors are. Mammalian species show a wide variety of sex behavior, but none displays a species-normal level of sexual activity if the anterior hypothalamus is destroyed. Likewise, no species of mammal becomes hyperphagic after damage to the lateral hypothalamic region.

Regulatory mechanisms in the hypothalamus control general functions like eating and drinking in about the same way in all mammals. And yet species-specific behavior is as real a phenomenon as class-common control mechanisms: dogs like stale bagels better than cats do. Fortunately, it is not hard to imagine how class-common hypothalamic centers can mediate species-specific behaviors. Central integrating mechanisms are far more conservative in evolution than receptor and effector elements. The processes for reflex coordination in the spinal shark, frog, and cat are very much the same, even though these species differ greatly in sensory and motor characteristics. We assume that the basic regulatory mechanisms of the hypothalamus have changed little in mammalian phylogeny and that different species evolved divergent input and output relations with the central regulating mechanism to permit selective and species-appropriate reactions to sign stimuli; and we also assume that they selected suitable fixed action patterns as they adopted to diverse niches. All mammals probably have similar sets of hypothalamic control centers that metaphorically order the organism to eat, to attack, etc. But the functional characteristics of the afferent and efferent systems associated with the centers differ in different species, to insure that a given behavior pattern occurs only when it is likely to produce results that favor the individual or her progeny.

The hypothalamic mechanisms for the control of behavior are thus imagined to consist of a class-common regulating device, innervated by variable, species-specific patterns of afferents and efferents. This schema seems also to characterize the functional organization of the telencephalic limbic system. Lesions in a given component of the limbic system like the hippocampus produce a wide variety of changes in the species-specific behaviors of different species of mammals, but underlying the heterogeneous set of particular symptoms of hippocampal insults, one can see a common feature, a reduction in the threshold for the initiation of behavior sequences (Isaacson, 1974).

Biopsychologists now rather freely generalize the results of studies on the hypothalamus across species. They are certainly correct in doing so, even when they deal with species-specific behaviors. There seems to be no reason why findings concerning the behavioral functions of the limbic system cannot be generalized across species as well. The fact that the class-common symptoms of damage to the amygdala and the hippocampus must be defined in much more abstract terms than the syndrome resulting from injuries to the vertromedial hypothalamic nucleus suggests, however, that we should perhaps be rather more cautious in generalizing about the behavioral effects of interventions in the limbic system than in the hypothalamus.

We have argued that neuropsychological results can often be generalized from one species to other species of mammals. It would be a gross error if the reader were to infer that this argument legitimatizes the trend to concentrate on rats and monkeys in behavioral biology. There are differences as well as similarities among the brains of mammals. The differences can be understood only if we determine the limits of interspecific generalizations and discover what behavioral peculiarities are associated with unusual brain characteristics. We cannot do this job with only rats and rhesus macaques.

5. SUMMARY

Some spontaneous behaviors are common to a large taxon, like the pattern of head scratching in Amniota. Others are observed only in a single species. Mammals display behaviors that range from species-specific to class-common.

All mammals have class-common behavioral capacities to cope with problems faced by every mammal, such as spatial orientation, sound localization, and learning. This fact suggested that class-common behaviors are mediated by class-common neural mechanisms, sufficiently similar to one another to permit valid generalizations across species. This view is supported by several recent ablation experiments.

There is no strong evidence for completely unique mechanisms for species-specific behavior patterns in the limbic system, indicating that worthwhile generalizations across species concerning the neural bases of species-specific behavior are also feasible.

The possibility of considerable generalization across species does not imply that neuroscientists can afford not to study a wide variety of species. It is as important to establish the limits of interspecific generality and to determine the behavioral significance of advances in brain structure as it is to establish broad generalizations across species.

6. REFERENCES

Alcock, J. *Animal behavior.* Sunderland, Mass.: Sinauer, 1975.

Brown, J. L. *The evolution of behavior.* New York: Norton, 1975.

Dewson, J. H. Preliminary evidence of hemispheric asymmetry of auditory functions in monkeys. In S. Harnad (Ed.), *Lateralization in the nervous system.* New York: Academic Press, 1977.

Dewson, J. H. Some behavioral effects of removal of superior temporal cortex in the monkey. *Proceedings of the sixth congress of the international primatology society.* New York: Academic Press, in press.

Divac, I. Frontal lobe system and spatial reversal in the rat. *Neuropsychologia,* 1971, *9,* 175–183.

Doty, R. W. Survival of pattern vision after removal of striate cortex in the adult cat. *Journal of Comparative Neurology,* 1971, *143,* 437–464.

Eibl-Eibesfeldt, I. *Ethology.* New York: Holt, Rinehart and Winston, 1970.

Forward, E., Warren, J. M., and Hara, K. The effects of unilateral lesions in sensorimotor cortex on manipulation by cats. *Journal of Comparative and Physiological Psychology,* 1962, *55,* 1130–1135.

on the vertebrate visual system. As he states, "As far back in the human past as there is a record, the supreme importance of vision and of its instrument, the eye, has been recognized." Up to 1800, for practical reasons, investigation was primarily directed to the eye and its diseases. Nevertheless, the role of the brain in visual-information processing was also fully appreciated. The fact that there were structural connections between the eyes and the brain, in the form of "nerves," "ducts," or "tubes," was established very early. However, up to the middle of the nineteenth century, knowledge of details was scanty and often inaccurate. The cerebral center for vision was almost invariably placed below the cerebral himespheres—in the lateral ventricles (Galen), the brain-stem (Willis), the pineal body (Descartes), and other sites.

One reason for this was technical in nature. The limitations inherent in gross anatomical study made it very difficult indeed to trace the visual pathways beyond the optic tract. But an even more important reason was of a conceptual nature. The dominating influence of Flourens' doctrine of the equipotentiality of the cerebral hemispheres made it seem pointless to look for a focal center for vision above the level of the thalamus.

However, Flourens' dogma was challenged by two contributions in the 1850s, one of an anatomical nature and the other consisting of experimental and clinical observations, and these laid the groundwork for the subsequent identification of a cortical center for vision. By means of careful dissection of fixed specimens, Gratiolet (1854) was able to demonstrate the optic radiations arising from the lateral geniculate nuclei and fanning out to the cortex of the occipital and parietal lobes. He described the radiations as "expansions of the optic nerve terminating in a specific region of the cortex of the hemispheres." A year later, Gratiolet's anatomical discovery was complemented by the observations of Panizza (1855), who established a rough correlation between lesions in the occipitoparietal area and visual impairment, both in human case material and in dogs subjected to experimental ablations. Panizza reported that bilateral destruction of this area resulted in complete blindness while unilateral damage caused blindness in the opposite eye. A clinicopathologic study by Chaillou (1863) of a patient with extensive destruction of the "posterior" lobes and concomitant visual impairment provided an additional bit of evidence in support of Panizza's correlation. Similarly, Meynert's (1869) description of the course of the optic radiations from the thalamic level to the occipital and temporal lobes partially substantiated the observations of Gratiolet.

A more intensive search for the site of the cortical center for vision, as well as for the other senses, followed upon the discovery of the motor area of the cortex by Fritsch and Hitzig (1870). Ferrier (1876, 1878, 1890) carried out a long series of studies involving both destruction and stimulation of different cortical areas in animals, primarily the monkey, and sought confirmation of his experimental findings in relevant clinical observations. He concluded that the angular gyrus was the site of the cortical visual center since its "unilateral destruction has the effect of causing temporary blindness of the opposite eye, while bilateral destruction causes total and permanent blindness in both eyes" (Ferrier, 1878, p. 122). Confronted by a substantial amount of contradictory evidence from the studies of other investigators, he later modified his position and conceded that the visual center occupied the territory of *both* the angular gyrus and the occipital lobes. But he still insisted that "the angular gyrus is the special region of clear or central vision of the opposite eye, and perhaps to some extent also of the eye on the same side" (Ferrier, 1886, p. 288). And he maintained that the occipital lobes "can be injured, or cut off bodily, almost up to the parieto-occipital fissure, on one or both sides simultaneously, without the slightest appreciable impairment of vision" (Ferrier, 1886, p. 273).

What could have led Ferrier to these inaccurate inferences? Given his crude surgical techniques, the suggestion by Starr (1884) and Schäfer (1888) that Ferrier had destroyed fibers of the underlying optic radiations in his angular gyrus ablations is probably correct. His notion that the opposite eye was affected by unilateral destruction of the angular gyrus rested on the conception (still held at the time by some experimentalists and clinicians including Charcot) that those retinogeniculate fibers which did not decussate at the optic chiasm crossed over to the opposite hemisphere though the colliculi so that the whole retina of a single eye was represented in a single lateral cortical area.

Studies by a number of experimentalists and clinicians in the 1870s and 1880s generated unassailable evidence that the locus of the cortical center for vision was to be found in the occipital lobes. The preeminent experimentalist of the period was the Berlin physiologist Hermann Munk, a painstaking investigator, whose studies on the dog and the monkey were technically and methodologically superior to those of most of his contemporaries. He was able to keep some of his operated animals alive for years and to study them thoroughly. Thus, he had the opportunity to note restitution of function, when it occurred, as well as certain peculiarities in visual behavior that could not be observed in the acutely operated animal. In 1876 he initiated a series of studies designed to elucidate the cortical basis of sensory and motor functions, the results of which were reported in detail in 16 lengthy communications (Munk, 1890).

With respect to vision, Munk demonstrated beyond reasonable doubt that, at least in dogs and monkeys, complete destruction of both occipital lobes produced permanent loss of vision, a condition which he designated as "cortical blindness." He also showed that complete destruction of a single occipital lobe produced a contralateral hemianopia and not blindness in the opposite eye, as supposed by Ferrier and others. Thus, he established that in the animals which he had studied the cortical "center" for vision was located in the occipital lobes.

Munk's early reports encountered a skeptical reception from other animal experimentalists, particularly on the part of antilocalizationists such as Goltz and close rivals such as Ferrier. But clinicians, already prepared by case reports such as those of Levick (1866) and Pooley (1877), which had raised the possibility of an association between hemianopia and occipital lobe disease, viewed his conclusions much more favorably. Only a year after the publication of Munk's first communication, Baumgarten (1878) described a patient with persistent left homonymous hemianopia and no other signs of brain disease in whom autopsy disclosed a large cyst in the right occipital lobe. He commented that, despite the clear association between the occipital lesion and the hemianopia, he would hesitate to infer a causal connection on the basis of a single case, if it were not for the observations of Munk, who "has been able to produce a lateral hemianopia (corresponding to our case) in monkeys by unilateral extirpation of the cortex of the occipital lobe." A year later, a very similar case was reported by Curschmann (1879). His patient, with a left homonymous hemianopia persisting until death, showed no other signs of brain disease. A focus of softening in the right occipital lobe was found on autopsy, leading Curschmann to conclude that his case confirmed Munk's correlation and to remark with some pride that "in view of the absence of other focal brain symptoms, it has the status of an experiment in man."

Within a few years, Munk's occipital localization of vision was widely accepted, although some of his more specific ideas proved to be incorrect. Reviewing Munk's work through 1883, Starr (1884) concluded that "the large number of animals used, the uniform results of the experiments in all cases, the length of time during which the symptoms persisted, and the minute care displayed in the observations combine to establish the truth of the conclusions reached." Starr added that "it remains for the pathologist to determine whether these facts which are true in the case of monkeys, are true also in the case of man." He proceeded to do this by means of a review of the relevant literature.

In fact, analyses of the evidence bearing on the question had already been published. The first of these was by Exner (1881) in his monograph on cortical localization of function in man. In his review of the findings in 167 autopsied cases reported in the literature through 1879, Exner distinguished between "absolute" cortical fields, lesions of which almost always produced a particular defect, and "relative" cortical fields, lesions of which produced the defect with notable frequency but not invariably. Thus, he classified a major part of the precentral gyrus as an absolute cortical field for motor function in the contralateral limbs since lesions in that area produced impairment in close to 100 percent of the cases. A larger surrounding territory was designated as a relative cortical field since lesions there produced contralateral motor impairment in 40–90 percent of the cases.

Although Exner's series was a large one, in only six cases were visual disturbances mentioned. (In contrast, no less than 100 cases presented with motor impairment of an upper extremity.) He was not able to identify an absolute cortical field for vision in that he found no area in which lesions always produced visual disturbances. However, he did find that lesions in a number of loci on the lateral and medial surfaces of the occipital lobes did produce impairment with frequencies ranging from 33 to 75 percent and hence he classified the occipital lobes as a relative field for vision. The highest frequency (60–75 percent) was associated with lesions in the superior part of the first occipital gyrus, leading to his designation of this area as the most "intensive" part of the relative cortical field for vision. Conversely, he found that lesions in the territory of the angular gyrus were associated with visual defect in only about 12 percent of the cases.

Insofar as vision was concerned, the weakness of Exner's review lay in the fact that even the very few cases with visual disturbance in his series were poorly described and of a heterogeneous character. [Neither Baumgarten's (1878) case nor that of Curschman (1879) was in-included in his series, although both were published before 1880.] His sparse data could show only that the occipital lobes appeared to be more important than other regions of the cerebral hemispheres in the mediation of visual function. The subsequent analyses of Marchand and Starr of the site of lesion in patients with hemianopic defects were far more informative and convincing.

Marchand (1882) reviewed 22 cases, 11 with a right hemianopic defect and 11 with a left hemianopic defect. Within each subgroup, autopsy study showed involvement of the opposite thalamus or optic tract in five cases, the lesions being for the most part tumors. In the remaining six cases in each subgroup, lesions in the opposite occipital lobe were invariably found, the majority of these being vascular in origin. Stressing the importance of small, circumscribed vascular lesions for the study of cerebral localization, Marchand described a patient with a complete left hemianopia following a stroke whom he studied in 1876. Autopsy disclosed only an area of necrosis in the right occipital lobe. The unsuspected absence of a lesion at the level of the thalamus or the optic tract was at the time quite puzzling and "only after Munk's discoveries did this case gain clarity and interest."

Starr's (1884) case material consisted of 32 cases presenting a right (15 cases) or left (17 cases) hemianopia, either in isolation or as part of an ensemble of deficits. With one exception, all the cases had come to autopsy, the pathology in the exceptional case having been described during the course of surgical intervention. Of the 32 cases, five involved unilateral lesions at the thalamic level, two of these being neoplastic lesions also extending into the occipital lobe. Thirteen cases of right hemianopia were found to have lesions in one of another part of the left occipital lobe. In two of these cases, the field defect had been the only permanent symptom. Similarly, a lesion of the right occipital lobe was found in 14 cases with a left hemianopia, as part of an ensemble of defects in nine, as the only symptom in four, and as the only permanent symptom in one case. Starr concluded that "anatomical research, physiological experiment, and pathological observation unite in assigning to the occipital lobes of the brain the function of sight. The right occipital lobe receives impressions from the right half of both eyes, and the left occipital lobe receives impressions from the left half of both eyes. The visual area of the brain lies in the occipital lobes."

2.2. Precise Localization of the Visual Center

From his ablation studies, Munk reached the conclusion that, although complete removal of the occipital lobes was required to produce cortical blindness (and complete removal of one lobe to produce a contralateral hemianopia), their upper convex surface represented the center of clearest vision. He proposed the idea that this area was the site of termination of the pathways from the foveal region of the retina but did not undertake any anatomical studies to demonstrate the point. This was as far as Munk was able to go and, as will be seen, a certain amount of confusion was engendered by his contention that lesions of the same area were also responsible for the production of another type of visual defect which he called "mindblindness." Munk, in 1879, was also the first investigator to propose that there was a fixed relationship between elements of the retina and corresponding loci in the occipital lobe.

The evidence that the primary cortical center for vision was to be found in the calcarine region of the mesial surface of the occipital lobes came from clinicopathologic correlations in patients with discrete lesions in that area. The first case of this type, reported by Huguenin (1881; Haab, 1882), concerned an 8-year-old tubercular girl who developed a left homonymous hemianopia during the course of an illness of 5 months' duration. She suffered from headache, convulsions, and general mental impairment, but showed no motor, auditory,

somatosensory, or speech defects. Autopsy disclosed two discrete neoplastic lesions, a small one in the left prefrontal area and a slightly larger
one on the mesial surface of the right occipital lobe. Since the small left
prefrontal lesion could be safely dismissed as the cause of the
hemianopia, it was evident that the mesial occipital tumor (Figure
3-1A) was the crucial lesion.

It was Haab (1882) who first raised the question of whether the
mesial, rather than the convex, region of the occipital lobes might be
the site of the cortical visual center. Commenting on the findings in
Huguenin's case, he remarked: "It is of interest to see that in this case
the tumor destroyed precisely the center of the cortical area in which
the stripe of Vicq d'Azyr is found. Has this peculiarly structured cortex
perhaps specific connections with the visual sense?" (Haab, 1882, p.
149). He went on to describe the findings in a second case which reinforced this possibility. It was that of a 61-year-old man with a left
homonymous hemianopia in whom autopsy study again disclosed a
lesion in the mesial area of the right occipital lobe. The visual field
defect and a slight awkwardness in moving the right arm and leg were
the only symptoms shown by this intelligent patient 5 months after a
stroke. The hemianopia persisted until the patient's death 3 years later.
The only lesion found on autopsy was an area of necrosis surrounding
the calcarine fissure in the right occipital lobe (Figure 3-1B).

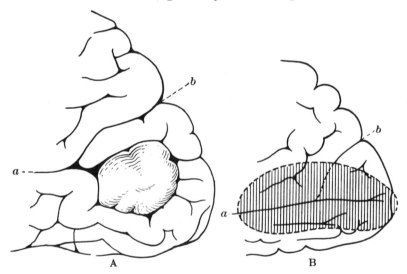

Figure 3-1.   (A) Side of lesion on the mesial surface of the right occipital lobe in the case
of Huguenin (1881); (B) in the case of Haab (1882). Both patients showed a left homonymous hemianopia during life.

An even more precise localization of the cortical visual center in a specific area of the occipital lobe was indicated by the subsequent case report of Hun (1887), describing a 57-year-old patient with a left homonymous inferior quadrantanopia of about 2 years' duration. The only finding on autopsy, apart from slight dilatation of the lateral ventricles, was a circumscribed atrophic area of cortex just above the calcarine fissure in the right occipital lobe, i.e., in the lower part of the cuneus.

> In this case there is a lesion which destroys the lower half of the right cuneus, and there is one constant symptom which is present during the whole course of the disease: a blindness limited to the lower left quadrant of the field of vision of each eye. In the absence of any other cerebral lesion the destruction of the lower half of the right cuneus must be regarded as the cause of the blindness in the lower left quadrant of each field of vision. . . . This case makes it probable that the fibres from the right upper quadrants of each retina terminate in the lower half of the right cuneus (Hun, 1887, pp. 144–145).

Hun's anatomic inference (or guess) that there was a topographic representation of the retinae onto the mesial surface of the occipital lobes was fully supported by subsequent investigators. Their work has been so well described by Brouwer (1936, pp. 459–482) and Polyak (1955, 179–203) that there is no point in reviewing it once again. It need only be pointed out that the leading investigators of the period, Wilbrand (1887, 1890; Wilbrand and Saenger, 1904, 1917) and Henschen (1890–1896), were primarily clinical researchers who correlated the perimetrically defined visual field defects shown by patients during life with autopsy findings. On the basis of an enormous case material, they were able to demonstrate that there was indeed a "cortical retina," as Henschen called it, on the mesial aspect of the occipital lobes, reflecting a point-to-point correspondence between the receptor surface and the cortical area.

Thus, clinicopathologic study of patients, rather than animal experimentation, provided the first indications of the locus and organization of the cortical visual center. The experimental demonstration that the calcarine region was the primary cortical end-station for vision was made by Minkowski (1911). He first showed that ablation of the cortical area on the convex surface that Munk had designated as the center for foveal vision produced no visual disturbances at all in the dog. He surmised that Munk's results were obtained because of inadvertent injury to the visual radiations which course directly under the cortex of the second and third occipital gyri, and in fact he showed by study of serial sections that, when an ablation presumably limited to the cortex did lead to visual defects, the radiations had been invariably injured. Minkowski went on to make complete and partial ablations of the striate area and found, in line with expectations, that complete bilateral destruction caused permanent blindness, complete unilateral ablation produced a contralateral hemianopia, and partial ablations of the superior and the inferior surface of the striate area produced an inferior and a superior hemianopia, respectively. Hence, he felt confident in concluding that the striate area constituted the cortical center for vision in the dog and that within this area there was a fixed correspondence between retinal loci and cortical loci.

2.3. Visual Agnosia

> If locus A_1 of the cerebral cortex of a dog is extirpated on both sides a peculiar disturbance in vision is noticeable 3–5 days after the injury, at a time when the inflammatory reaction has passed and no abnormality of hearing, smell, taste, movement, and sensation in the animal is present. The dog moves quite freely and easily indoors as well as in the garden without bumping against a single object. If obstacles are placed in his path, he regularly goes around them or, if a detour is not possible, he overcomes them adroitly, e.g., by crawling under a stool or carefully climbing over the man's foot or the animal's body which obstructs his path. But now the sight of people whom he had always greeted joyfully leaves him cold, as does the company of other dogs with whom he used to play. He may be so hungry and thirsty that he is overactive; yet he no longer looks for food in the part of the room where he used to find it. And if the bowl of food and bucket of water are placed directly in his path, he repeatedly goes around them without paying attention to them. Food presented to him visually evokes no response as long as he does not smell it. A finger or fire brought close to the eye no longer makes him blink. The sight of a whip, which invariably used to drive him into a corner, no longer frightens him at all. He had been trained to present the ipsilateral paw when one waved a hand in front of an eye. Now one can wave one's hand indefinitely, the paw remains at rest until one says, "paw." And there are other observations of this nature. There can be no doubt about their interpretation. As a result of the extirpation, the dog has become mindblind, i.e., he has lost the visual ideas which he possessed, his memory images of previous visual perceptions, so that he does not know or recognize what he sees. However, the dog sees. Visual sensations reach consciousness and the stage of perception. They make it possible for ideas about the presence, form, and location of external objects to arise so that new visual ideas based on new memory images of the visual perceptions can be acquired.

Thus Munk (1878, pp. 162–163; 1890, pp. 21–22) described for the first time the condition to which he gave the name "mindblindness," and which later came to be designated as "visual agnosia" or "optic agnosia." Concomitantly, he offered an explanation for the condition.

The animal had lost his "memory images" of previously perceived stimuli. Consequently, he could not relate current experience to past experience and hence failed to grasp the "meaning" of a perceived stimulus.

But Munk found that mindblindness was only a temporary condition. Within a few weeks, the dog once again could recognize his master and other dogs and once again responded in a normal fashion to them. His explanation was that during the course of postoperative experience, new memory images were laid down in parts of the occipital cortex other than locus A_1. It will be recalled that Munk had specified that locus A_1 was the cortical center for foveal vision as well as the depository of memory images.

Munk's concept received a mixed reception. The fact that mindblindness appeared after a relatively superficial lesion in the very same area that subserved foveal vision and that it was a temporary condition made it seem probable that the animal's impaired behavior was due simply to loss of central vision. His notion that the mindblind dog was reduced to the status of a puppy without a store of visual memory images who could now deposit new images in another part of the occipital cortex seemed quite farfetched. Even his assumption that the mindblind dog's behavior was clearly deviant was questioned. Minkowski (1911), having removed Locus A_1 from dogs without finding either a loss of central vision or signs of "mindblindness," remarked that he had often observed normal dogs to behave "unintelligently" in the face of visual stimuli, showing no response to the brandishing of a whip or sticking their paw in a piece of burning wood.

Consequently a substantial number of investigators, the earliest of whom was Mauthner (1881), interpreted mindblindness as the product of defective central vision perhaps coupled with postoperative mental blunting. For example, Siemerling (1890) studied a patient with mindblindness and was able to demonstrate a reduction in both visual acuity and color sensitivity which he concluded was responsible for the impairment in visual recognition.

But Munk's concept of mindblindness was accepted by other clinicians who observed a similar condition in some of their patients. Wilbrand (1887) and Lissauer (1890) described such patients who did not recognize objects or persons despite seemingly adequate visual acuity, and they related the condition to focal disease of the occipital lobes. Wilbrand agreed with Munk in attributing the defect to a loss of visual memory images but deviated from his thinking by postulating the existence of a discrete occipital cortical area, separate from the center for visual perception, which he designated the "visual memory field."

For his part, Lissauer (1890) not only presented a detailed description of the behavior of a patient with mindblindness but also offered a thoughtful discussion of the mechanisms that might be operating to produce the defect. The complete act of recognition involves two processes. The first is apperception, i.e., the conscious perception of an object, person, or event, implying the integration of the received sensory data into a unity or entity. The second process is the linking of the content of the perception with past experiences, implying associative activity and conferring meaning on the perception. Theoretically a patient might be rendered mindblind by a defect in one or the other mechanism. In practice, every patient suffering from mindblindness probably suffers from defects in both mechanisms because of the intimate interactive relationship between them. However, the severity of impairment in each might differ significantly. Thus, Lissauer felt that his patient exhibited a primarily associative type of mindblindness since a number of test performances indicated that he had excellent visual discriminative capacity.

One of the points made by Freud (1891) in his monograph on aphasia was the necessity for distinguishing between defects in naming objects and defects in recognizing them if clarity of thinking about the aphasic disorders was to be achieved. He therefore proposed that the term "agnosia" be employed to denote impairment in recognition within the context of adequate basic sensory capacity. His suggestion was generally adopted and "mindblindness" was discarded in favor of "visual agnosia" or "optic agnosia."

Up to this time, the structural characteristics of the occipital lobes and their connections with other hemispheric regions had received little attention. This gap was now filled by detailed anatomic study. Smith (1907) distinguished between morphologically differentiated striate and extrastriate occipital cortex, subdividing the latter into parastriate and peristriate areas. Brodmann (1909) similarly divided extrastriate cortex into an area 18 immediately surrounding striate cortex (area 17) and an outlying preoccipital area 19, a parcellation roughly corresponding to Smith's classification. At the same time, beginning with the work of Flechsig (1901), the connections of the occipital lobes with other cortical areas were investigated. Short association fibers connect area 17 with areas 18 and 19, from which arise longer association tracts leading to other parts of the cerebral hemispheres. These findings provided an anatomical framework for inferences about the lesional basis for disturbances in visual performance. Area 17 was the center for elementary visual experience. Elaboration of that experience into meaningful percepts required the functional integrity of areas 18 and 19, for these regions were the essential link between the primary visual center and the rest of the cortex. Thus, visual agnosia could be conceived as the outcome of lesions in area 18 and 19 which prevented the transmission and eventual integration of information arriving in area 17.

The concept of visual agnosia has had a checkered career since its introduction by Munk and the early studies of human subjects. On the one hand, the "reductionist" interpretation of Mauthner and Siemerling that the disorder is not a higher-level impairment in perceptual integration, association, or memory but only the expression of basic sensory deficit has been supported by some outstanding experimentalists and clinical investigators. The issue is, of course, whether or not the agnosic animal or patient does in fact have at his disposal the sensory information necessary for an accurate cognitive response. For example, Pavlov (1927, 1928) interpreted the mindblindness of Munk not as a higher-level psychological impairment but simply as loss of the capacity to make fine visual discriminations, and he suggested that the classical formula, "the dog sees but does not understand," should be reversed to read, "the dog understands but does not see sufficiently well" (Pavlov, 1927, p. 343). Similarly, Bay (1950, 1953, 1954) contended that visual agnosia in patients is explainable in terms of certain defects in visuosensory capacity, these defects typically occurring within the context of general mental impairment which itself hampers the process of drawing conclusions on the basis of inadequate visual information. He placed particular stress on alterations in rate of sensory adaptation as the defect which may underlie the type of behavior called "visual agnosia." Critchley (1964) and Bender and Feldman (1965) also have advanced the view that visual agnosia is essentially the outcome of defective sensory capacity coupled with an overall decline in intellectual level. The "reductionists" have supported their position by citing the fact that practically every patient with visual agnosia is found to have *some* type of visual impairment, such as a field defect, inadequate visual scanning, or a disturbance in ocular fixation.

But the concept of visual agnosia as a "higher-level" disorder was fully accepted by other clinical investigators who described different subtypes of visual agnosia. The rather gross disability shown by Munk's dogs and Lissauer's patient was designated as "visual object-agnosia" while less pervasive disabilities involving one or another aspect of visual perception such as "visual form agnosia," "facial agnosia," and "visuospatial agnosia" were singled out for special study. Countering the argument that these disorders merely represent a partial impairment in basic sensory capacity, the "antireductionists" have pointed to the innumerable cases of severe visual defect that do not show the perceptual–integrative or associative disturbances characteristic of the agnosic patient.

3. THE METHOD OF DOUBLE SENSORY STIMULATION

3.1. Jacques Loeb

In 1884, the physiologist Jacques Loeb, who had worked with Goltz in Strasbourg, published a paper on the visual disturbances that follow experimental ablations of the brain in dogs. In it and two subsequent papers (Loeb, 1885, 1886), he described for the first time the responses of operated animals to double bilateral visual stimulation. Having noted that the most frequent immediate effect of unilateral destruction of one cerebral hemisphere is to produce a contralateral hemiamblyopia in which the animal is completely nonresponsive to visual stimulation on that side, he then described the course of recovery from the defect. In the first stage, the dog still does not perceive objects brought slowly into the affected field of vision but may respond to oscillating objects or to those that are rapidly introduced into the field. Further recovery of function then occurs.

> The intensity of stimulus in the crossed visual half-field, which is necessary to elicit a reaction on the part of the dog, decreases steadily. After a time, if a single piece of meat is presented to the dog, he will react to it, even if it is not moved. In addition, when the meat is moved or thrown to the right, the dog follows it just as he would if it were moved or thrown to the left. It would appear from these tests that a visual disturbance is no longer present. However, if two pieces of meat are suddenly presented simultaneously to the dog, one in the right and the other in the left visual field, the animal who has been operated in the left hemisphere will without exception take the piece of meat to the left (Loeb, 1886, p. 294).

He then pointed out that such an impairment in response to double visual stimulation may be the only functional outcome of a less destructive cerebral lesion.

> These findings record the course of a rather severe hemiamblyopia from the time of operation to the restitution of visual capacity; however, after superficial lesions and favorable conditions of operation and recovery, the initial disturbance is not as severe as here described. In the majority of cases, only the last described stage is present from the very beginning: the dog takes single pieces of meat under all conditions and favors that situated on the side of the lesion only upon simultaneous presentation of two pieces of meat (Loeb, 1886, pp. 275–276).

Seeking a physiological explanation of this pattern of responsiveness in which stimulation in the affected field is perceived when it is presented in isolation but not reacted to when presented in combination with concurrent stimulation in the healthy field, Loeb postulated that a unilateral hemispheric lesion produced impaired conduction in the involved neural pathways. As a consequence, the reactions mediated by these pathways are slower and weaker than those mediated by the neural connections of the intact hemisphere. In support of this interpretation, he cited the observation that if, under a condition of double stimulation, the intensity of the stimulus in the affected field is augmented to a sufficient degree, it would be perceived along with the stimulus to the healthy field.

3.2. Clinical Application

Loeb demonstrated the behavior of his dogs to the clinical neurologist Hermann Oppenheim, who immediately applied the method of double sensory stimulation to patients with brain disease and found some who showed the predicted pattern of responsiveness (Oppenheim, 1885). Thus, two patients who perceived tactile stimulation on their affected side when it was presented in isolation failed to perceive it in combination with stimulation on the healthy side. Another patient showed failure to respond to tactile or visual stimuli when each was paired with corresponding stimulation on the healthy side. Still another patient showed failure to respond adequately to double simultaneous tactile or auditory stimulation. Confirming Loeb's observations on dogs, Oppenheim also reported that augmentation of the intensity of the stimulus on the affected side could lead to the normal perception of both stimuli on the part of a patient.

Finding that the procedure was of clinical value in an occasional case, Oppenheim adopted it as a diagnostic maneuver and described it in his famous textbook of neurology.

> In certain cerebral diseases, which lead to unilateral sensory disturbances, I have often employed the following method of examination: two symmetrical locations on both sides of the body are simultaneously stimulated with touching by a brush or by pinpricks; under these conditions it happens that the patient invariably perceives only the stimulus which has been applied to the healthy side, while with single stimulation he feels every stimulus on the affected side. We shall designate this mode of examination as the method of double stimulation (Oppenheim, 1898, p. 51).

Subsequently the method of double sensory stimulation was utilized for investigative purposes in patients with suspected unilateral lesions by a few neurologists. Poppelreuter (1917) designated defective responsiveness to double visual stimulation as a "hemianopic weakness of attention." Thiébaut and Guillaumat (1945) called the deficit a "relative hemianopsia." The phenomenon was studied in detail by Bender and his co-workers (Bender and Teuber, 1946; Bender, Teuber and Battersby, 1950; Bender, 1952; Bender and Feldman, 1952), who showed that it occurred in the different sensory modalities, gave it the name of "extinction," and described the diverse forms it may take. It was possible to show with human patients, who could give a verbal report of their experience, that partial extinction of response in the double stimulation paradigm may occur, i.e., the patient perceives the stimulus on the affected side or field but experiences it as weaker than when the stimulus is presented in isolation. Bender called this phenomenon "obscuration."

Utilizing a method of subjective magnitude estimation, Benton and Levin (1972) were able to produce the "obscuration" response in normal subjects by appropriate manipulation of the relative strength of competing tactile stimuli. Another type of deviant response, originally described by Jones (1907), was a tendency on the part of patients with unilateral lesions to report that both limbs had been touched when in fact stimulation had been applied only to the ipsilateral limb.

Eighty years after Loeb's pioneer studies, extinction to bilateral sensory stimulation was once again investigated experimentally in animals by Schwartz and Eidelberg (1968). Having been trained to respond differentially to electrical stimulation of the right, left, and both hands, monkeys were subjected to unilateral parietal and frontal ablations. Postoperatively a tendency to respond to double tactile stimulation as if single stimulation had been delivered to the hand ipsilateral to the side of lesion was observed. Daily fluctuations in the relative frequency of extinction responses, noted by Bender in patients, were also noted. Moreover, some animals showed the phenomenon of "synchiria" reported by Jones in patients, i.e., they responded to single stimulation of the limb ipsilateral to the side of the lesion as if double stimulation had been applied.

4. CONCLUDING COMMENTS

This sketch of the successive stages in the development of investigative work on two topics in the area of brain lesion research indicates how the experimental and clinical approaches interacted to advance understanding of the specific problem. As was mentioned earlier in the chapter, the initial observations were made on animals and these provided the impetus for analogous and more refined study of human subjects. In turn, the results of clinical study led to more detailed experimental investigation in animals. Thus, Munk's conclusion that the cortical mechanisms mediating visual function were located in the occipital lobes received a much more favorable reception from clinicians than from his fellow experimentalists, whose own preconceptions hindered acceptance. In contrast, as Marchand and others pointed out, clinicians found Munk's results helpful in explaining previous observations, the significance of which had not been at all clear. Once Munk's experiments showed clinicians where to look for the cortical lesions producing visual impairment, they took full advantage of the experiments of nature that came their way and they were able to go far beyond the experimentalists of the period in establishing precise anatomical–behavioral correlations. Given this background of knowledge, Minkowski could once again investigate the problem in greater depth and provide experimental confirmation of the clinical correlations.

Is it the rule that the interplay of experimental and clinical research on a brain–behavior problem is likely to be initiated by observations in animals? There is probably no such rule. The choice of a starting point in recounting the history of investigative work on a particular topic is largely determined by one's perception of whose work was particularly influential in determining the direction of subsequent research. With respect to vision, the experiments of Ferrier and Munk certainly meet this criterion and, hence, one regards them as pioneers. But their efforts were surely inspired by the discovery of the excitable motor cortex by Fritsch and Hitzig, who, on their part, cited earlier clinical observations relating discrete paralyses to focal brain lesions in support of the principle of cortical localization of motor function.

As early as 1874, Jackson advanced the concept that the posterior area of the right hemisphere subserved visual recognition and visual memory in human subjects. Subsequently, he published a case report in support of it (Jackson, 1876). Ferrier was quite familiar with Jackson's ideas along these lines and indeed referred to them as "hypotheses deserving consideration and further investigation" (Ferrier, 1878, p. 119). Thus, one could consider that Jackson was the "real" pioneer in pointing to a posterior representation of visual function or even Panizza (1855), whose early contribution seems to have been completely ignored at the time of its publication. Attention was called to it only after the publication of Munk's research (cf. Tamburini, 1880). And Panizza reported both experimental findings and clinical observations to make his point.

Thus, it seems rather fruitless to attempt to determine a starting point in an absolute sense and to ask whether this was represented by animal experimentation or clinical observation. The important fact is that, generally speaking, both the experimentalists and the clinicians kept themselves informed about developments in the others' field and took full advantage of these developments.

5. REFERENCES

Baumgarten, P. Hemiopie nach Erkrankung der occipitalen Hirnrinde. *Centralblatt für die Medicinischen Wissenschaften,* 1878, *16,* 369–371.

Bay, E. *Agnosie und Funktionswandel.* Berlin: Springer-Verlag, 1950.

Bay, E. Disturbances of visual perception and their examination. *Brain,* 1953, *76,* 515–550.

Bay, E. Optische Faktoren bei den räumlichen Orientierungsstörungen. *Deutsche Zeitschrift für Nervenheilkunde,* 1954, *171,* 454–459.

Bender, M. B. *Disorders in perception.* Springfield, Ill.: Charles C. Thomas, 1952.

Bender, M. B., and Feldman, D. S. Extinction of taste sensation on double simultaneous stimulation. *Neurology,* 1952, *2,* 195–202.

Bender, M. B., and Feldman, M. The so-called "visual agnosias." *Proceedings, VIII International Congress of Neurology,* 1965, 153–156.

Bender, M. B., and Teuber, H. L. Phenomena of fluctuation, extinction and completion in visual perception. *Archives of Neurology and Psychiatry,* 1946, *55,* 627–658.

Bender, M. B., Teuber, H.-L., and Battersby, W. S. Discrimination of weights by men with penetrating lesions of parietal lobes. *Transactions of the American Neurological Association,* 1950, *75,* 252–255.

Benton, A. L., and Levin, H. S. An experimental study of "obscuration." *Neurology,* 1972, *22,* 1176–1181.

Brodmann, K. *Vergleichende Lokalisationslehre der Grosshirnrinde.* Leipzig: J. A. Barth, 1909.

Brouwer, B. Chiasma, Tractus opticus, Sehstrahlung und Sehrinde. In O. Bumke and O. Foerster (Eds.), *Handbuch der Neurologie.* Vol. 6. Berlin: Springer-Verlag, 1936.

Chaillou, F. H. Ramollissement multiple du cerveau. *Bulletin de la Société Anatomique de Paris,* 1863, *8* (2nd Ser.), 70–73.

Critchley, M. The problem of visual agnosia. *Journal of the Neurological Sciences,* 1964, *1,* 274–290.

Curschmann, H. Die lehre von der Hemianopsie und von den cerebralen Centren des Gesichtssinnes. *Centralblatt für Praktische Augenheilkunde,* 1879, *3,* 181–182.

Exner, S. *Untersuchungen uber die Localisation der Functionen in der Grosshirnrinde des Menschen.* Wien: Wilhelm Braunmüller, 1881.

Ferrier, D. *The localisation of cerebral disease.* London: Smith, Elder and Co., 1878.

Ferrier, D. *The functions of the brain.* London: Smith, Elder and Co., 1876; 2nd Ed., 1886.

Ferrier, D. *The Croonian lectures on cerebral localisation.* London: Smith, Elder and Co., 1890.

Flechsig, P. Developmental (myelogenetic) localisation of the cerebral cortex in the human subject. *Lancet,* 1901, *2,* 1027–1029.

Freud, S. *Zur Auffassung der Aphasien.* Leipzig und Wien: Deuticke, 1891.

Fritsch, G., and Hitzig, E. Ueber die elektrische Erregbarkeit des Grosshirns. *Archiv für Anatomie, Physiologie und Wissenschaftliche Medizin* (Leipzig), 1870, 300–332.

Gratiolet, P. Note sur les expansions des racines cérébrales du nerf optique et sur leur terminaison dans une région determinée de l'écorce des hémisphères. *Comptes Rendus de l'Académie des Sciences,* Paris, 1854, *29,* 274–278.

Haab, O. Ueber Cortex-Hemianopie. *Klinische Monatsblätter für Augenheilkunde,* 1882, *20,* 141–153.

Henschen, S. E. *Klinische und anatomische Beiträge zur Pathologie des Gehirns,* Parts 1–3 Upsala: Almquist and Wiksell, 1890–1896.

Huguenin, G. Ueber Hemiopie. *Korrespondenz-Blatt für Schweizer Aerzte,* 1881, *11,* 43–44.

Hun, H. A clinical study of cerebral localization, illustrated by seven cases. *American Journal of the Medical Sciences,* 1887, *93,* 140–168.

Jackson, J. H. On the nature of the duality of the brain. *Medical Press and Circular,* 1874 (reprinted in *Brain,* 1915, *38,* 80–103).

Jackson, J. H. Case of large cerebral tumour without optic neuritis and with left hemiplegia and imperception. *Royal Ophthalmic Hospital Reports,* 1876, *8,* 434–444.

Jones, E. The precise diagnostic value of allochiria. *Brain,* 1907, *30,* 490–532.

Levick. Abscess of brain. *American Journal of the Medical Sciences,* 1866, *52,* 413–414.

Lissauer, H. Ein Fall von Seelenblindheit nebst einem Beitrag zur Theorie derselben. *Archiv für Psychiatrie und Nervenkrankheiten,* 1890, *21,* 222–270.

Loeb, J. Die Sehstörungen nach Verletzung der Grosshirnrinde. *Pfluger's Archiv für die Gesamte Physiologie,* 1884, *34,* 67–172.

Loeb, J. Die elementaren Störungen einfacher Functionen nach oberflächlicher, umschriebener Verletzung des Grosshirns. *Pfluger's Archiv für die Gesamte Physiologie,* 1885, *37,* 51–56.

Loeb, J. Beiträge zur Physiologie des Grosshirns. *Pflüger's Archiv fur die Gesamte Physiologie,* 1886, *39,* 265–346.

Marchand, F. Beitrag zur Kenntnis der homonymen bilateralen Hemianopsie und der Faserkreuzung im Chiasma opticum. *Graefe's Archiv für Ophthalmologie,* 1882, *28,* 63–96.

Mauthner, L. *Gehirn und Auge.* Wiesbaden: Bergmann, 1881.

Meynert, T. Beiträge zur Kenntnis der centralen Projection der Sinnesoberflächen. *Sitzungsberichte der Kaiserlichen Akademie der Wissenschaften, Mathematisch-Naturwissenschaftliche Classe,* Wien, 1869, *60,* 547–566.

Minkowski, M. Zur Physiologie der corticalen Sehsphäre. *Deutsche Zeitschrift für Nervenheilkunde,* 1911, *41,* 109–118.

Munk, H. Weitere Mittheilungen zur Physiologie der Grosshirnrinde. *Archiv für Anatomie und Physiologie,* 1878, *2,* 162–178.

Munk, H. Weiteres zur Physiologie der Sehsphäre der Grosshirnrinde. *Archiv für Anatomie und Physiologie,* 1879, *3,* 581–592.

Munk, H. *Ueber die Functionen der Grosshirnrinde.* Berlin: August Hirschwald, 1890.

Oppenheim, H. Ueber eine durch eine klinisch bisher nicht verwerthete Untersuchungsmethode ermittelte Form der Sensibilitätsstörung bei einseitigen Erkrankungen des Grosshirns. *Neurologisches Zentralblatt,* 1885, *4,* 529–533.

Oppenheim, H. *Lehrbuch der Nervenkrankheiteu fur Aerzte und Studirende,* II Aufl. Berlin: Karger, 1898.

Panizza, B. Osservazioni sul nervo ottico. *Giornale, Istituto Lombardo di Scienze e Lettere,* 1855, *7,* 237–252.

Pavlov, I. P. *Conditioned reflexes.* London: Oxford University Press, 1927.

Pavlov, I. P. *Lectures on conditioned reflexes.* New York: International Publishers, 1928.

Polyak, S. *The vertebrate visual system.* Chicago: University of Chicago Press, 1955.

Pooley, T. R. Rechtseitige binoculare Hemiopie bedingt durch eine Gummigeschwulst im linkeren hinteren Gehirnlappen. *Archiv für Augen und Ohrenheilkunde,* 1877, *6,* 27–29.

Poppelreuter, W. *Die psychischen Schädigungen durch Kopfschuss im Kriege 1914–1916: die Störungen der niederen und höheren Sehleistungen durch Verletzungen des Okzipitalhirns.* Leipzig: Voss, 1917.

Schäfer, E. A. Experiments on special sense localisation in the cortex cerebri of the monkey. *Brain,* 1888, *10,* 362–380.

Schwartz, A. S., and Eidelberg, E. "Extinction" to bilateral simultaneous stimulation in the monkey. *Neurology,* 1968, *18,* 61–68.

Siemerling, E. Ein Fall von sogenannter Seelenblindheit nebst anderweitigen cerebralen symptomen. *Archiv für Psychiatrie und Nervenkrankheiten,* 1890, *21,* 284–299.

Smith, G. E. New studies on the folding of the visual cortex and the significance of the occipital sulci in the human brain. *Journal of Anatomy,* 1907, *41,* 198–207.

Starr, M. A. The visual area in the brain determined by a study of hemianopsia. *American Journal of the Medical Sciences*, 1884, *87*, 65–83.

Tamburini, A. Rivendicazione al Panizza della scoperta del centro visivo corticale. *Revista Sperimentale di Freniatria e Medicina Legale*, 1880, *6*, 153–154.

Thiébaut, F., and Guillaumat, L. Hémianopsie relative. *Revue Neurologique*, 1945, *77*, 129–130.

Wilbrand, H. *Die Seelenblindheit als Herderscheinung und ihre Beziehungen zur homonymen Hemianopsie*. Wiesbaden: J. F. Bergmann, 1887.

Wilbrand, H. *Die hemianopischen Gesichtsfeld-Formen und das optische Wahrnehmungszentrum*. Wiesbaden: J. F. Bergmann, 1890.

Wilbrand, H, and Saenger, A. *Die Neurologie des Auges*. Vol. 3, 1904, Vol. 7, 1917. Wiesbaden: J. F. Bergmann.

PART III

ANATOMICAL RESPONSE TO CNS INJURY

4

Lesion Experiments:
Some Anatomical Considerations

THOMAS A. WOOLSEY

1. INTRODUCTION

Until quite recently, the selective lesion technique was the principal tool for experimental neuroanatomy. This approach to the understanding of the structure and the neuronal connectivity of the nervous system has its foundation in clinical neurology. Thus, by carefully correlating functional and behavioral deficits in living patients with pathology in the nervous system examined after death, the "functions" subserved by many of the principal tracts were determined. Indeed, by these correlations the functional organization within several areas of the brain of man was determined (e.g., Jackson, 1958; Holmes, 1918).

Anatomists, like neurophysiologists and psychologists, soon found it profitable to introduce surgical lesions into experimental animals (which do not necessarily suffer the sequellae of syphilis and war). Advantage was taken of a variety of neuronal and glial responses to this experimental *pathology* to determine the anatomical organization of the nervous system. These changes are observed by a variety of neuroanatomical methods and in particular a number of techniques have been developed to demonstrate selectively degeneration of components of the nervous system.

Careful workers were quick to realize that, from an anatomical point of view, the lesion methods were open to a number of interpre-

THOMAS A. WOOLSEY • Department of Anatomy and Neurobiology. Washington University School of Medicine, St. Louis, Missouri 63110.

tive difficulties. Not the least of them is that the structure of the nervous system is inordinately complex (a source of fascination for some) and that with few exceptions it is anatomically impossible to interfere with one functional group of neurons without inadvertently damaging portions of others. The solution to this problem has been achieved largely by damaging a particular target from several surgical approaches (e.g., Domesick, 1972). In the analysis, the investigator, like the clinician, "subtracts out" those features not common to all cases involving the target, hoping to eliminate most of the fibers of passage. Nevertheless, cautious investigators remain concerned that even this stratagem can be misleading (e.g., Guillery, 1970c).

Fortunately, as our understanding of cell biology has grown, a number of experimental neuroanatomical methods have become available which are based upon the *physiological* properties of neurons. Thus, "anterograde" (Cowan, Gottlieb, Hendrickson, Price, and Woolsey, 1972) and "retrograde" techniques (LaVail and LaVail, 1972) for tracing axonal connections, while not without interpretive difficulties, have already shown their value in experimental neuroanatomy and have helped to clarify data based on experimental lesions.

It would be out of place if not impossible to review the entire anatomical experience with lesions here. The tack which I shall take is simply to highlight a number of observations and problems which should be borne in mind when attempting to correlate behavioral findings with lesions placed in specific anatomical locales. A number of more detailed reviews will be cited to which reference can be made for fuller details. For technical details see the article by Wolf, Stricker, and Zigmond (1978) in this volume.

2. THE ANATOMICAL ORGANIZATION OF THE BRAIN: GENERAL CONSIDERATIONS

There are two principal cell types in the nervous system, *neurons* and *neuroglia*, which are originally embryological derivatives of the neuroepithelium and the neural crest in the central and peripheral nervous systems, respectively (Langman, 1975). The functional properties of the nervous system are usually attributed to the neurons by virtue of their long processes, the axons and dendrites, which establish the well-known specific connectivity of brain by an enormous number of articulations known as *synapses*. The glia are usually considered the "supporting" elements of the brain. The two principal types of glia in the CNS are the astrocytes which form the "intercellular matrix" and the oligodendrocytes which myelinate CNS axons. In the periphery the Schwann cells myelinate and cover axons as well as encapsulating the somata of the peripheral ganglion cells (Bunge, 1970). Fibrous elements provide support. In addition, in the CNS there is a third glial cell type—the microglia—the embryological origin and functions of which are at present unclear (Skoff, 1975; Skoff, Price, and Stocks, 1976*a,b*).

A casual glance at a fresh brain, one stained for cell bodies (Figure 4-1A) or one stained for fibers (Figure 4-1B), shows an apparent segregation of nervous system components into cell groups—gray matter—and axonal pathways—white matter. The grey matter, however, is not exclusively composed of neuronal cell bodies but also of the axons of those cells, terminals of distant cells projecting to that region, and glia. A slightly different organization is found in the white matter. With very few exceptions the fiber tracts, also containing glia, of the brain are not homogeneous in their axonal composition. For this reason it is rare that a fiber pathway, even in the spinal cord, is as discrete and precisely localized as one is led to believe by the anatomical diagrams found in the textbooks (compare Carpenter, 1976, with Lawrence and Kuypers, 1968*a,b*).

While the nervous system is unique in the complexity of the interrelationships of its cellular components, it has a number of characteristics in common with the other body tissues. For lesion experiments, the most important of these is blood supply: arterial and venous. Compromise of the blood supply to the brain or its parts results in a complex sequence of cellular phenomena which may result in swelling or *edema* and in extreme cases cell death of the deprived region (Florey, 1970; Stern, 1972). When edema is present in soft tissues in a closed compartment such as the skull (Miller and Adams, 1972) or anterior tibial compartment (Hoopes and Jabaley, 1973), there is a positive feedback in that as the swelling progresses systemic blood pressure is insufficient to supply the bordering tissues, etc., until the blood supply to the large portion of the compartment is severely compromised.

Finally, the central nervous system is continuously bathed in a fluid—the cerebral spinal fluid (CSF)—which is actively produced by the choroid plexus into the ventricular system of the brain. This enters the space around the central nervous system—the subarchnoid space—by apertures at the base of the cerebellum after flowing through the ventricular system. If the continuity with the subarchnoid space is broken, the continued secretion of CSF will inflate the ventricular system compressing the brain against the skull, and lead to hydrocephalus (Milhorat, 1972).

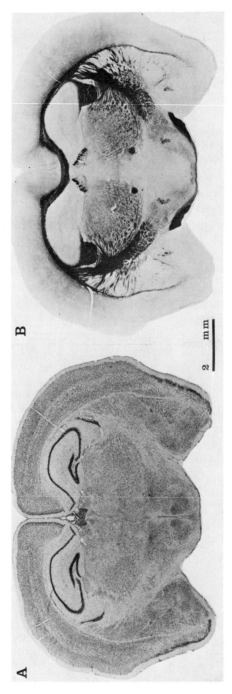

Figure 4-1. Frontal sections through the mouse brain at approximately the same level to show cellular and fiber components. *A.* Neuronal cell bodies are stained to show the disposition of gray matter. The level is through the thalamus in which several nuclear groups can be seen. 50 μm frozen section, Thionin. *B.* Myelinated fibers are stained to show the disposition of the white matter. Note that the stain demonstrates some areas not stained in *A.* 50 μm frozen section, stained with Hematoxylin (Jebb and Woolsey, 1977).

3. GROSS ANATOMICAL CONSIDERATIONS

In lesions a number of considerations are of importance which follow from the above discussion. First, it is necessary to assess each specimen for evidence of unsuspected neuronal damage consequent to the inadvertent interruption of a vessel (Adams and Victor, 1977). Chronic venous congestion is likely to result if one of the dural venous sinuses is entered or sufficiently irritated to promote a clot (Krayenbühl, 1967). In man a number of findings are related to venous sinus thrombosis such as seizures, paralysis, and difficulties of mentation. The interruption or partial severing of an artery can "lesion" a much larger territory than intended, and if the target is deep this may not be appreciated until post-mortem examination.

Another problem is that the introduction of a lesion may interfere with the normal circulation of the CSF. This has been documented in a study in which the behavioral consequences of a total cerebellectomy were being examined. The authors noted that a number of specimens had developed hydrocephalus (Wirth and O'Leary, 1974). Since this condition when uncorrected is associated, among other things, with retarded mental development in humans (Milhorat, 1972), it is not unreasonable to expect that it might alter behavior in animals. If hydrocephaly is unsuspected, it could conceivably lead to a confusion of the results. These are several non-neural (in the sense of injury to the chosen target) factors which must be assessed by routine and thoughtful anatomical examination of experimental specimens.

Most workers in the field will be familiar with the necessity for the corrections applied in placing deep lesions stereotaxically. But it is always important to confirm these either physiologically at the time the lesion is made or anatomically in the specimen. What may not be so widely appreciated is that when dealing with inbred laboratory animals, there can be significant interstrain differences within a species (Wahlsten, Hudspeth, and Bernhardt, 1975). Finally, when a cortical area of known functional properties is to be damaged, it is good to obtain some physiological information prior to placement of lesions. Although the brains of some adult rodents are sufficiently constant to omit this step, in human neurosurgery the use of surface landmarks alone to define a cortical locus has long been known to be inadequate (Penfield and Boldry, 1937). Indeed, until quite recently the variability in the location of homologous portions of the cat auditory cortex along the "constant" ectosylvian gyrus was not fully appreciated (e.g., Merzenich, Knight, and Roth, 1975; Zeki and Sandman, 1976; see Figure 4-2).

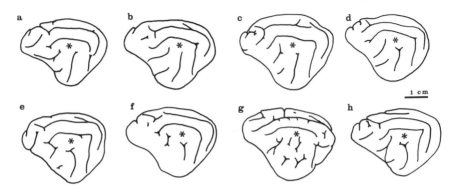

Figure 4-2. To show the variability in sulcal patterns in the cerebral cortex of the cat. The position of tonotopically equivalent points on the ectosylvian gyrus (*) showed considerable variation. Adapted from Merzenich, *et al.,* 1975.

4. NEURONAL RESPONSE TO INJURY

The nucleus and perikaryon of the neuron are essential to the maintenance of its processes. If the axon of a cell is severed by a lesion, the portion of the axon beyond the cut will degenerate (anterograde or Wallerian degeneration, Waller, 1850). The response of the parent cell is more variable, from little morphological change to death (retrograde neuronal degeneration). In different animals and neuronal systems, both responses occur at variable rates (Van Crevel, 1958; Grafstein, 1975).

For large tracts, it is possible to assess an anterograde response anatomically using Nissl and myelin stains. While hardly optimal, in Nissl preparations a tract will become compressed and gliotic (see below). Fiber stains are preferable since the myelin loss shows up very clearly (e.g., see Fig. 1, Woolsey, Gorska, Wetzel, Erickson, Earls, and Allman, 1972). Both of these stains are simple and usually routine in most laboratories. In addition, they are the principal staining methods which can be consistently applied to specimens in which lesions have been placed months and years before. The obvious disadvantage of the myelin stain is that it does not demonstrate unmyelinated fibers.

Several specific stains have been developed over the years to reveal degenerating axons and their coverings. The first of these is a stain for degenerating myelin sheaths developed by Marchi in the last century (Swank and Davenport, 1935). Following World War II a number of procedures were devised to demonstrate degenerating axoplasm. For a long time the most popular of these techniques was the method published by Nauta and Gygax in 1954. The Nauta methods, when used carefully, clearly revealed degenerating fibers, and it is on this method that much of our current knowledge of neuronal connectivity is based. In 1967 Fink and Heimer introduced a modification of the Nauta method, of which there are now a number of variants, which would also selectively stain degenerating axonal terminals (for a review, see Heimer, 1970).

With the advent of the electron microscope, it was observed that serving an axon would produce a number of recognizable changes (Guillery, 1970b). These are generally placed in two categories: the neurofilamentous reaction in which the axons and terminals of severed fibers accumulated enormous numbers of neurofilaments and the electron dense reaction in which cut axons became electron dense following a lesion (e.g., Laatsch and Cowan, 1967; Jones and Rockel, 1973). In both electron microscopy (EM) and light microscopy (LM) the specific response is reported to progress from the cut toward the terminals, a sequence that may correlate with failure to drive synapses (Miledi and Slater, 1970).

From the degeneration methods it is known that pathways differ in the rate at which they degenerate and that degeneration in similar pathways in different species may proceed at different paces (e.g., Murray and Grafstein, 1969, versus Guillery, 1970a). In addition, if the anatomical effects of a specific lesion are assessed by, say, the Nauta and EM methods, the time course for each can differ (Jones and Powell, 1968, 1969). Of interest here is that, with the possible exception of the Marchi method, many anatomically demonstrable consequences of a lesion can be appreciated only in the first week or so following surgery, a time usually too short for the assessment of behavioral changes. Nevertheless, if a particular lesion is being introduced into a number of animals, it may be advisable to take several specimens as "anatomical" controls in which degenerating fibers are specifically demonstrated.

Transection of a neuron's axon can also produce a number of changes in the parent soma. These were first observed with Nissl stains and have now been documented in a number of sites in the nervous system. Generally, a neuron will exhibit the so-called chromatolytic response in which the perikaryon swells, the nucleus becomes eccentrically located, and the Nissl substance is dissipated (the chromatolysis, e.g., Grafstein, 1975). This response, which, depending on the system under study, may take days or weeks, is eventually resolved either by complete degeneration of the soma (Figure 4-3c, e) or recovery of a normal cytoplasmic organization. As with the phenomenon of Wallerian degeneration, the retrograde response varies considerably in its severity and time course from system to system and in different species.

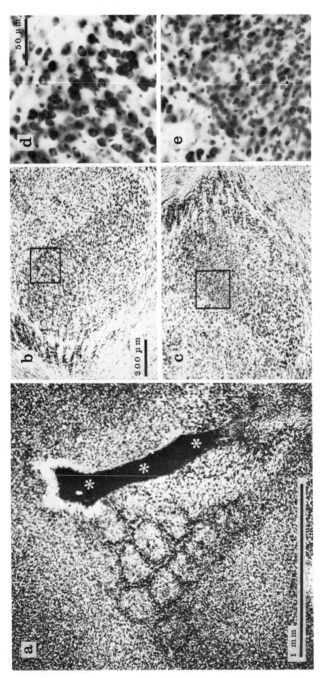

Figure 4-3. To show the location of a cortical lesion in a cytoarchitectonic field and the consequent retrograde cell degeneration. *a.* Tangential section in the plane of cortical layer IV from the right hemisphere of the mouse. Specific barrels (Rows B,C,D, and E) have been damaged (Woolsey and Van der Loos, 1970) by an aspiration lesion. The animal survived two weeks. Note the intense gliosis at the lesion site (*). The presence of cytoarchitectonic markers—the barrels—locate the lesion accurately. Thionin, 75 μm, celloidin. *b.* Low-power transverse section through the thalamus at the level of the ventrobasal complex—VB on the normal left side. Thionin, 50 μm, celloidin. Inset locates *d.* *c.* Section of thalamus on right side to show retrograde neuronal degeneration in VB. Preparation and magnification same as *b.* Inset marks location of field shown in *e.* *d.* Higher power to show normal appearance of VB neurons shown in *d.* In comparison to neurons shown in *d,* many neurons have undergone degeneration following a cortical lesion. Smaller nuclei are astrocytic.

considerably more advanced at birth than a hamster. An example of the importance of the age of an animal at the time a lesion is placed comes from our own work on the mouse. In Figure 4-4 are examples of three different animals which had the nerves to certain whiskers on the face damaged at different postnatal ages. There is a profound effect on the cellular organization in the sensory pathway subserving these tactile structures: in the thalamus, which is two synapses away from the peripheral damage, and in the cortex, which is at least three synapses away. Anatomically, the effects of the same experimental procedure differ systematically depending upon the age of the animal at the time of the experiment. We interpret these changes as alterations in the normal pattern of development (Woolsey and Wann, 1976; Anderson and Woolsey, 1977).

Schneider's (1973) work on the hamster visual system is an excellent example of the profound effect that lesions in the developing brain can have upon its consequent development. The removal of the superior colliculus of one side results in a number of abnormal patterns of connectivity of the optic tract. He has several examples in which these fibers connect with the remaining superior colliculus with maladaptive results. On the basis of their behavior the animals apparently interpret an object moving toward the nose as moving away from it, a behavior which can be explained in part by the patterns of connections that the optic fibers establish.

Another difficulty arises from the fact that, even among mammals, there are significant species differences in the details of organization of the nervous system. For example, the fibers of the cortical spinal tracts in the primate are located in the lateral funiculus of the spinal cord while in the rodent they are located in the dorsal column (Barnard and Woolsey, 1956). Probably based upon connectivity (compare cat, Shatz, 1975; with primate, Hubel, Weisel, and LeVay, 1977; geniculo-cortical pathways), size, niche, etc., the anatomical responses to lesions in the same functional systems may be quite different. The behavioral dissimilarities following "similar" lesions in different species are also quite striking (e.g., Wirth and O'Leary, 1974; Woolsey, Gorska, Wetzel, Erickson, and Allman, 1970; Woolsey, et al., 1972). Thus, great caution must be exercised in translating data from an animal for which anatomical data are available to ones where they are not.

Earlier we alluded to intraspecies differences which were related to the genetic strain of the animal. These can affect the gross disposition of neuronal structures and certain sensory systems. There are now examples of genetically related alterations of neuronal structure and central pathways. For example, Guillery and his colleagues (Guillery, 1974) have shown that there is an abnormality in the pattern of crossing of

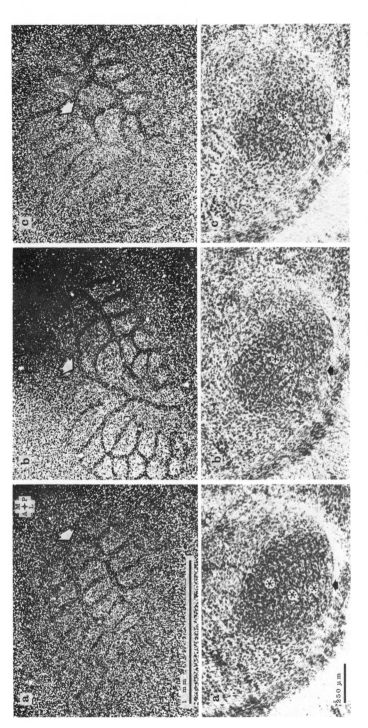

Figure 4-4. To show the altered organization of somatic sensory cortex and VB thalamus consequent to damage of mouse somatosensory periphery at different postnatal ages. *a*. Normal barrel field in a section tangential to the cortex. Row C is marked with an arrow. Thionin, 75 μm, celloidin. M, medial; L, lateral; A, anterior; P, posterior. *a'*. Normal disposition of "barreloids" in the thalamus (Van der Loos, 1976). The plane of section is oblique but approximates horizontal. Thionin, 50 μm, celloidin. Arrow and asterisks (*) mark row *c*. *b*. Barrel field of an animal in which the middle row of whiskers was damaged on the first day of life. Note the absence of the middle row of barrels. Thionin, 75 μm, celloidin. *b'*. VB of the animal shown in *b*. The barreloids are also abnormally organized with middle row being absent. Thionin, 50 μm, celloidin. *c*. Barrel field of an animal in which the middle row of whiskers was damaged on the third day of life. Note that the middle row of barrels is abnormal but not as severely affected as in *b*. Thionin, 75 μm, celloidin. *c'*. VB of the animal shown in *c*. The barreloids are affected but not to the extent shown in *b'*. Thionin, 50 μm, celloidin. *a*, *b*, *c* and *a'*, *b'*, *c'* all to same magnification. Orientation as in *a*.

optic fibers at the optic chiasm in albino animals. Too many fibers from an eye project to the opposite side of the brain and as a consequence these animals are behaviorally and functionally abnormal. The defect has even been described in the common laboratory white rat. Other animals, principally mice, have a number of other genetically related abnormalities from the absence of a corpus callosum (Sidman, Green, and Appel, 1965) to profound disorganization of the cortical mantle (Caviness, 1976). While these represent extreme examples, for the albinos at least, neuroanatomy has pointed to a previously unsuspected alteration in the anatomy of an animal having abnormal behavioral correlates which might be incorrectly attributed to a lesion rather than a structural defect.

7. SUMMARY AND COMMENTS

I have attempted to review briefly the anatomical experience with experimental lesions of the nervous system. The emphasis has been on phenomena which are likely to be of importance in the interpretation of the behavioral consequences of lesion experiments, on complications which are of considerable importance in evaluating specimens, and on the principal anatomical methods which can be used to correlate structural changes with behavioral changes. As an anatomist, my bias is clearly to encourage all workers to attempt to obtain reliable histological controls for their experiments.

This is not to say that neuroanatomy is the final court in which experimental cases are decided. Nothing could be farther from the truth. In fact, in relation to cytoarchitectonics, the anatomical work has been in many instances misleading (see Lorente de Nó, 1938). But if we, as neurobiologists, are ever to understand the most important manifestation of brain function in the behavior of the organism, we must take advantage of the multidisciplinary approach. Of necessity, this means that investigators of the anatomical persuasion must occasionally become behaviorists (Guillery, Casagrande, and Oberdorfer, 1974) and vice versa (Diamond, 1976).

ACKNOWLEDGMENT

This work was supported by NIH Grant NS10244.

8. REFERENCES

Adams, R. D., and Victor, M. *Principles of neurology.* New York: McGraw-Hill, 1977, pp. 496–561.

Anderson, J. R., and Woolsey, T. A. Effects of early whisker damage on the thalamus of the mouse: negative evidence for "competition" in the somatosensory system. *Neuroscience Abstracts,* 1977, *3,* 475.

Barnard, J. W., and Woolsey, C. N. Study of localization in corticospinal tracts of monkey and rat. *Journal of Comparative Neurology,* 1956, *105,* 25–50.

Blier, R. Retrograde transsynaptic cellular degeneration in mammillary and ventral tegmental nuclei following limbic decortication in rabbits of various ages. *Brain Research,* 1969, *15,* 365–393.

Bunge, R. P. Structure and function of neuroglia: some recent observations. In F. O. Schmitt (Ed.), *The neurosciences: Second study program.* New York: Rockefeller, 1970, pp. 782–797.

Cajal, S. R. *Neuron theory or reticular theory?* (Translated by M. U. Purkiss and C. A. Fox). Madrid: Consejo Superior de Investigationes Científicas, 1954.

Carpenter, M. B. *Human neuroanatomy.* Baltimore: Williams and Wilkins, 1976, p. 270.

Caviness, V. S., Jr. Patterns of cell and fiber distribution in the neocortex of the reeler mutant mouse. *Journal of Comparative Neurology,* 1976, *170,* 435–448.

Cowan, W. M. Anterograde and retrograde transneuronal degeneration in the central and peripheral nervous system. In W. J. H. Nauta and S. O. E. Ebbesson (Eds.), *Contemporary research methods in neuroanatomy.* New York: Springer, 1970, pp. 217–251.

Cowan, W. M., Gottlieb, D. I., Hendrickson, A. E., Price, J. L., and Woolsey, T. A. The autoradiographic demonstration of axonal connections in the central nervous system. *Brain Research,* 1972, *37,* 21–51.

Diamond, I. T. Organization of the visual cortex: comparative anatomical and behavioral studies. *Federation Proceedings,* 1976, *35,* 60–67.

Domesick, V. B. Thalamic relationships of the medial cortex in the rat. *Brain, Behavior and Evolution,* 1972, *6,* 457–483.

Fink, R. P., and Heimer, L. Two methods for selective silver impregnation of degenerating axons and their synaptic endings in the central nervous system. *Brain Research,* 1967, *4,* 369–374.

Florey, H. W. *General pathology.* Philadelphia: Saunders, 1970.

Fry, F. J., and Cowan, W. M. A study of retrograde cell degeneration in the lateral mammillary nucleus of the cat, with special reference to the role of axonal branching in the preservation of the cell. *Journal of Comparative Neurology,* 1972, *144,* 1–24.

Grafstein, B. The nerve cell body response to axotomy. *Experimental Neurology,* 1975, *48,* 32–51.

Guillery, R. W. The laminar distribution of retinal fibers in the dorsal lateral geniculate nucleus of the cat: a new interpretation. *Journal of Comparative Neurology,* 1970a, *138,* 339–368.

Guillery, R. W. Light- and electron-microscopical studies of normal and degenerating axons. In W. J. H. Nauta and S. O. E. Ebbeson (Eds.), *Contemporary research methods in neuroanatomy.* New York: Springer, 1970b, pp. 77–105.

Guillery, R. W. Discussion of paper. In W. J. H. Nauta and S. O. E. Ebbesson (Eds.), *Contemporary research methods in neuroanatomy.* New York: Springer, 1970c, p. 250.

Guillery, R. W. Binocular competition in the control of geniculate cell growth. *Journal of Comparative Neurology,* 1972, *144,* 117–127.

Guillery, R. W. Visual pathways in albinos. *Scientific American,* 1974, *230,* No. 5, 44–54.

Guillery, R. W., Casagrande, V. A., and Oberdorfer, M. D. Congenitally abnormal vision in Siamese cats. *Nature,* 1974, *252,* 195–199.

Guth, L. History of central nervous system regeneration research. *Experimental Neurology,* 1975, *48,* 3–15.

Heimer, L. Bridging the gap between light and electron microscopy in the experimental tracing of fiber connections. In W. J. H. Nauta and S. O. E. Ebbesson (Eds.), *Contemporary research methods in neuroanatomy.* New York: Springer, 1970, pp. 162–172.

Holmes, G. Disturbances of vision by cerebral lesions. *British Journal of Ophthalmology,* 1918, *2,* 353–384.

Hoopes, J. E., and Jabaley, M. E. Soft tissue injuries of the extremities. In W. F. Ballinger, R. B. Rutherford, and G. D. Zuidema (Eds.), *The management of trauma.* Philadelphia: Saunders, 1973, pp. 496–527.

Hubel, D. H., Weisel, T. N., and LeVay, S. Plasticity of ocular dominance columns in monkey striate cortex. *Philosophical Transactions of the Royal Society London, B,* 1977, *278,* 377–409.

Jackson, J. H. On the anatomical and physiological localization of movements in the brain. In J. Taylor (Ed.), *Selected writings of John Hughlings Jackson,* Vol. I. New York: Basic Books, 1958, pp. 37–76.

Jebb, A. H., and Woolsey, T. A. A simple hematoxylin method for myelin in frozen sections: a modification of Mahon's method. *Stain Technology,* 1977, in press.

Jones, E. G., and Powell, T. P. S. The projection of the somatic sensory cortex upon the thalamus in the cat. *Brain Research,* 1968, *10,* 369–391.

Jones, E. G., and Powell, T. P. S. An electron microscopic study of the mode of termination of cortico-thalamic fibres within the sensory relay nuclei of the thalamus. *Proceedings of the Royal Society, B,* 1969, *172,* 173–185.

Jones, E. G., and Rockel, A. J. Observations on complex vesicles, neurofilamentous hyperplasia and increased electron density during terminal degeneration in the inferior colliculus. *Journal of Comparative Neurology,* 1973, *147,* 93–118.

Kerr, F. W. L. Structural and functional evidence of plasticity in the central nervous system. *Experimental Neurology,* 1975, *48,* 16–31.

Krayenbühl, H. A. Cerebral venous and sinus thrombosis. *Clinical Neurosurgery,* 1967, *14,* 1–24.

Laatsch, R. H., and Cowan, W. M. Electron microscopic studies of the dentate gyrus of the rat. II. Degeneration of commissural afferents. *Journal of Comparative Neurology,* 1967, *130,* 241–262.

Langman, J. *Medical embryology.* Baltimore: Williams and Wilkins, 1975.

LaVail, J. H., and LaVail, M. M. Retrograde axonal transport in the central nervous system. *Science,* 1972, *176,* 1416–1417.

Lawrence, D. G., and Kuypers, H. G. J. M. The functional organization of the motor system in the monkey. I. The effects of bilateral pyramidal lesions. *Brain,* 1968*a, 91,* 1–14.

Lawrence, D. G., and Kuypers, H. G. J. M. The functional organization of the motor system in the monkey. II. The effects of lesions of the descending brainstem pathways. *Brain,* 1968*b, 91,* 15–36.

LeGros Clark, W. E., and Penman, G. C. The projection of the retina in the lateral geniculate body. *Proceedings of the Royal Society, B,* 1934, *114,* 292–313.

Liu, C. N., and Chambers, W. W. Intraspinal sprouting of dorsal root axons. *Archives of Neurology and Psychiatry,* 1958, *79,* 46–61.

Lorente de Nó, R. Architectonics and structure of the cerebral cortex. In J. F. Fulton (Ed.), *Physiology of the nervous system.* London: Oxford University Press, 1938, pp. 291–327.

Merzenich, M. M., Knight, P. L., and Roth, G. L. Representation of cochlea within primary auditory cortex in the cat. *Journal of Neurophysiology,* 1975, *38,* 231–249.

Miledi, R., and Slater, C. R. On the degeneration of rat neuromuscular junctions after nerve section. *Journal of Physiology (London),* 1970, *207,* 507–528.

Milhorat, T. H. *Hydrocephalus and the cerebrospinal fluid.* Baltimore: Williams and Wilkins, 1972.

Miller, D., and Adams, H. Physiopathology and management of increased intracranial pressure. In M. Critchley, J. L. O'Leary, and B. Jennett (Eds.), *Scientific foundations of neurology.* Philadelphia: F. A. Davis, 1972, pp. 308–324.

Murray, M., and Grafstein, B. Changes in the morphology and amino acid incorporation of regenerating goldfish optic neurons. *Experimental Neurology*, 1969, *23*, 544–560.

Nauta, W. J. H., and Gygax, P. A. Silver impregnation of degenerating axons in the central nervous system: a modified technique. *Stain Technology*, 1954, *29*, 91–93.

Penfield, W., and Boldrey, E. Somatic motor and sensory representation in the cerebral cortex of man as studied by electrical stimulation. *Brain*, 1937, *60*, 389–443.

Rose, J. E., and Woolsey, C. N. Cortical connections and functional organization of the thalamic auditory system of the cat. In H. F. Harlow and C. N. Woolsey (Eds.), *Biological and biochemical bases of behavior*. Madison: University of Wisconsin Press, 1958, pp. 127–150.

Schneider, G. E. Early lesions of superior colliculus: factors affecting the formation of abnormal retinal projections. *Brain, Behavior and Evolution*, 1973, *8*, 73–109.

Seddon, H. *Surgical disorders of the peripheral nerves*. Edinburgh: Churchill Livingstone, 1975.

Shatz, C. Ocular dominance columns in the cat's visual cortex. *Neuroscience Abstracts*, 1975, *1*, 56.

Sidman, R. L., Green, M. C., and Appel, S. H. *Catalog of the Neurological Mutants of the Mouse*. Cambridge, Massachusetts: Harvard University Press, 1965.

Skoff, R. P. The fine structure of pulse labeled ³H-thymidine cells in degenerating rat optic nerve. *Journal of Comparative Neurology*, 1975, *161*, 595–612.

Skoff, R. P., Price, D. L., and Stocks, A. Electron microscopic autoradiographic studies of gliogenesis in rat optic nerve. I. Cell proliferation. *Journal of Comparative Neurology*, 1976*a*, *169*, 291–312.

Skoff, R. P., Price., D. L., and Stocks, A. Electron microscopic autoradiographic studies of gliogenesis in rat optic nerve. II. Time of origin. *Journal of Comparative Neurology*, 1976*b*, *169*, 313–334.

Sperry, R. W. Optic nerve regeneration with return of vision in anurans. *Journal of Neurophysiology*, 1944, *7*, 56–69.

Sperry, R. W. The problem of central nervous reorganization after nerve regeneration and muscle transposition. *Quarterly Review of Biology*, 1945, *20*, 311–369.

Stern, W. E. The cerebral edema. In M. Critchley, J. L. O'Leary, and B. Jennett (Eds.), *Scientific foundation of neurology*. Philadelphia: F. A. Davis, 1972, pp. 289–296.

Swank, R. L., and Davenport, H. A. Chlorate-osmic-formalin method for staining degenerating myelin. *Stain Technology*, 1935, *10*, 87–90.

Valverde, F. Rate and extent of recovery from dark rearing in the visual cortex of the mouse. *Brain Research*, 1971, *33*, 1–11.

Van Crevel, H. *The rate of secondary degeneration in the central nervous system: An experimental study in the pyramid and optic nerve of the Cat*. Leiden: E. Ijdo N. V., 1958.

Van der Loos, H. Barreloids in mouse somatosensory thalamus. *Neuroscience Letters*, 1976, *2*, 1–6.

Wahlsten, D., Hudspeth, W. J., and Bernhardt, K. Implications of genetic variation in mouse brain structure for electrode placement by stereotaxic surgery. *Journal of Comparative Neurology*, 1975, *162*, 519–532.

Waller, A. Experiments on the section of the glossopharyngeal and hypoglossal nerves of the frog, and observations of the alterations produced thereby in the structure of their primitive fibres. *Philosophical Transactions*, 1850, *140*, 423–469.

Wirth, F. P., and O'Leary, J. L. Locomotor behavior of decerebellated arborial mammals—monkey and raccoon. *Journal of Comparative Neurology*, 1974, *157*, 53–86.

Wolf, G., Stricker, E. M., and Zigmond, M. J. Brain lesions: Induction, analysis, and the problem of recovery of function. In S. Finger (Ed.), *Recovery From Brain Damage: Research and Theory*. New York: Plenum, 1978.

Woolsey, C. N., Gorska, T., Wetzel, K., Erickson, T. C., and Allman, J. Patterns of localization in the "motor" cortex of the dog. *Physiologist*, 1970, *13*, 348.

Woolsey, C. N., Gorska, T., Wetzel, A., Erickson, T. C., Earls, F. J., and Allman, J. M. Complete unilateral section of the pyramidal tract at the medullary level in *Macaca mulatta. Brain Research*, 1972, *40*, 119–123.

Woolsey, T. A. Somatosensory, auditory and visual cortical areas in the mouse. *Johns Hopkins Medical Journal*, 1967, *121*, 91–112.

Woolsey, T. A. Organization of corticothalamic projections in the mouse. *Anatomical Record*, 1972, *172*, 429.

Woolsey, T. A., and Van der Loos, H. The structural organization of layer IV in the somatosensory region (SI) of mouse cerebral cortex. *Brain Research*, 1970, *17*, 205–242.

Woolsey, T. A., and Wann, J. R. Areal changes in mouse cortical barrels following vibrissal damage at different postnatal ages. *Journal of Comparative Neurology*, 1976, *170*, 53–66.

Zeki, S. M., and Sandman, D. R. Combined anatomical and electrophysiological studies on the boundary between the second and third visual areas of rhesus monkey cortex. *Proceedings of the Royal Society London, B*, 1976, *194*, 555–562.

Brain Lesions: Induction, Analysis, and the Problem of Recovery of Function

GEORGE WOLF, EDWARD M. STRICKER, AND MICHAEL J. ZIGMOND

1. INTRODUCTION

The ablation of tissue is a traditional approach to the study of its function, with regard to both peripheral structures and elements within the central nervous system. For many years this was the principal technique used by neuropsychologists in their studies of brain–behavior relationships, and it remains, in many ways, the most simple of the various approaches that are in common use. In this chapter we will discuss some of the basic techniques that are used and problems that occur when brain lesions are produced by (a) an electrode used to destroy all tissue at the target site, (b) a knife used specifically to disjoin fiber tracts, or (c) chemicals administered intracranially in order to destroy selectively certain types of neurons. Then we will discuss some prob-

GEORGE WOLF • Division of Natural Sciences, State University of New York, Purchase, New York 10577 **EDWARD M. STRICKER** • Department of Psychology, University of Pittsburgh, Pittsburgh, Pennsylvania 15260 **MICHAEL J. ZIGMOND** • Department of Biology, University of Pittsburgh, Pittsburgh, Pennsylvania 15260 Supported by NIH grants NS-12514 (to G.W.) and MH-20620 (to M.J.Z. and E.M.S.). The authors are thankful to Robin Kaplan for graphic work and Gregory Kapatos for histochemical analysis. Dr. A. Sclafani graciously lent assistance in the review of the mechanical lesions.

lems in assessing the effects of lesions, with special attention paid to those that are caused by recovery of function within residual elements of the damaged system.

2. INDUCTION OF LESIONS

2.1. Electrolytic Lesions

The term *electrolytic* is used here to denote lysis or destruction of cells by an electrical process. Such lesions are commonly induced by means of either direct current (DC) or radio frequency (RF) current. The term *electrolytic* is sometimes used to denote DC procedures only, while the terms *electrocoagulative* or *thermocoagulative* are used to denote RF procedures.

Electrolytic lesions are made in deep brain structures by passing current through stereotaxically inserted needle electrodes which are insulated except for a small area at the tip. The current density is sufficient to produce tissue destruction only within a limited region around the exposed tip. DC is thought to destroy tissue through a combination of factors including disruption of charged molecules in the cells, alteration of tissue pH, and liberation of gases or metal ions. RF produces lesions by generating high temperatures which coagulate the tissue around the tip of the electrode, although other factors, such as those associated with the local production of water vapor, are probably also involved (see Rowland, 1966, for a more extensive discussion of the mechanisms by which lesions are produced by electrical currents).

A special type of DC lesion results when anodal current is passed through stainless-steel or copper electrodes. In such cases, ferric or cupric ions are deposited. A wide variety of acute behavioral and physiological effects have been attributed to irritative actions of the deposited metallic ions, and these effects can be confounded with effects due to tissue destruction (e.g., Rolls, 1970; Whishaw and Robinson, 1974; Gold, 1975).

There are also specific morphological peculiarities of ion-depositing electrolytic lesions (Cox, Gisi, and Wolf, 1977). Figure 5-1 shows lesions produced by two deposit-free procedures (Figure 5-1*A* and *B*) in comparison to a lesion produced by anodal DC through a stainless-steel electrode (Figure 5-1*C*). The annulus of pathologic tissue surrounding the central cavity or core of amorphous necrotic material is much narrower in the deposit-free lesions. The broad annulus in the lesion produced by anodal DC through a stainless-steel electrode is presumably due to the deposited ferric ions, which cause a gradual necrosis of cells beyond the region of electrolytic destruction. It is also im-

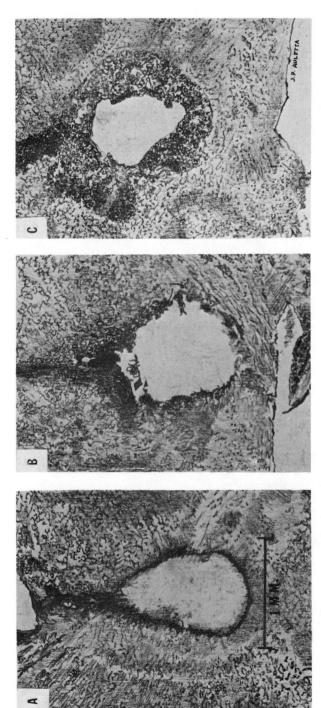

Figure 5-1.   Microprojector illustrations of parasagittal sections through lesions in the brain stem of rats. (A) Anodal DC through platinum-iridium electrode. (B) RF through stainless-steel electrode. (C) Anodal DC through stainless-steel electrode. (From Cox et al., 1977.)

portant to note that the ions do not readily invade white matter so that dense fiber tracts passing through the annular region tend to be spared. It may be that diffuse fibers or fine fascicles passing through the annulus are also spared, but this has not yet been determined.

The production of lesions by passing anodal DC through stainless-steel electrodes has been used extensively. The ready availability of fine, rigid, stainless-steel needles or wires and the highly reliable relationship between amount of current passed and lesion size have promoted the use of this procedure. Moreover, ion-depositing lesions may be used to great advantage when one wants to minimize damage to white matter within or adjoining a target area of gray matter, so long as the acute irritative effects do not influence subsequent observations.

On the other hand, both functional and morphological data indicate that, for total and unambiguous destruction of brain tissue, deposit-free electrolytic procedures are generally preferable to those which deposit toxic ions. Cathodal DC and RF do not cause metallic erosion and thus may be used with stainless-steel electrodes for production of deposit-free lesions. Fine wires made of relatively inert alloys with high tensile strength, such as platinum-iridium, also can be used for production of essentially deposit-free lesions, even with anodal DC. However, deposit-free electrolytic lesioning methods have been shunned by many workers because of inconsistency of size or shape of the lesions. This problem results from the sporadic reduction or complete blockage of current flow through the electrode–tissue interface, presumably due to the formation of gases around the electrode tip. When this happens the electrode insulation is put under increased stress and may break at one or more points along the shaft, thereby resulting in accessory lesions. Problems of inconsistent current flow can be minimized by increasing the size of the exposed electrode tip and reducing current intensity.

Thus, it is possible to produce lesions of relatively constant size with deposit-free DC (Cox *et al.*, 1977) or RF procedures (LeVere and Nicholson, 1969). Furthermore, the reliability of RF lesions can be increased. In at least one case this has been accomplished by coupling a thermistor to the lesioning electrode for monitoring the temperature of the target tissue (Pecson, Roth, and Mark, 1969). Of the three deposit-free procedures, we have obtained the best overall results with anodal DC passed through a platinum-iridium electrode (for important details see Cox *et al.*, 1977).

2.2. Mechanical Lesions

Fine disjunctions of fiber tracts can be made by means of a retractable wire knife (e.g., Albert, 1969; Sclafani, 1971; Gold, Kapatos, and

Carey, 1973). The "blade" is a length of fine (about 150 μ in diameter), resilient wire which is retracted inside the shaft of a metal cannula. A bend at the tip of the cannula causes the wire, when extended, to emerge roughly perpendicular to the shaft after it is lowered to the target site. The entire assembly is then lowered through the target site to produce a slender incision. An implantable assembly which allows the cut to be made in a freely moving animal has also been employed (Hamilton and Timmons, 1976).

Retractable knives are especially useful for disjoining diffuse fiber systems such as the medial forebrain bundle. Such diffuse systems generally have a broad trajectory so that a spherical lesion large enough to encompass their cross-sectional extent would destroy a large volume of the bed nucleus. However, while diffusely coursing axons are readily severed by the wire, compact fiber bundles (white matter) are less amenable to sectioning because they are relatively elastic in consistency and tend to be deflected rather than severed. When such bundles are round in cross section, they can be readily disjoined with negligible accessory damage by precisely positioned electrolytic lesions (Krieckhaus, 1964). Alternatively, broad regions of white matter can be transected with a wire knife it it is abruptly passed through the tissue. For example, a spring-loaded carrier which causes the knife to be briskly snapped downward has been used to sever the fornix between hippocampus and septum (Hamilton, Worsham, and Capobianco, 1973). Olton (1975) has described an alternative procedure for transecting broad regions by passing RF between two electrodes which span the region. Finally, a special knife which can be rotated after insertion into the brain to circumsect a specific region completely has been devised and used with great advantage to disjoin the hypothalamus from the brain stem (Ellison, 1972).

2.3. Chemical Lesions

Over the past 10 years, methods have been developed which permit the destruction of neuronal elements characterized by the transmitter which they utilize rather than, or in addition to, their anatomical location. These procedures involve the use of unstable, synthetic analogues of the biogenic amines, such as 6-hydroxydopamine (or its precursor, 6-hydroxydopa), 6-aminodopamine, 5,6-dihydroxytryptamine, and 5,7-dihydroxytryptamine (Figure 5-2). Use of such drugs began with the demonstration that 6-hydroxydopamine (6-HDA), administered directly into brain tissue (Ungerstedt, 1968) or via the cerebroventricular system (Bloom, Algeri, Groppetti, Revuelta, and Costa, 1969; Uretsky and Iversen, 1970), would deplete brain areas of the ca-

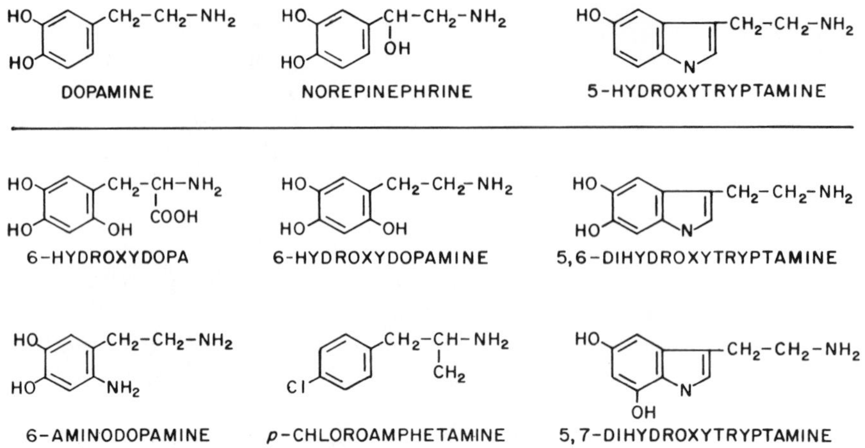

Figure 5-2. Structures of the biogenic amines and of some of the structural analogues used to produce specific chemical lesions.

techolamines (CA), norepinephrine (NE) and dopamine (DA), with little or no loss of other neurotransmitters.

Like many of the other agents, 6-HDA readily oxidizes to yield peroxides and quinones.* In sufficient concentration, 6-HDA apparently will produce irreversible damage to all nerve cells. However, since this compound is selectively transported into catecholaminergic nerve terminals (Heikkela and Cohen, 1971), it is often possible to limit most of the damage primarily to these cells (Figure 5-3). The ratio of specific to nonspecific damage produced by 6-HDA will depend on several variables, including the purity of the initial solution, its concentration, and the area into which it is injected. For example, since the high-affinity uptake system by which 6-HDA is concentrated resides primarily in the terminal region, specific effects are more easily produced there than in the area of the cell body where little specific uptake takes place. Likewise, low concentrations of 6-HDA administered into regions of dense innervation will favor specific damage, while high concentrations placed in areas with little catecholaminergic innervation will produce relatively greater nonspecific effects. When anatomical specificity is not required, nonspecific damage can be minimized by administering 6-HDA into the cerebrospinal fluid by way of the lateral ventricles or the cisterna magna. In young animals in whom a blood–brain

---

* In order to prevent its breakdown prior to use, 6-HDA must be stored as a dry powder at below 0°C under an inert gas and should be used within several months. Once in solution, it should be used immediately, although its stability may be increased by keeping it on ice and adding 1% ascorbic acid.

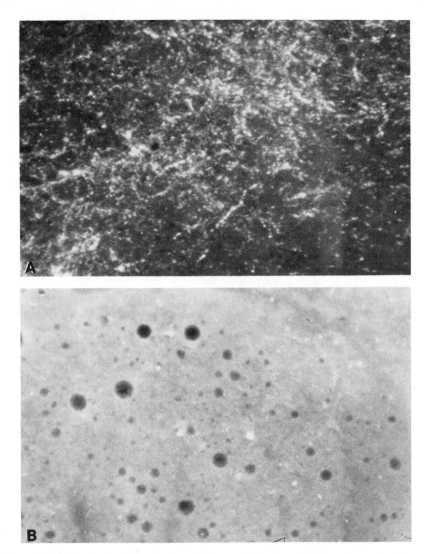

Figure 5-3.   Histological examination of damage following 6-hydroxydopamine. Shown is a 30-μm section through the lateral septal nucleus of the rat prepared by exposing the unperfused material to buffered glyoxylic acid and then visualizing fluorophores derived from endogenous catecholamines by fluorescent microscopy (Lindvall and Björklund, 1974). (*A*) Untreated control. (*B*) Four days after the intraventricular administration of 20 μl 6-HDA containing 250 μg to a rat pretreated with pargyline (50 mg/kg). This is about the maximal dose that can be given without producing considerable nonspecific effects, the pargyline apparently potentiating the effects of the 6-HDA by blocking its catabolism by monoamine oxidase.

barrier has not yet developed, systemic administration can be used as well (6-HDA does not cross the blood–brain barrier in adults). The species being studied probably also plays a role in determining specificity. For example, while intraventricular injection of 6-HDA produces little nonspecific damage in the rat, such damage can be considerable in the monkey.

Despite its ability to act selectively on catecholaminergic neurons, the issue of specificity among those neurons is an important one. There are a number of anatomically distinct catecholaminergic projections, each of which may subserve a different function. Because of the close proximity of their cell bodies and axons, it may be impossible to limit the effects of 6-HDA to a single catecholaminergic pathway, even with the most localized injections. It is not always possible to restrict the effects of this neurotoxin to neural pathways utilizing a single catecholamine. Pretreatment of rats with desmethylimipramine (DMI, administered i.p.) blocks the transport of 6-HDA into noradrenergic neurons, limiting damage to dopaminergic cells. However, an equally successful blockade of the effects of 6-HDA on dopaminergic elements is not yet available. While relatively small doses of 6-HDA administered into the cerebrospinal fluid can produce selective depletions of NE amounting to 40–50% of control values, larger NE depletions always are associated with considerable DA depletions as well. As a result, in functional studies of noradrenergic damage using 6-HDA-treated rats, animals with comparable DA depletions (produced by giving 6-HDA together with DMI) are often used as controls.

Other chemical treatments which have been used to destroy catecholaminergic terminals include 6-hydroxydopa and 6-aminodopamine. 6-Hydroxydopa acts by being converted to 6-HDA by the ubiquitous enzyme, *l*-aromatic amino acid decarboxylase. However, unlike 6-HDA, 6-hydroxydopa is an amino acid. As a result, it is possible to affect the brain with a systemic route of administration. On the other hand, nonspecific damage can be expected to be more severe since 6-hydroxydopa is a substrate for the general carrier system for endogenous neutral amino acids. 6-Aminodopamine is also reported to be somewhat less specific than 6-HDA, although it has been used to destroy noradrenergic neurons with little effect on DA. Like 6-HDA, it appears to act through its cytotoxic oxidation products.

In 1971, an hydroxylated derivative of serotonin, 5,6-dihydroxytryptamine, was introduced, soon to be followed by another serotonin analogue, 5,7-dihydroxytryptamine (5,7-DHT) (Baumgarten and Lachenmayer, 1972). While these agents given alone also destroy noradrenergic neurons, the combination of 5,7-DHT and DMI has been used to produce permanent loss of serotonin in rats with no detectable loss of norepinephrine or dopamine. Another synthetic compound which appears to selectively destroy serotonergic cells is p-chloroamphetamine (Harvey, McMaster, and Yunger, 1975; Sanders-Bush, Bushing, and Sulser, 1975), although the mechanism of its effect is unknown at present.

3. ANALYSIS OF NEUROLOGICAL EFFECTS OF LESIONS

3.1. Histological Analysis

We have discerned two major problems in the histologic analysis of electrolytic lesions. The first concerns problems in determining the extent of tissue damage, and the second concerns the transformation of histologic data into a form which is amenable to visual and/or quantitative analysis.

The morphological characteristics of lesions change as a function of postoperative survival time. Over the first few postoperative days the annulus surrounding the central cavity of electrolytic lesions changes from a chromophobic to an intensely stained appearance in Nissl-stained material. Generally, the boundary between pathologic and normal tissue is quite distinct, especially in the case of deposit-free lesions, and is clearly apparent in simple Nissl-stained sections. However, one occasionally encounters cases in which the transition between pathologic and normal tissue is more gradual and indistinct. Infections and infarcts may produce varying degrees of indistinct pathology in tissue adjoining a lesion site. Also, ambiguous areas or uncertain degrees of pathology are sometimes found within the broad annulus produced by toxic ions.

Since the boundaries of electrolytic lesions are generally quite distinct, objective and accurate estimation of the extent of primary tissue damage presents no problem as long as the shapes and sizes of the lesions have not undergone significant modification. However, a more difficult problem is encountered when one attempts to determine the original extent of tissue damage after long postoperative periods. A progressive contraction of the lesion commences about one week postoperatively and continues for several months thereafter. The lesion may shrink to as little as 20% of its initial size as the central cavity collapses and its convex perimeter becomes flattened or irregularly indented. The gliotic annulus around the central cavity also contracts during this time (Wolf and DiCara, 1969), and the shapes of brain structures adjoining the lesion become distorted due to ingression into the receding lesion area (Figure 5-4).

Probably the most accurate reconstruction of the original extent and placement of a contracted lesion can be gained by determining the volumes of intact remnants of surrounding structures invaded by the lesion. While this procedure by itself provides data for correlative analysis, it can also be utilized to determine the original volume of the lesion by subtracting the volumes of the intact remnants from the normal volumes of these structures. A simple and accurate procedure for determining volumes of brain structures from serial sections has been described elsewhere (Wolf, 1971). Unfortunately, many nuclei have indistinct boundaries, thus making it very difficult to determine residual volumes after structural distortion. In such cases one may have to be content with determining specific tissue damage in a sample of subjects which are sacrificed prior to the onset of structural distortion.

The second problem of analyzing lesion data involves the conversion of microscopic information contained in histologic material to a form which is readily accessible to visual analysis and numerical transformation. The first step toward this end is commonly achieved by making photomicrographs of the sections or by tracing outline diagrams of the lesions and surrounding structures from projected enlargements of the sections. The photos or drawings can be viewed in toto in conjunction with numerical values for the dependent variables to gain an overall view of anatomical–behavioral relationships. The photos or drawings can also be used to calculate lesion volumes by the procedure noted before.

It is not uncommon to encounter apparently contradictory findings on specific lesion effects by different researchers. Presumably many of these conflicting findings are due to differences in the size, shape, placement, or variability of the lesions, but the nature of these differences often cannot be ascertained due to the paucity of histologic data in the reports. Histologic data are not as readily or completely amenable to reduction by averaging processes as are the unidimensional data of the dependent variables.

Figure 5-5 shows four common procedures for graphic presentation of lesion data—a representative photomicrograph, overlays of individual lesion boundaries on an atlas diagram, the common area of destruction, and individual projection drawings. We favor the projection drawings because the boundaries of the lesions and of adjacent structures can be depicted at a very low level of magnification to allow efficient presentation of individual data so that relationships between lesion variability and the dependent variable can be studied. While the

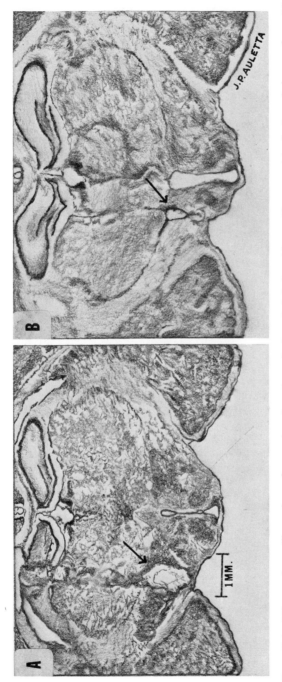

Figure 5-4. Microprojector illustrations of coronal sections through electrolytic lesions (denoted by arrows) in the hypothalamus of rats. (*A*) One week after operation. (*B*) Two months after operation. Note contraction of lesion and concomitant expansion of ventricle and distortion of left hypothalamus. (From Cox *et al.*, 1977.)

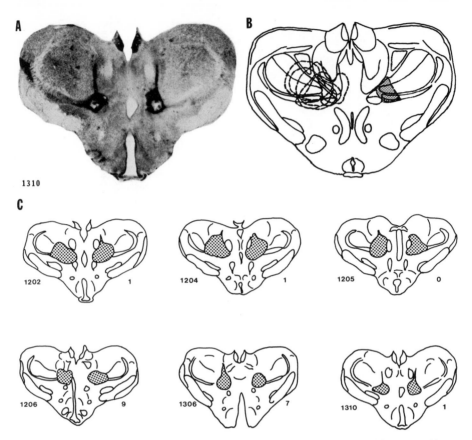

Figure 5-5. Four common methods for depicting histologic lesion data. (*A*) Photomicrograph of section with lesions representative of those shown in the six projection drawings below. (*B*) Section traced from stereotaxic atlas. On the left side the dashed lines represent the perimeters of each of the left lesions shown in the projection drawings. On the right side the shaded area represents the region of common overlap of each of the right lesions shown in the projection drawings. (*C*) Projection drawings of sections near the centers of lesions (shaded areas) in each of six brains. The number to the left of each section identifies the rat and the number to the right gives the rat's score on a critical dependent variable.

other three procedures are useful for summarizing results, they are not optimal for providing evidence of lesion–effect relationships. It should also be noted that the common procedure of depicting lesions by tracing them on atlas diagrams allows for a wide margin of error when the lesions are contracted and surrounding structures are distorted.

Histologic verification of knife cuts can be accomplished quite simply. When the brain is sectioned perpendicular to the cut, the area of

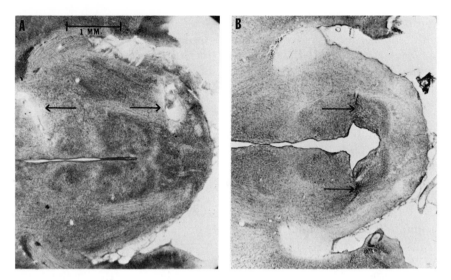

Figure 5-6.   Photomicrographs of horizontal sections through coronal cuts (denoted by arrows) in hypothalamus of rats made via encephalotome described by Sclafani (1971). (*A*) One day after operation. Note that the anterior cut is finer than the posterior cut, which apparently ruptured a blood vessel. (*B*) Several months after operation. Note that cuts have healed leaving only a fine line of gliosis and a local expansion of the ventricle. (Section *B* from Sclafani and Berner, 1977).

destruction appears first as a narrow cleft and, after healing, as a thin line of gliosis (Figure 5-6). While the thin scar resulting from a knife cut may diminish in length and breadth, it will not cause a major shift in adjoining structures as do large spherical lesions. On the other hand, inadvertent transection of blood vessels can result in considerable accessory necrosis as well as subtle alterations in structure and function of distant tissue. Also, one must take account of the possible regeneration of fibers across a cut during prolonged postoperative survival periods (Marks, 1972).

3.2. Neurochemical Analysis

Damage to monoaminergic neurons—whether produced by chemical or other means—cannot be properly assessed via conventional histological techniques, since their axons are often thin and unmyelinated and detection of degenerative changes is difficult. However, there are several alternative procedures which are satisfactory. For example, various means are available for visualizing the transmitters or related enzymes. For example, many neurotransmitters (the biogenic amines) can be converted to a fluorophore. Alternatively, it is often possible to bind biosynthetic enzymes (e.g., tyrosine hydroxylase, dopamine-β-hydroxylase, phenylethanolamine-N-methyltransferase) to a complex containing a specific antibody and some material which can be visualized at the light or electron microscope level. Although these procedures provide the advantage of precise anatomical localization (e.g., Ungerstedt, 1971a; Lindvall and Björklund, 1974), at best they permit only a semiquantitative measure of damage (Kopin, Palkovits, Kobayashi, and Jacobowitz, 1974). Much greater sensitivity and precision can be obtained through the use of biochemical analyses. Methods are now available which permit the detection of many transmitters in quantities as low as 10–100 pg (Iversen, Iversen, and Snyder, 1975). These can be used in combination with microdissection methods (Palkovits, 1973; Zigmond and Ben-Ari, 1976) to permit a precise determination of transmitter loss. Nevertheless, even these methods, like the histochemical localization of amines, are measuring transmitter loss, not degeneration. Thus, it is sometimes possible to confuse a temporary inhibition of synthesis or storage with degenerative changes. As a result, in contrast to the analysis of more traditional types of lesions (see above), analyses of chemical lesions are sometimes best carried out

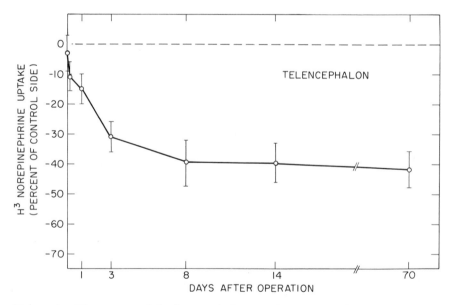

Figure 5-7.   Time course of the decrease in ^{3}H-norepinephrine uptake in synaptosome-rich homogenates prepared from animals sustaining an electrolytic lesion of the lateral hypothalamus. (From Zigmond et al., 1971.)

weeks or months after the lesion has been produced. Unfortunately, this may not provide a safeguard against a second problem, distinguishing between a loss in transmitter content due to degenerative changes and a loss of transmitter in intact neurons which is secondary to degenerative changes in an input pathway. One alternative is to use *in vitro* chemical procedures to obtain an index of the number of high-affinity uptake sites for specific transmitters, a measure which appears to reflect degenerative changes in nerve terminals (Figure 5-7; Zigmond, Chalmers, Simpson, and Wurtman, 1971; Kuhar, 1973).

4. RECOVERY OF FUNCTION: A PROBLEM IN THE ANALYSIS OF LESIONS

A general problem in analysis of the effects of brain lesions results from recovery of function. For example, extensive DA depletions produced by intraventricular 6-HDA treatment results in akinesia and catalepsy in rats (Ungerstedt, 1971b; Zigmond and Stricker, 1972). Nevertheless, if animals are maintained by intragastric intubations of liquid nutrients, they gradually exhibit seemingly normal movement and behavioral patterns, including the ability to maintain themselves by voluntary food and water consumption. This recovery of function occurs despite the fact that DA depletions are permanent (Zigmond and Stricker, 1973; Stricker and Zigmond, 1974).

We have been particularly interested in studying this apparent paradox, and have considered several explanations for it (Zigmond and Stricker, 1974; Stricker and Zigmond, 1976). (1) The initial deficits may be due to DA depletions, while resumption of feeding may result from functional recovery within the damaged pathway that is not detectable by conventional measurements of amine concentration. (2) The initial deficits may be due to DA depletions, but resumption of feeding may result from transfer of function formerly served by DA to other neurochemical pathways. (3) The initial deficits may not be causally related to observed DA depletions but to another, as yet unknown effect of the lesions that is more temporary.

The third hypothesis cannot yet be ruled out, although the concentrations of other putative neurotransmitter substances in the brain are not changed by this 6-HDA treatment. Moreover, we have observed that the initial deficits can be reinstated by further reduction of central dopaminergic function, either by increasing the size of the lesions, by inhibiting DA biosynthesis, or by blocking DA receptors (Zigmond and Stricker, 1973; Stricker and Zigmond, 1976; Heffner, Zigmond, and Stricker, 1977). These results suggest the possibility that recovery from

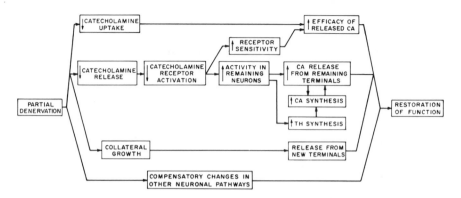

Figure 5-8.   A model for recovery of function within central catecholamine-containing neurons following subtotal damage. Immediately following the lesion, net CA release will be reduced, reflecting the proportion of undamaged neurons that remain. Even though the loss of uptake sites will increase the efficacy of released amine, net decreases in receptor stimulation should occur and lead to increased CA release from residual neurons. This increased turnover should be accompanied by increases in CA synthesis. Prolonged stimulation should increase the neurons' capacity for CA biosynthesis (e.g., through the induction of tyrosine hydroxylase) and thus progressively raise their capacity for sustained increases in CA turnover, while enhanced sensitivity of the postsynaptic membrane should increase the effectiveness of the released CA and further promote the recovery of function. A decrease in the affinity of residual terminals for CA, collateral growth from intact axons, regeneration of the damaged fibers, and adjustments within systems containing other neurotransmitters that are functionally interrelated with the central CA systems might also contribute to the recovery of function, although the nature of the stimulus for these processes is unknown. (From Stricker and Zigmond, 1976.)

the initial deficits following extensive depletion of brain DA is dependent on compensatory processes occurring within the damaged systems. The proposed sequence of events is summarized in Figure 5-8.*

Several lines of evidence support this concept of recovery. First, 6-HDA-treated rats are considerably more sensitive than vehicle-injected controls to the functional impairments that result from α-methyltyrosine, an inhibitor of tyrosine hydroxylase (the rate limiting enzyme in the biosynthesis of catecholamines) (Zigmond and Stricker, 1973; Heffner, Zigmond, and Stricker, 1977). This increased sensitivity is highly correlated with the degree of depletion of striatal DA (Zigmond and Stricker, 1974). Since CA depletion after the inhibition of tyrosine hydroxylase is dependent on the rate of turnover within the neurons, these data suggest that lesion-induced depletions of brain cat-

_____

* In addition to these processes, recovery of function might be aided by the reversal of certain secondary effects of electrolytic lesions—e.g., vasomotor changes, hemorrhage, edema, the proliferation of glial cells—which might have contributed to the initial deficits, and by repletion of catecholamines within central neurons that are depleted by 6-HDA injections in the absence of any ultrastructural damage.

echolamines are accompanied by an increase in CA turnover and synthesis rates in the remaining neurons. This hypothesis is further supported by recent measurements of DA synthesis in rats following damage to the nigro-striatal dopaminergic fibers (Agid, Javoy, and Glowinski, 1973). Second, the uptake of exogenous CA into the telencephalon decreases after the 6-HDA treatment (Uretsky and Iversen, 1970). This decrease may result from a reduced affinity of the residual terminals for amine as well as a reduction in number of axon terminals (Zigmond and Stricker, 1974). Assuming that the released transmitter is normally inactivated by being taken up into surrounding aminergic neurons, these changes should lead to an increase in the availability of CA at the postsynaptic receptor. This effect may account for the increased sensitivity of 6-HDA-treated animals to dopa (a precursor in the biosynthesis of DA, which is converted to DA in the brain) (Schoenfeld and Uretsky, 1973; Stricker and Zigmond, 1976). Third, there is an increase in the amount of motor activity that is elicited by apomorphine (a direct-acting dopaminergic agonist) in 6-HDA-treated rats which are depleted of telencephalic DA by at least 85–90% (Schoenfeld and Uretsky, 1972; Thornburg and Moore, 1975; Stricker and Zigmond, 1976). This effect is accompanied by an increase in the responsiveness of striatal adenylate cyclase to DA and probably reflects a change in the postsynaptic membrane (Zigmond and Stricker, 1975).

These observations have three important implications for the analysis of the effects of lesions. First, most measurements of behavioral deficits in lesioned animals may seriously underestimate the functional significance of the lesioned structure, since compensatory changes in residual neurons may be able to maintain function despite extensive and irreversible damage. In the case of catecholaminergic projections, a number of processes appear to be available to allow immediate compensation for the neuronal destruction. For example, basal DA synthesis rate is normally only a small fraction of maximal biosynthetic capacity, and thus a large and rapid increase in DA turnover from the residual neurons should be possible after a lesion-induced increase in demand. Only when need exceeds the capacity of such short-term processes should gross behavioral changes appear. This prediction is consistent with the absence of conspicuous behavioral impairments in human Parkinsonian patients until 75–90% of striatal DA has been lost (Hornykiewicz, 1973) and may also explain why early studies utilizing 6-HDA, which left 20–40% of DA terminals intact, failed to detect any significant behavioral effects.

Second, compensatory changes may conceal subtle compromises in function. These impairments presumably result from the neurochemical compensations that permit recovery of function. For example, it has been hypothesized that animals with fewer catecholominergic neurons should be proportionately less tolerant of strong sensory stimuli than intact animals, because the residual catecholaminergic neurons would have already increased their rate of DA turnover and thus have less reserve capacity for a further increase when a stimulus provoked additional release. Consequently, intense stimuli might increase neuronal activity so much that CA synthesis could not keep up with release and subsequent degradation, CA levels in the terminal would be depleted, and the resultant decrease in receptor stimulation would reestablish akinesia and catalepsy (Stricker and Zigmond, 1976). In other words, because of the considerable compensation that is possible within the residual neurons, degeneration of central catecholaminergic fibers may go unnoticed until some stressful incident precipitates prominent symptoms. In fact, such "traumatic Parkinsonism" is a well-known clinical phenomenon (Schwab and England, 1968). Similarly, animals bearing extensive damage to central catecholaminergic projections, which appear to behave normally in the neutral laboratory setting, consistently respond poorly following experimental treatments involving the abrupt onset of severe challenges to homeostasis, such as hypovolemia, cold stress, or hypoglycemia (Stricker and Zigmond, 1974; Stricker, Friedman, and Zigmond, 1975; Stricker, 1976). On the other hand, these animals respond more normally if they have been pretreated with drugs that would increase either tyrosine hydroxylase activity (Zigmond, Volz, Friedman, and Stricker, 1976) or the sensitivity of postsynaptic receptors to released CA (Stricker and Zigmond, 1976).

Third, lesions of specific brain areas may not reveal the function of those structures but of distant sites, due to interruption of fibers of passage. For example, all of the functional impairments observed after 6-HDA-induced DA depletions also are observed following electrolytic lesions of the lateral hypothalamic area (e.g., Ungerstedt, 1971*b*; Zigmond and Stricker, 1972, 1973; Fibiger, Zis, and McGeer, 1973; Breese, Smith, Cooper, and Grant, 1973; Stricker and Zigmond, 1974), which also transect the ascending dopaminergic projections. Thus, it may be that the profound initial deficits, the gradual recovery of function, and the curious residual deficits that characterize the well-known "lateral hypothalamic syndrome" (Teitelbaum and Epstein, 1962; Epstein, 1971) actually result, in large part, from disruption of dopaminergic fibers rather than from damage to hypothalamic tissue *per se* (Stricker and Zigmond, 1976).

5. SUMMARY

Physiological psychology continues to show its evolutionary roots in neurology by maintaining the traditional use of the lesion approach in the study of behavior. Recent advances in the induction of electrolytic and mechanical brain lesions and the histological analysis of their effects have enhanced the usefulness of these familiar procedures. Biochemical and neuropharmacological techniques and analyses also have become available in the last few years, and they already have produced clear gains in elucidating the anatomy of the central nervous system, and in promoting an understanding of recovery of function as well as such diverse central processes as those that are involved in the control of sleep and arousal, blood pressure, temperature regulation, motivated ingestive behaviors, and various clinical disorders. That so much has been accomplished so rapidly leads us to characterize the 1970s as the beginning of a new era in brain research, which will eventuate in the development of new drugs and biochemical approaches providing unparalleled opportunities for neuropsychologists to study brain function.

6. REFERENCES

Agid, Y., Javoy, F., and Glowinski, J. Hyperactivity of remaining dopaminergic neurones after partial destruction of the nigro-striatal dopaminergic system in the rat. *Nature (London), New Biology,* 1973, *245,* 150–151.

Albert, D. J. A simple method of making cuts in brain tissue. *Physiology and Behavior,* 1969, *4,* 863–864.

Baumgarten, H. G., and Lachenmayer, L. Chemically induced degeneration of indoleamine-containing nerve terminals in rat brain. *Brain Research,* 1972, *38,* 228–232.

Bloom, F. E., Algeri, S., Groppetti, A., Revuelta, A., and Costa, E. Lesions of central norepinephrine terminals with 6-OH-dopamine: Biochemistry and fine structure. *Science,* 1969, *166,* 1284–1286.

Breese, G. R., Smith, R. D., Cooper, B. R., and Grant, L. D. Alterations in consumatory behavior following intracisternal injection of 6-hydroxydopamine. *Pharmacology, Biochemistry and Behavior,* 1973, *1,* 319–328.

Cox, J. R., Gisi, J. M., and Wolf, G. Deposit free electrolytic lesions: Methodologic and histologic observations. *Physiology and Behavior,* 1977, *18,* 969–973.

Ellison, G. The use of microknives in brain lesion studies and the production of isolated brain-stem islands. In R. D. Myers (Ed.), *Methods in psychobiology.* Vol. 2 London: Academic Press, 1972.

Epstein, A. N. The lateral hypothalamic syndrome: Its implications for the physiological psychology of hunger and thirst. In E. Stellar and J. M. Sprague (Eds.), *Progress in physiological psychology.* Vol. 4. New York: Academic Press, 1971.

Fibiger, H. C., Zis, A. P., and McGeer, E. G. Feeding and drinking deficits after 6-hydroxydopamine administration in the rat: Similarities to the lateral hypothalamic syndrome. *Brain Research,* 1973, *55,* 135–148.

Gold, R. M. Anodal electrolytic brain lesions: How current and electrode metal influence lesion size and hyperphagiosity. *Physiology and Behavior,* 1975, *14,* 625–632.

Gold, R. M., Kapatos, G., and Carey, R. J. A retracting wire knife for stereotaxic brain surgery made from a microliter syringe. *Physiology and Behavior,* 1973, *10,* 813–816.

Hamilton, L. W., and Timmons, C. R. Knife cuts while you wait: A simple and inexpensive procedure for producing knife cuts in freely moving animals. *Physiology and Behavior,* 1976, *16,* 101–103.

Hamilton, L. W., Worsham, E., and Capobianco, S. A spring loaded carrier for transection of fornix and other large fiber bundles. *Physiology and Behavior,* 1973, *10,* 157–159.

Harvey, J. A., McMaster, S. E., and Yunger, L. M. *p*-Chloroamphetamine: Selective neurotoxic action in brain. *Science,* 1975, *187,* 841–843.

Heffner, T. G., Zigmond, M. J., and Stricker, E. M. Effects of dopaminergic agonists and antagonists on feeding in intact and 6-hydroxydopamine-treated rats. *Journal of Pharmacology and Experimental Therapeutics,* 1977, **201,** 386–399.

Heikkela, R., and Cohen, G. Inhibition of biogenic amine uptake by hydrogen peroxide: A mechanism for toxic effects of 6-OHDA. *Science,* 1971, *172,* 1257–1258.

Hornykiewicz, O. Parkinson's disease: From brain homogenate to treatment. *Federation Proceedings, Federation of American Societies for Experimental Biology,* 1973, *32,* 183–190.

Iversen, L. L., Iversen, S. D., and Snyder, S. H. (Eds.), *Handbook of psychopharmacology.* Section 1, Vol. 1. New York: Plenum Press, 1975.

Kopin, I. J., Palkovits, M., Kobayashi, R. M., and Jacobowitz, D. M. Quantitative relationship of catecholamine content and histofluorescence in brain of rats. *Brain Research,* 1974, *80,* 229–236.

Krieckhaus, E. E. Decrements in avoidance behavior following mammillothalamic tractotomy in cats. *Journal of Neurophysiology,* 1964, *27,* 753–767.

Kuhar, M. J. Neurotransmitter uptake: A tool in identifying neurotransmitter-specific pathways. *Life Sciences,* 1973, *18,* 1623–1634.

LeVere, T. E., and Nicholson, L. A. A simple method for producing discrete subcortical lesions using radio-frequency currents. *Behavior Research Methods and Instrumentation,* 1969, *4,* 150–152.

Lindvall, O., and Björklund, A. The organization of the ascending catecholamine neuron systems in the rat brain as revealed by the glyoxylic acid fluorescence method. *Acta Physiologica Scandinavica,* 1974, Supplementum *412,* 1–48.

Marks, A. F. Regenerative reconstruction of a tract in a rat's brain. *Experimental Neurology,* 1972, *34,* 455–464.

Olton, D. S. Technique for producing directionally specific brain lesion with radio frequency current. *Physiology and Behavior,* 1975, *14,* 369–372.

Palkovits, M. Isolated removal of hypothalamic or other brain nuclei of the rat. *Brain Research,* 1973, *69,* 449–450.

Pecson, R. D., Roth, D. A., and Mark, V. H. Experimental temperature control of radio frequency brain lesion size. *Journal of Neurosurgery,* 1969, *30,* 703–707.

Rolls, B. J. Drinking by rats after irritative lesions in the hypothalamus. *Physiology and Behavior,* 1970, *5,* 1385–1394.

Rowland, V. Stereotaxic techniques and the production of lesions. In L. Martini and W. F. Ganong (Eds.), *Neuroendocrinology.* Vol. 1. New York: Academic Press, 1966.

Sanders-Bush, E., Bushing, J. A., and Sulser, F. Long-term effects of *p*-chloroamphetamine and related drugs on central serotonergic mechanisms. *Journal of Pharmacology and Experimental Therapeutics,* 1975, *192,* 33–41.

Schoenfeld, R. I., and Uretsky, N. J. Altered response to apomorphine in 6-hydroxydopamine-treated rats. *European Journal of Pharmacology,* 1972, *19,* 115–118.

Schoenfeld, R. I., and Uretsky, N. J. Enhancement by 6-hydroxydopamine of the effects of dopa upon the motor activity of rats. *Journal of Pharmacology and Experimental Therapeutics,* 1973, *186,* 616–624.

6

Age, Brain Damage, and Performance

DAVID JOHNSON AND C. ROBERT ALMLI

1. AGE–BRAIN DAMAGE RELATIONSHIPS

Intensive investigation of the research literature reveals two relatively consistent results with respect to the effects of brain damage upon behavior. The first is that, following brain damage, the long-term deficits in behavior are rarely as severe as the initial or short-term deficits. In other words, a certain degree of recovery or sparing of function typically occurs following neural trauma (Stein, Rosen, and Butters, 1974). Superimposed upon this general principle, the research literature also frequently reveals that brain damage sustained early in life is often associated with less deleterious effects upon behavior than are found for similar brain damage sustained by the more mature animal. This notion is exemplified by the differential language deficits which follow trauma to neural language regions in young, as opposed to mature, humans. When such neural trauma is sustained early in life, relatively normal language capacity is eventually achieved; however, similar neural damage leads to severe and persistent language difficulties when inflicted in more mature humans. The notion that the infant brain displays greater "plasticity" than the adult brain has almost achieved the status of a principle. We will discuss this issue in the remainder of this chapter in an attempt to determine the validity of the infant plasticity notion.

Contrary to the notion that the infant brain has more capacity for recovery from neural trauma than the adult brain is the growing body

DAVID JOHNSON AND C. ROBERT ALMLI • Department of Psychology, Ohio University, Athens, Ohio 45701

of evidence which suggests that the infant brain is more susceptible (i.e., more vulnerable) than the adult brain to a variety of pathological conditions (Brazier, 1975). For example, nutritional, hormonal, and environmental deficiencies lead to greater neural and behavioral abnormality when the deficiencies are experienced early in life as opposed to later in life. These results would not be expected if the infant brain had a generally enhanced capacity for recovery or sparing of function.

Thus, the infant brain is simultaneously characterized as showing enhanced plasticity yet greater vulnerability as compared to the mature brain. Although resolution of this apparent contradiction is not obvious, the greater vulnerability demonstrated by the infant brain may be considered the first evidence questioning the general notion of enhanced plasticity of the infant brain. Alternatively, nutritional, hormonal, and environmental deficiencies most likely depress or arrest brain growth, thereby involving the entire brain, whereas traumatic brain injury may not produce such widespread brain dysfunction. The capacity for growth is an important factor in understanding the effects of infant brain damage, and we will frequently return to the "growth" issue in the remainder of the chapter.

1.1. The Age Factor

One of the major considerations when studying the effects of brain damage, and the subsequent degree of recovery from such damage, is the *age* or *maturation level* of the animal at the time of neural insult. Development reflects a process, beginning with conception and ending with death. In between these two endpoints is the dynamic continuum through the neonatal, pre- and postweaning, juvenile, early-, middle-, and late-adulthood, and senescence phases of life. To make the blanket assumption that the brain, or the behavior, of animals is homologous through this continuum is to ignore the facts of life.

The evaluation of performance following brain damage, when brain damage is sustained at different ages, requires the consideration of a number of factors. Critical research and meaningful interpretation of research results for age–brain damage relationships requires some specification of the following: the degree to which the behavior under study is homologous across ages, the degree to which experience and environmental interaction is altered across ages, and the degree to which the brain and/or the brain region under study is homologous across ages.

The behavior of animals is not necessarily homologous across the animals' lifespan, and therefore the behavioral capacity of an animal at the time of neural destruction is one factor which should be considered in studies where brain damage is inflicted in animals at different ages. Realistic comparisons between early and late brain damage can be meaningful only when both age groups have similar behaviors at the time they sustain neural trauma. For example, weanling rats consume food and water in an adultlike manner, and lateral hypothalamic destruction in weanling rats yields feeding and drinking deficits nearly identical to those produced in adults with similar neural destruction (Almli and Golden, 1974). Since infants and adults display homologous consummatory behaviors, the effects of brain damage for both age groups can be studied immediately following such damage. Furthermore, such homologous behaviors allow longitudinal analysis. On the other hand, what does it mean when infant animals sustain damage to a neural area, and upon maturing, are tested for DRL or delayed-alternation performance? Would it be wise to suggest that destruction of that brain region, in and of itself, produced the DRL performance deficits, or is the situation more complicated? We suggest the latter. The fact that the animal sustained brain damage during infancy automatically precludes "normal" ontogeny, a condition which is not paralleled when brain damage is sustained later in life. Thus, the infant brain-damaged and adult brain-damaged animals may share similar neural destruction; however, they obviously have not shared an equivalent ontogenetic interaction with their environments. The role of "experience" is too often neglected in studies of the effects of brain damage upon performance of complex cognitive behaviors. The environmental interaction variable is also a factor to be considered in situations in which behaviors are homologous across the lifespan; however, in this case the behavioral capacity can be studied immediately following brain destruction, rather than after long delays as in the case of nonhomologous behaviors.

Another factor which is often neglected in the brain-damage literature is that during the lifespan of an animal relatively drastic changes are taking place in the brain. The assumption of homologous brain tissue across the developmental continuum ignores the well-documented facts of ontogenetic growth and differentiation of the brain. The developing brain may be characterized as showing various degrees of morphological, biochemical, and electrophysiological maturity and, hence, immaturity. Even within a given age group, we must be aware of the fact that the entire brain does not show equivalent maturity across different neural regions (Vernadakis and Weiner, 1974). Although simplistic, development of the brain seems to be characterized by a caudal-to-rostral developmental sequence. Brain stem regions mature earlier, in terms of morphological, biochemical, and electrophysiological char-

acteristics, than do neocortical regions. Also, interconnections between
different brain regions do not develop in a homogenous fashion: the
development of cortical–thalamic fiber systems seem to precede the development to transcortical fiber systems.

Thus, the developing brain has been shown to be characterized by
growth and differentiation, which, after plateauing during adulthood,
begins a degenerative descent through senescence. When brain damage
is sustained by animals at different ages, the behavioral deficits (or lack
of deficits) which result must be considered as being superimposed
upon this dynamic (i.e., growth and differentiation) continuum. The
behavioral effects of "early" versus "late" neural destruction may be
more closely related to the "dynamic" nature of the neural area at the
time of destruction, than to the neural area *per se*.

The "behavioral capacity" and "neural maturation" factors discussed above for age–brain damage relationships warrant increased attention when interspecies comparisons are added to an already complex situation. It is well-known that different species of animals can be
characterized by differential patterns of maturation for both neurological and behavioral characteristics. For example, guinea pigs are quite
precocious at birth and develop rapidly, whereas rats and hamsters are
altricial during the neonatal period. If the problems of interspecies
comparisons faced by comparative psychologists can be overcome and
homologous behavior patterns can be experimentally documented
across selected species, then interspecies comparisons for age–brain
damage relationships may become a means by which we can obtain
some degree of control over the "experience–maturation" factor involved in studies concerned with the effects of early brain damage.
However, until these conditions are met, interspecies comparisons of
brain damage–age phenomena require cautious interpretation.

A final factor to be closely considered is that of sex of the animal
under study. The fact that males and females are different hardly
requires documentation, yet the ever-increasing evidence suggesting
differences in male and female brains requires our strict attention.
These sex differences may be found to underlie differential patterns of
neural development and, further, may underlie differential behavioral
propensities for males and females. For example, amygdaloid destruction sustained by infant rats leads to delayed puberty for females, while
males' puberty is unaffected (Relkin, 1971). On the other hand, lateral
hypothalamic destruction sustained by preweanling rats yields permanent body-weight deficits for males, while females show only transitory
body-weight depression (Almli and Golden, 1976a). Further experimentation may very well reveal sex differences for the effects of brain
damage upon cognitive abilities as well.

In summary, research concerned with age–brain damage relationships must deal with the following factors: (1) the behavioral capacity of the animal throughout its lifespan, (2) the maturation level of the brain, or more specifically the neural region, at the time of neural insult, and (3) the differential effects upon environmental interaction and experience when brain damage is sustained at different ages. These factors become more complex when interspecies and intersex comparisons are made for age–brain damage relationships. Thus, when one is studying the effects of brain damage across different ages, one enters a situation which is fraught with complex interactions, and the results of our studies require cautious interpretation and strict avoidance of overgeneralization.

1.2. Mechanisms of Recovery

Most brain damage that produces behavioral deficits is followed by some degree of improvement in performance with time, and a host of theories or mechanisms have been proposed to account for this phenomenon (Stein *et al.*, 1974). Most of these theories or mechanisms have been advanced for brain damage sustained by the mature animal, yet there seems to be an inherent assumption that these mechanisms may be even more effective in situations where brain damage is sustained by the immature animal. As these theories or mechanisms are discussed at length in other chapters, we will present them only briefly here. Some of the mechanisms proposed to account for the time-attenuating effects of brain damage upon performance are: (1) von Monakow's diaschisis theory, which suggests a temporary traumatic disruption of neural organization and integration, (2) substitution theory, which suggests a neural redundancy for maintaining functional capacity by a secondary neural system, (3) vicariation or equipotentiality theory, in which brain regions not specialized for a specific function subsume the function of the damaged tissue, (4) regeneration theory, new growth in damaged neurons, (5) collateral sprouting, new growth in undamaged neurons adjacent to destroyed neural tissue, (6) denervation supersensitivity, increased sensitivity to transmitter substance by neurons which have lost innervation as a result of brain damage, and (7) behavioral strategy change, where different environmental (internal and external) cues are utilized to maintain function.

The degree to which the above mechanisms play a role in the recovery-of-function phenomena is of course subject to current debate. However, if any of these mechanisms underlies recovery of function, we might expect these factors to operate differentially throughout the lifespan of the animal when brain damage is sustained at different ages. In this context, it does not seem illogical that the developing animal may have an advantage, as its nervous system is characterized as dynamic with respect to growth and differentiation. This advantage may then be translated into an enhanced "recovery" potential for brain damage sustained early in life, at which time destruction of more dynamic brain regions leads to greater recovery, while damage to less dynamic regions leads to attenuated recovery.

Due to the dynamic nature of the developing brain, it has been easy to accept (1) the notion that brain damage sustained early in life is followed by enhanced recovery of function as compared to brain damage sustained by the mature animal and (2) that this enhanced recovery of function is mediated by some form of neural reorganization (e.g., mechanisms 1–6, above). In the remainder of the chapter we shall document numerous examples where destruction of a variety of brain regions during early life does *not* yield enhanced recovery of function for many types of behaviors. In addition, while there is considerable documentation of neural reorganization following brain damage, the idea that neural reorganization underlies recovery of function has not been overwhelmingly supported. For example, Schneider (1973) has demonstrated that neural reorganization *does* occur following brain damage in infant hamsters; however, the anomalous neural connections often result in *abnormal* behavior patterns. In addition, most research demonstrating collateral sprouting (Lynch and Cotman, 1975; Raisman and Field, 1973) has used subcortical brain regions of adult animals, where recovery of function following brain damage is least impressive.

Thus, while some form(s) of neural reorganization or growth may ultimately account for recovery of function following the infliction of brain damage during early life, we must be cautious lest we be blind to alternative explanations; i.e., whereas neural reorganization may eventually be shown to account for recovery of function for some brain region–behavior relationships, other brain region–behavior relationships may reflect recovery of function via some form of behavioral adjustment.

1.3. Regional Brain Differences

With respect to adult animals, it is often noted that the probability of recovery of function occurring following brain damage is related to the brain region destroyed and the behavior under study. In general, there is a tendency for greater recovery of function following cortical destruction, and there also is a tendency for greater recovery of gross behaviors as opposed to more specific behaviors (Stein *et al.*, 1974). Goldberger (1974) has noted that recovery from brain damage is greater for those brain regions which are nontopographically arranged and thus possess diffuse overlap of efferent and afferent projections. Such brain regions are referred to as being "loosely coupled," and an example would be association cortex. In contrast, for precise point-to-point, topographically organized neural areas, the probability of recovery following damage is decreased. These brain regions are characterized as "tightly coupled," and the primary motor cortex and subcortical regions would be examples.

The principles of "tight" and "loose" coupling may be related to the maturational level of specific brain regions; we may conceive of a situation in which some brain regions are loosely coupled early in life, with maturational tightening of the coupling of the brain region. Such developmental changes in the coupling of certain neural regions may underlie situations in which brain damage sustained during early life yields enhanced recovery of function as compared to similar neural destruction sustained by mature animals. However, the development from loose to tight coupling of a brain region may also underlie the frequently observed phenomena of delayed behavioral deficits which sometimes occur when brain regions are damaged during early life.

1.4. Delayed Effects Following Brain Damage

One of the most perplexing results found when brain damage is sustained during infancy is that many behavioral deficits do not become manifest until after considerable time has elapsed. In other words, behavioral deficits are not apparent following brain damage, but sometime later in the lifespan of the animal the behavioral deficiencies develop and then persist. Such results are obviously contrary to notions of enhanced recovery of function for brain damage inflicted in young animals, and these results also cast doubt upon notions that neural reorganization underlies recovery of function.

"Delayed" behavioral deficits following brain damage sustained during early life have been shown to occur for a variety of brain region–behavior relationships and are found for a variety of species, e.g., dorsolateral cortex in monkeys affects delayed alternation tasks (Goldman, 1971, 1972, 1974); lateral preoptic area in rats affects drinking behavior (Almli, Golden, and McMullen, 1976); pyramidal tract in monkeys affects fine control of movement (Lawrence and Hopkins, 1970).

Goldman (1971, 1972, 1974) has suggested that delayed effects following brain damage sustained at an early age may be related to the degree of functional maturity of the brain region–behavior relationship under study. More specifically, if a neural area has not yet become functionally committed to a specific behavior at the time neural destruction is inflicted (i.e., the brain area is functionally immature), then destruction of that brain region does not yield behavioral deficits. However, with maturation, as that brain region would normally become committed to the behavior in question, deficits in behavior of the brain-damaged animal become manifest. This conceptualization of delayed lesion effects would suggest that the functional maturity of a brain region–behavior relationship could be evaluated with the brain-lesion technique. Thus, if brain damage during early life yields immediate behavioral deficits, such results would suggest that the brain region–behavior relationship under study had achieved functional maturity at that time. Further, if damage to a neural area early in life yields an initial sparing of function, followed later by the development of behavioral deficits, these results would suggest that the brain region–behavior relationship would have achieved functional maturity at the time the behavioral deficits first appeared. Finally, if damage to a neural area during early life produced no behavioral deficits, while damage to that same area later in life yielded permanent behavioral deficits (Kolb and Nonneman, 1976), a late development of functional maturity may also be indicated.

The delayed effect following brain damage sustained in early life is intriguing and may very well represent an indication of the development of functional maturity of a brain region–behavior relationship. However, we should seek confirmation of the functional maturity of a brain region with more positive techniques such as morphological, biochemical, and electrophysiological analyses.

In summary, the recovery-of-function model for evaluating the effects of brain damage sustained by animals at different ages has served its purpose and now leads us into forced catagorization and overgeneralization. As an alternative, the notions of functional maturity and tight versus loose coupling of brain region–behavior relationships are stimulating in that the lesion technique and anatomical, biochemical, and electrophysiological techniques can be used together for confirmation of results. With this alternative we now have a theoretical basis for predicting the effects of brain damage when such damage is sustained by animals at different ages.

2. SELECTED STUDIES OF AGE–BRAIN DAMAGE RELATIONSHIPS

Having presented what we feel are the most relevant theoretical considerations, we will now review selected infant-brain-damage studies with some comment on how these findings relate to the above theoretical considerations.

First, we should note the uneasy yet inextricable relationship between the historical development of the concepts of "localization of function" and "recovery of function." Recovery-of-function studies have not been attempted until investigators could at least generally agree on a behavioral syndrome following a particular lesion in adult animals (localization of function). At the same time, the phenomenon of recovery has been used by investigators from Flourens (1824) to Lashley (1929) to LeVere (1975) to challenge definitive localization of function concepts.

Studies of age–brain damage relationships are generally dated from the early work of Kennard (1936), although the work of Soltmann (1876) predates Kennard's work. From 1936 until the early 1960s age–brain damage studies concentrated on the effects of cortical lesions sustained in infancy versus adulthood. Study of the effects of subcortical lesions in infant animals awaited the proliferation of studies on the effects of subcortical lesions in adult animals. By 1960 the effects of hypothalamic, amygdaloid, hippocampal, septal, or thalamic lesions in adults were sufficiently documented to allow comparisons of infant versus adult damage at subcortical levels.

Because of the chronology of events there has been a strong tendency to conceptualize recovery of function in terms of cerebral organization, particularly cortical brain damage versus subcortical brain damage. There are, however, several problems with this conceptualization. For example, cortical structures are generally less mature in infancy than are more caudal brain structures. It also should be noted that behaviors studied following cortical lesions are often qualitatively different from behaviors studied following subcortical lesions. Cognitive tasks are quite different from specific sensorimotor functions, which also differ from regulatory functions. One might expect "regulatory processes" to be more permanently affected by hypothalamic lesions in infancy than would "delayed recall" following cortical lesions in infancy. Within the cortical level, sensory and motor functions seem more liable following neural destruction than associative-type function. There has been a great variety of results (recovery, partial recovery, or no recovery) across tasks, areas of destruction, species, etc. It might be less confusing if we could more precisely define the underlying variables (e.g., maturation, loose versus tight coupling) rather than fall back on less precise cortical versus subcortical distinctions.

2.1. Decortication during Infancy

The first widely referenced studies of the effects of infant brain damage are those of Kennard (1936, 1938, 1940, 1942). Generally, she reported that precentral lesions in infant monkeys resulted in relatively minor motor disturbance in adulthood, whereas similar lesions in adult animals produced profound motor deficits. Most investigators citing her work (particularly in introductory sections of research papers) overlook certain other of her results. Kennard reported that the discrepancy between infant lesion and control animals increased during development, primarily as a result of increased coordination of motor function in the normal animals. While "forced grasping," for example, continued in infant operates, voluntary control was making its appearance in normal animals. Spasticity became more apparent in infant-operate animals with advancing age, although never reaching the severity observed in animals operated upon as adults. In fact, the matured infant-lesion animals were quite similar behaviorally to animals fully recovered from pyramidal lesions (Goldberger, 1974). The prominent difference between infant-lesion and adult-lesion animals in Kennard's studies seems to be the absence of the traumatic, acute effects of the precentral lesion (diaschisis) in infant operates. It is also worth noting that the effects of precentral lesions in infancy became more noticeable with age, when the damaged area would have been assuming control of voluntary coordination. This is the first instance reported in the literature where ontogenetic encephalization of function and age at the time of observation clearly interact with the infant-lesion procedure to produce a delayed-onset deficit. This result seems clearly related to the delayed effects recently reported by Goldman (1971, 1972, 1974).

Kennard (1938) also published results which relate to the recovery process we have called "substitution" and "growth." Unilateral precentral lesions placed in infant monkeys resulted in contralteral motor effects which, while not completely absent, were much less severe than when similar unilateral lesions were produced in adult monkeys. When, as adults, the contralateral precentral area was destroyed, a profound bilateral motor deficit was observed. Thus, it would seem that substitute tissue (presumably the contralateral precentral area) in the infant brain can more readily assume functions which would normally be controlled by the destroyed tissue.

Subsequent to Kennard's work, a series of experiments was published which reported that cortical lesions in adults produced more severe deficits than cortical lesions in infant animals. Tsang (1937) found maze performance in rats to be less severely impaired following decortication in infancy than following similar decortication in adults. Beach (1938) reported that cortical lesions in infant rats resulted in less severe disruption of sexual behavior than did cortical lesions in adult rats. Benjamin and Thompson (1959, roughness discrimination) and Akert, Orth, Harlow, and Schiltz (1960, delayed response learning) have also reported results which generally support the notion of enhanced recovery following cortical lesions in infancy.

Research on sparing of function following destruction of visual cortex has produced inconsistent results. Wetzel, Thompson, Horel, and Meyer (1965) reported that pattern discrimination was not as severely disrupted following destruction of the visual cortex in infancy as when the damage was produced in adults. However, cats in this experiment frequently bumped into objects in their path. Doty (1971) has reported that when prestriate cortex and area 17 are destroyed in infant animals, the visual-discrimination deficit is permanent. Some experiments which report visual sparing following destruction in infancy also report that the lateral geniculate nucleus has not completely degenerated.

Other studies using a variety of tasks have reported little or no sparing following decortication in infancy. Brooks and Peck (1940) report that lesions of the sensorimotor cortex in rats leads to deficits in the placing response regardless of age at the time of surgery. Kling and Tucker (1967) found recovery on a delayed-response task, but no recovery on a delayed-alternation task. Harlow, Blumquist, Thompson, Schiltz, and Harlow (1968) reported that delayed response learning was not affected by lesions at 5 months of age; however, the effects of decortication at 12 months of age were more severe than the effects of decortication at 18 or 24 months of age. Goldman, Rosvold, and Mishkin (1970) have reported that, following destruction of the orbital cortex, infant-lesion animals were impaired on a delayed-response task when compared to control animals but were not as severely affected as animals receiving lesions as adults.

Although this is not an exhaustive review, the studies cited above present little support for the idea that cortical brain damage in infancy is routinely followed by enhanced recovery. The evidence from studies of subcortical damage in infants is even more damning to this overgeneralization.

2.2. Subcortical Destruction during Infancy

During the last 15 years, it has become possible and fashionable to study the effects of subcortical lesions sustained during infancy. The results of subcortical studies were initially interpreted in terms of the expectation of recovery which had developed over the years from work with cortical lesions in infancy. It is apparent now, however, that simple conceptualizations will no longer suffice. Indeed, the failure of recovery reported in so many studies involving subcortical lesions has given impetus to a reconsideration of past concepts of recovery.

Amygdalectomies in kittens (Kling, 1962, 1965) and infant monkeys (Green and Kling, 1966) failed to produce the most prevalent aspects (severe unresponsiveness) of the Klüver–Bucy (1939) syndrome. It is not surprising that hypersexuality was not observed in the prepubescent monkey, and the lack of hypersexuality during this period of development should not be taken as evidence of recovery. Some of the animals in Kling's studies did display aberrant sexual behaviors, but not until the onset of sexual maturity. Amygdalectomies in adults produce marked alterations in social behavior (Jonason and Enloe, 1971). It is quite possible that altered social behavior through development might, in some unspecified manner, alter an animal's sexual responsiveness. Thompson, Schwartzbaum, and Harlow (1969) also point out that the animal's familiarity with the testing environment has a marked impact upon recovery following amygdalectomy in monkeys.

In a major study on the effects of hippocampal lesions in infant cats, Isaacson, Nonneman, and Schmaltz (1968) report a wide variety of results. Their results suggest that the structural integrity of the dorsal hippocampus was to some extent reformed following disruption by the lesion in infancy. Such neural reorganization might result since, at the time the lesion is produced, the hippocampus is characterized by cell division and migration (growth). Behaviorally, the DRL and reversal learning deficits which are characteristic following hippocampal destruction in adults are not evident for infant-lesion cats; however, the infants displayed a rather marked and lasting impairment on a passive avoidance task.

Brunner and Altman (1974) have reported the effects of x-irradiation on the developing hippocampus when nearly 85% of all granular cells were destroyed. These investigators found scant evidence of behavioral recovery although they used a variety of behavioral tests. Brunner and Altman emphasized the need to insure that animals in both experimental and control groups be comparable, and they have suggested the following: (1) equal recovery periods for animals treated in infancy versus adulthood and (2) experimental and control animals to be tested over the same range of ages. However, even if recovery periods are equivalent in time, how does one know that the infant system does not "recover" more substantially with equivalent postlesion intervals?

Recent research in our laboratory (Johnson, unpublished) has suggested that ventral hippocampal lesions produced in infancy result in no effect when animals are tested at 30 days of age on a two-way conditioned avoidance task. However, if testing is conducted at 45 or 60 days of age, lesions sustained in infancy result in marked facilitation of conditioned avoidance response (CAR) learning in comparison to age-mate controls. At 30 days of age, lesion and normal animals display an abnormally high efficiency on the CAR task; however, this effect continues only in animals with hippocampal lesions. The rat with a hippocampal lesion in infancy, at least on the CAR task, displays yet another instance of the delayed-onset phenomenon. Brunner and Altman (1974) also report CAR facilitation in their study of hippocampal x-irradiation, when testing was conducted beyond 30 days of age.

Studies of the effects of septal lesions in both infant and adult animals have consistently reported alterations in performance across a variety of behaviors (Gittis and Hothersall, 1974; McMullen and Almli, 1975; Johnson, Bieliauskas, and Lancaster, 1973; Schoenfeld, Hamilton, and Gandelman, 1974; Johnson, 1972). DRL behavior is equally hampered by septal lesions in infancy or adulthood, and conditions which enhance recovery in infants or adults, such as long recovery periods (Johnson, *et al.,* 1973) or the opportunity for the animal to engage in mediating behavior (Gittis and Hothersall, 1974), have similar impacts on infant-lesion or adult-lesion animals.

Septal lesions also enhance CAR acquisition (Johnson, 1972; Schoenfeld *et al.,* 1974) regardless of age at the time of lesion. In contrast to the results following hippocampal lesions in infancy, pilot work (Johnson, unpublished) indicates that the CAR enhancement following septal lesions seems to be present even if animals are tested at 30 days of age. Furthermore, enhanced social behavior has been observed following septal destruction regardless of age at the time of lesion (Johnson, 1972), and such extensive social contact during development would, in and of itself, have an impact on a variety of performance variables. Finally, McMullen and Almli (1975) have shown that, as in adults, septal destruction during infancy results in chronic hyperdipsia, which persists through adulthood.

It is curious that septal lesions in infancy and adults should yield such equivalent behavioral alteration. This might be an artifact of the location and relative isolation of the septum from surrounding structures. One can rather confidently state that the entire septum has been destroyed with minimal damage to adjacent structures. In contrast, attempts to destroy the hippocampus bilaterally are usually accompanied by incomplete destruction, damage to a variety of adjacent structures, and differential lesion size bilaterally. Thus, the limited potential for recovery from septal damage may be related to more thorough destruction, but, more likely, these results may indicate early septal maturation.

When tectal lesions were produced in young hampsters (Schneider, 1973), orientation to visual stimuli was not lost as was the case when similar damage was produced in adult animals. Schneider reports abnormal growth of the retinotectal system in these animals, and suggests that such axonal sprouting may be responsible for recovery. However, the brain-damaged hamsters display abnormal behavior.

Research involving caudate lesions in infant animals has indicated that delayed-response and delayed-alteration deficits are present if lesions are produced in juvenile or adult monkeys (Goldman, 1972). Unilateral caudate lesions in infant rats have been observed to produce locomotor dysfunctions (hyperactivity) similar to the results following unilateral caudate lesions in adult animals (Johnson and Becker, 1973). Goldman (1974) argues that the functional relationship between caudate and frontal cortical areas was the determining factor in experiments dealing with recovery from frontal cortical lesions. In young animals, the caudate area mediates the behavior in question, and cortical lesions produced no deficit at that time. As function would have been assumed by the damaged cortical area, performance deficits became manifest.

Almli and his students have been investigating the effects of early subcortical brain damage upon the ontogeny of regulatory and sensorimotor capacity. Bilateral lateral hypothalamic area (LHA) lesions in infancy result in complete cessation of suckling (aphasia and adipsia?) even if the lesions are produced at 7–10 days of age (Almli and Golden, 1976a, 1974). Some of these animals survive when tube fed, but it is 50 days or more before such rats maintain survival via voluntary feeding and drinking. Specific feeding and drinking challenges administered to the infant operates throughout development indicate that regulatory deficiencies are permanent. This pattern of results is essentially the same as that observed following LHA lesions in adults, and, if anything, the animals that survive recover regulatory behaviors more slowly than animals with LHA lesions in adulthood. Almli, McMullen, and Golden (1976) have also demonstrated that LHA units display basal firing rates similar to adult LHA units, and furthermore that the percent of LHA-osmosensitive units is similar to that found in adults. Thus, on the basis of electrophysiological and lesion evidence, the LHA appears to be mature and functioning by the end of the first week of life.

Unilateral lesions in the LHA of infant animals (Almli and Golden, 1976b) are followed by mild and transitory deficits. If at 150 days of age the contralateral LHA is destroyed, dramatic regulatory deficits are reinstated. These results (Almli and Golden, 1976b), like those discussed above (Kennard, 1938), demonstrate that the intact contralateral neural structure has the potential to maintain function following loss of neural tissue on one side of the brain.

In an effort to expand the scope of the investigations of neural ontogeny of regulatory and sensorimotor phenomena, Almli and his students have recently reported that, similar to adults: (1) lateral preoptic lesions in infant rats result in abnormalities in drinking behavior

(Almli, Golden, and McMullen, 1976), (2) substrantia nigra lesions in infancy yield sensorimotor and regulatory deficits (Almli and Fisher, 1977), and (3) midbrain and pontine gustatory lesions result in severe and persistent sensory and regulatory deficits (Almli and Hill, 1977). All of these effects are similar, if not identical, to the effects of analogous lesion treatments in adult animals.

2.3. Early Spinal Transection

Finally, we will discuss the effects of thoracic spinal transection in neonatal versus weanling rats. Stelzner, Ershler, and Weber (1975) report that reflex ontogeny in the distal segment of the cord of the rat is less disrupted by removal of supraspinal influences at 1–4 days of age than at 21–26 days of age. They suggest that as the interconnections between levels of the CNS develop, the acute impact of transection (spinal shock–diaschisis) becomes more pronounced.

3. THE FUTURE: AGE–BRAIN DAMAGE RELATIONSHIPS

3.1. Overview

Throughout this review of age–brain damage relationships, two of the most pervasive results were (1) lack of the tramatic (diaschisis) effects of brain damage on infant animals following surgery and (2) evidence of delayed onset of deficit phenomenon. These results are reported in studies investigating the effects of early-lesion treatments at the spinal, subcortical, and cortical levels of organization, and each is probably related to the ontogeny of encephalization.

Most studies of the age–brain damage relationship have catagorized results into "recovery of function–no recovery of function" classifications. From a survey of the literature it is apparent that following infant brain damage some degree of recovery of function ensues in almost every study; however, this is also true for studies involving brain damage in adult animals. In some studies, recovery of function seems more complete following brain damage in infancy than when similar brain damage was produced in adult animals, whereas in other studies, evidence of enhanced recovery following the infant-lesion treatment is minimal. In between these extremes are examples of recovery on some tasks and little recovery on others. These complex results require more than a simple "recovery–no recovery" conceptual framework. Organizing results in terms of brain hierarchies (e.g., cortical versus subcortical) is also not satisfactory, as regional dichotomies mask other relevant variables, such as task complexity, functional maturity of a neural system, and loose versus tight coupling.

After defining what we felt to be the most cogent variables for age–brain damage relationships, we had difficulty in assessing the relevance of any particular study to these variables. In part, this is because these variables have frequently been used in *post hoc* explanations of results. One encounters statements, for example, that recovery may have been facilitated by the development of alternative strategies. We are not familiar with a single study, however, which was designed to determine if this occurs. The many conflicting results might not be so confusing if investigators designed research to answer hypotheses currently used in a *post hoc* manner. Goldman and Almli, for example, answer questions relating to functional maturity of brain regions, because their experimental designs specifically relate to that hypothesis.

3.2. Research Considerations

In this final section we would like to point out some of the problems which are encountered when conducting research, or evaluating research reports, on age–brain damage relationships. These problems have been with us in the past, and in most cases the problems are difficult to deal with. Nevertheless, we must gear our efforts toward their resolution before age–brain damage relationships can be understood fully.

When brain damage is sustained during early life, the brain damage and surgical trauma may interact to produce alteration in the ability of the animal to maintain normal nutritional and environmental–social relationships. These secondary effects of early brain damage have the potential to effect performance alteration on a variety of tasks. Physical and experiential variables have, to a great extent, been ignored in favor of "main effects" within the "recovery–no recovery" and "localization" models. Advancement of knowledge in the age–brain damage field requires some documentation and/or control for nutritional and experience variables, especially when brain damage is sustained in early life.

Many research studies in the age–brain damage field utilize designs whereby brain damage is inflicted at an early age, while performance evaluation is delayed until the animals mature. In addition, the effects of early brain damage upon some behavior is often studied without knowledge of the normal ontogeny of the behavior in question. The weaknesses of the above designs emphasize the need for longitudinal research in this area. Longitudinal analysis would serve to increase our understanding of the ontogeny of behavior, as well as divulging the time-course of behavioral alteration following early brain damage. This approach would decrease emphasis upon the unwarranted assumption that one can control for infant versus adult brain damage by utilizing equal postlesion recovery periods. Neglect of longitudinal analysis has left us with too great a dependence upon "infant versus adult brain damaged" comparisons.

Some of the research associated with comparing adult brain-damaged animals with mature infant operates is obviously biased. The infant operates rarely have the advantage of the equivalent of a "culture free" testing situation, as most testing procedures have been developed using normal intact adult animals. In this sense, we are testing infant operates in an adult world. Furthermore, as evidenced by many research designs, motivational equivalence between infant and adult operates is assumed. A longitudinal approach avoids these problems by forcing creative efforts in the design of testing and motivational procedures which would "evolve" with the developing brain-damaged animal. We then would be evaluating *behavioral capacity* of infant operates, as opposed to merely determining whether or not the infant operate shows behavioral equivalence to the adult.

Reliance upon singular testing procedures has, probably more than anything else, led us into perpetuation of the "recovery of function–no recovery" conceptualization for age–brain damage relationships. Singular testing procedures lead to singular explanations of research results. Fortunately, there is a trend for research of age–brain damage relationships to include multiple tasks in evaluating performance. More often than not, performance is altered for some tasks and not for others, and these results indicate that age–brain damage phenomena require more than simple explanations.

Finally, early-brain-damage studies typically are characterized by relatively long time lapses between infliction of brain damage and subsequent histological analysis of the damaged neural tissue. These extended time periods make specification of the damaged tissue difficult at best. For example, there may be filling in (or shrinking) of the damaged area, ventricular dilation or collapse, and so on. In other words, it is often nearly impossible to document precisely which neural tissue is destroyed and which is intact. We are in dire need of research which specifies the gross and molecular changes which take place within the brain following both early and late infliction of brain damage. Fortunately, this research is forthcoming.

The list of problems above is not meant to be exhaustive but is intended to highlight some of the more important considerations which must be made in order to enhance our understanding of age–brain damage relationships. It should be obvious, if the intent of the present chapter is realized, that the notion of "enhanced plasticity" of the infant brain may be due to our tunnel vision, which has been manifest in our experimental designs. With respect to early brain damage, we have looked for enhanced recovery and we have found it. This brings to mind the frequently quoted statement by Alfred Binet, "Tell me what you are looking for and I will tell you what you will find."

4. REFERENCES

Almli, C. R., and Fisher, R. S. Infant rats: Sensorimotor ontogeny and effects of substantia nigra destruction. *Brain Research Bulletin*, 1977, in press.

Almli, C. R., and Golden, G. T. Infant rats: Effects of lateral hypothalamic destruction. *Physiology and Behavior*, 1974, *13*, 81–90.

Almli, C. R., and Golden, G. T. Preweanling rats: Recovery from lateral hypothalamic damage. *Journal of Comparative and Physiological Psychology*, 1976a, *90*, 1063–1074.

Almli, C. R., and Golden, G. T. Serial lateral hypothalamic destruction: Infancy and adulthood. *Experimental Neurology*, 1976b, *53*, 646–662.

Almli, C. R., and Hill, D. L. Infant rats: Effects of central gustatory and reticular formation destruction upon the ontogeny of sensorimotor and regulatory behaviors. *Neuroscience Abstracts*, 1977.

Almli, C. R., Golden, G. T., and McMullen, N. T. Ontogeny of drinking behavior of preweanling rats with lateral preoptic damage. *Brain Research Bulletin*, 1976, *1*, 437–442.

Almli, C. R., McMullen, N. T., and Golden, G. T. Infant rats: Hypothalamic unit activity. *Brain Research Bulletin*, 1976, *1*, 543–552.

Akert, K., Orth, O. S., Harlow, H. F., and Schiltz, F. Learned behavior of rhesus monkeys following neonatal bilateral prefrontal lobotomy. *Science*, 1960, *132*, 1944–1945.

Beach, F. A. The neural basis of innate behavior: II. Relative effects of partial decortication in adulthood and infancy upon maternal behavior of the primaparous rat. *Journal of Genetic Psychology*, 1938, *53*, 109–148.

Benjamin, R. M., and Thompson, R. F. Differential effects of cortical lesions in infant and adult cats on roughness discrimination. *Experimental Neurology*, 1959, *1*, 305–321.

Brazier, M. A. B. (Ed.), *Growth and development of the brain. Nutritional, genetic, and environmental factors*. Vol. 1. International Brain Research Organization Monograph Series. New York: Raven Press, 1975.

Brooks, C. M., and Peck, M. E. Effects of various cortical lesions on development of placing and hopping reactions in rats. *Journal of Neurophysiology*, 1940, *3*, 66–73.

Brunner, R. L., and Altman, J. The effects of interference with the maturation of the cerebellum and hippocampus on the development of adult behavior. In D. G. Stein, J. J. Rosen, and N. Butters (Eds.), *Plasticity and recovery of function in the central nervous system*. New York: Academic Press, 1974.

Doty, R. W. Survival of pattern vision after removal of striate cortex in the adult cat. *Journal of Comparative Neurology*, 1971, *33*, 93–02.

Flourens, P. Recherches expérimentals sur les propriétés et les fonctions du système nerveux dans les animaux vertèbres. Paris: Chez Crevot, 1824. Translated by G. von Bonin (Ed.), *The cerebral cortex*. Springfield: Charles C Thomas, 1960.

Gittis, A., and Hothersall, D. DRL performance of juvenile rats with septal lesions. *Physiological Psychology*, 1974, *2*, 38–42.

Goldberger, M. E. Recovery of movement after CNS lesions in monkeys. In D. G. Stein, J. J. Rosen, and N. Butters (Eds.), *Plasticity and recovery of function in the central nervous system.* New York: Academic Press, 1974.

Goldman, P. S. Functional development of the prefrontal cortex in early life and the problem of neuronal plasticity. *Experimental Neurology, 1971, 32,* 366–387.

Goldman, P. S. Developmental determinants of cortical plasticity. *Acta Neurobiologica,* 1972, *32,* 495–511.

Goldman, P. S. An alternative to developmental plasticity: Heterology of CNS structures in infants and adults. In D. G. Stein, J. J. Rosen, and N. Butters (Eds.), *Plasticity and recovery of function in the central nervous system.* New York: Academic Press, 1974.

Goldman, P. S., Rosvold, E. H., and Mishkin, M. Evidence for behavioral impairment following prefrontal lobectomy in the infant monkey. *Journal of Comparative and Physiological Psychology,* 1970, *70,* 454–463.

Green, P. C., and Kling, A. Effect of amygdalectomy on affective behavior in juvenile and adult macaque monkeys. *Proceedings of the 75th Annual Convention of the American Psychological Association,* 1966, 93–94.

Harlow, H. F., Blumquist, A. J., Thompson, C. I., Schiltz, K. A., and Harlow, M. K. Effects of induction-age and size of frontal lobe lesions on learning in rhesus monkeys. In R. L. Isaacson (Ed.), *The Neuropsychology of Development: A Symposium,* New York: John Wiley and Sons, 1968.

Isaacson, R., Nonneman, J., and Schmaltz, L. W. Behavioral and anatomical sequelae of damage to the infant limbic system. In R. L. Isaacson (Ed.), *The neuropsychology of development: A symposium,* New York: John Wiley and Sons, 1968.

Johnson, D. A. Developmental aspects of recovery of function following septal lesions in the infant rat. *Journal of Comparative and Physiological Psychology,* 1972, *78,* 331–348.

Johnson, D. A., and Becker, T. M. Development of open-field activity in the rat following caudate lesions in infancy. *Bulletin of the Psychonomic Society,* 1973, *1,* 331–332.

Johnson, D. A., Bieliauskas, L., and Lancaster, J. DRL training and performance following anterior, posterior, or complete septal lesions in infant rats. *Physiology and Behavior,* 1973, *11,* 661–669.

Jonason, K. R., and Enloe, L. J. Alterations in social behavior following septal lesions and amygdaloid lesions in the rat. *Journal of Comparative and Physiological Psychology,* 1971, *75,* 286–301.

Kennard, M. A. Age and other factors in motor recovery from precentral lesions in monkeys. *American Journal of Physiology,* 1936, *115,* 138–146.

Kennard, M. A. Reorganization of motor function in the cerebral cortex of monkeys deprived of motor and premotor areas in infancy. *Journal of Neurophysiology,* 1938, *1,* 477–497.

Kennard, M. A. Relation of age to motor impairment in man and in subhuman primates. *Archives of Neurology and Psychiatry,* 1940, *44,* 377–397.

Kennard, M. A. Cortical reorganization of motor function. Studies on series of monkeys of various ages from infancy to maturity. *Archives of Neurology and Psychiatry,* 1942, *48,* 227–240.

Kling, A. Amygdalectomy in the kitten. *Science,* 1962, *137,* 429–430.

Kling, A. Behavioral and somatic development following lesions of the amygdala in the cat. *Journal of Psychiatric Research,* 1965, *3,* 263–273.

Kling, A., and Tucker, T. J. Effects of combined lesions of frontal granular cortex and caudate nucleus in the neonatal monkey. *Brain Research,* 1967, *6,* 428–439.

Klüver, H., and Bucy, P. C. Preliminary analysis of functions of the temperal lobes in monkeys. *Archives of Neurological Psychiatry,* 1939, *42,* 979–1000.

Kolb, B., and Nonneman, A. J. Functional development of prefrontal cortex in rats continues into adolescence. *Science,* 1976, *193,* 335–336.

Lashley, K. S. *Brain mechanisms and intelligence.* Chicago: University of Chicago Press, 1929.

LeVere, T. E. Neural stability, sparing, and behavioral recovery following brain damage. *Psychological Review,* 1975, *82,* 344–358.

Lynch, G., and Cotman, C. The hippocampus as a model for studying anatomical plasticity of the adult brain. In R. Isaacson and K. Pribram (Eds.), *The Hippocampus,* Vol. I. New York: Plenum Press, 1975.

McMullen, N. T., and Almli, C. R. Longterm hyperdipsia following septal destruction in infant rats. Paper presented at the Psychonomic Society, Denver, 1975.

Raisman, G., and Field, P. M. A quantitative investigation of the development of collateral reinnervation after partial deafferentiation of the septal nuclei. *Brain Research,* 1973, *50,* 241–264.

Relkin, R. Absence of alteration in puberal onset in male rats following amygdaloid lesioning. *Endocrinology,* 1971, *88,* 1272–1274.

Schneider, G. E. Early lesions of superior colliculus: Factors affecting the formation of abnormal retinal projections. *Brain, Behavior and Evolution,* 1973, *8,* 73–109.

Schoenfeld, T. A., Hamilton, L. W., and Gandelman, R. Septal damage during the maturation of inhibitory responding: Effects in juvenile and adult rats. *Developmental Psychobiology,* 1974, *7,* 195–205.

Soltmann, O. Experimentelle Studien über die Functionen des Grosshirne der Neugeborenen. *J b. F. Kinderheilk. (n. F.),* 1876, *9,* 106–148.

Stein, D. G., Rosen, J. J., and Butters, N. (Eds.). *Plasticity and recovery of function in the central nervous system.* New York: Academic Press, 1974.

Stelzner, D. J., Ershler, W. B., and Weber, E. D. Effects of spinal transection in neonatal and weanling rats: Survival of function. *Experimental Neurology,* 1975, *46,* 156–177.

Thompson, C. I., Schwartzbaum, J. S., and Harlow, H. F. Development of social fear after amygdalectomy in infant rhesus monkeys. *Physiology and Behavior,* 1969, *4,* 249–254.

Tsang, Y. C. Maze learning in rats hemidecorticated in infancy. *Journal of Comparative Psychology,* 1937, *24,* 221–254.

Vernadakis, A., and Weiner, N. (Eds.), *Drugs and the developing brain.* Vol. 8, *Advances in behavioral Biology.* New York: Plenum Press, 1974.

Wetzel, A. B., Thompson, V. E., Horel, J. A., and Meyer, P. M. Some consequences of perinatal lesions of the visual cortex in the cat. *Psychonomic Science,* 1965, *3,* 381–382.

7

Lesion Momentum and Behavior

STANLEY FINGER

1. CLINICAL OBSERVATIONS

In 1836 Marc Dax wrote a short manuscript in which he specifically associated aphasia with lesions of the left cerebral hemisphere. His paper was intended for presentation at a regional medical congress at Montpellier (Joynt and Benton, 1964). There is no evidence, however, that Dax actually attended the conference (Broca himself made personal inquiries), and it was not until 1865 that the manuscript was published by his son, Gustav Dax, also a physician. By this time Marc Dax had been dead for 28 years and Broca's key papers (1861, 1863, 1865) already had been published.

The Dax memoir, translated into English by Joynt and Benton (1964), begins with six specific examples of loss of "memory for words" but not of "memory for things" after left hemispheric damage. These observations were made between 1800 and 1814 and Dax states that between then and 1836:

> I have continued to collect similar observations, more than forty in number at the present time, without encountering a single exception during this long period of time. Even if some exceptions should appear in the future they would not invalidate the rule as they would be small in number. . . . A true exception, which I have not seen as yet, would be an impairment of memory for words resulting from a disease that was confined to the right hemisphere (p. 852).

STANLEY FINGER • Department of Psychology, Washington University, St. Louis, Missouri 63130

In the very same paragraph the following sentence also appears:

> I would not even regard as an exception a disease of the left hemisphere
> without an alteration of speech, particularly if the disease were slight *or if it*
> *had developed slowly* (p. 852). (Italics added.)

Thus, Dax probably preceded Broca in associating speech disturbances with left hemispheric lesions, although his specific thoughts concerning cerebral dominance for language were not made public until a
later date (1865; see also G. Dax, 1865). Of importance for the present
thesis, however, is the fact that Dax made reference to the distinct possibility that slow-growing lesions may have less deleterious effects on
behavior than lesions with rapid onset. Further, this possibility is stated
in such a way that one is inclined to suspect that by the 1830s this phenomenon was already a widely accepted fact of clinical medicine.

More than 100 years later, Riese (1950) opened one of the last
chapters in his *Principles of Neurology* with the following remark:

> The time a lesion needs for originating, growing and spreading, is an
> essential element in cerebral localization. Sudden changes such as traumata,
> vascular accidents, etc., are most likely to produce symptoms, although
> sometimes only temporary ones. . . . this chronological factor has not been
> given the full credit it deserves in our attempts to correlate lesions with
> symptoms, though as early as 1761 Morgagni mentioned brain lesions of
> slow onset not associated with paralysis, and though in 1841 Hall made the
> statement that tumors of the brain "when developed slowly," may exist with
> scarcely any symptom (p. 138).

The term "momentum of lesions," which is sometimes used to
describe phenomena such as these, can be traced to Jackson (1879). He
frequently used *mv* (mass × velocity) to refer to it (see Joynt, 1970).
Jackson (1879, 1894) asserted that the rapidity of growth of a lesion
must be considered when attempting to understand symptomatology.
He noted that deficits resulting from sudden hemorrhages usually were
more striking than those due to slowly developing softenings of the
brain. He also observed, however, that symptoms tended to be more
permanent when they eventually emerged in slow-growing cases.

Von Monakow, Jackson's contemporary who is best known for his
doctrine of diaschisis (neural shock), also had a more than passing interest in cases of brain damage without noticeable symptoms. In 1897
he suggested that intracerebral hemorrhage without coma was possible
provided that bleeding was slow, and in 1914 he reemphasized the position that aphasia may be absent with slowly growing tumors in Broca's
area. As pointed out by Riese (1950), the majority of the "negative"
cases (brain damage without symptoms) that von Monakow collected

from the literature and his own material involved slowly growing tumors.

In the second quarter of the present century Head (1926) stated:

> . . . in all attempts to correlate the site of structural changes with defects of functions it must never be forgotten that the severity and acuteness of the lesion exert an overwhelming effect on the manifestations (p. 441).

Similar words were reechoed by Riese (1948) in his case studies on neurological patients with similarly localized lesions differing in speed of development:

> Sudden lesions, i.e., those of greatest momentum, are most likely to produce aphasia, though only transitory in uncomplicated cases. In lesions of slow momentum, speech may be preserved either throughout the whole history, or, at least, for a long time (p. 75).

Hence, some effects of lesion momentum are long-recognized clinical phenomena. Furthermore, the rate of lesion development is one of a number of factors which can be invoked to account for intersubject variability on a wide variety of neurological and behavioral tests designed to identify and localize brain damage. Nevertheless, in part because the principle is very difficult to assess under controlled conditions with human patient populations, it is discussed in minimal detail and is rarely referenced in most current textbooks and clinical monographs.

2. ANIMAL MODELS

The fact that behavioral scientists can perform experiments on laboratory animals such as rats, cats, and monkeys permits the assessment of lesion-momentum phenomena in controlled settings. Unlike clinical neurologists, however, laboratory researchers have been more concerned with bilateral damage in a given cortical or subcortical area than with the spread of a lesion to adjacent loci on the same side of the brain. In addition, while clinical patients typically have penetrating brain wounds, strokes, or tumors, laboratory animals generally are subjected to limited aspirative ablations or electrolytic lesions aimed for well-defined target zones that can be verified histologically immediately after testing. Nevertheless, there is reason to believe that the animal studies will lead to greater clarification and increased understanding of the effects displayed by the patient population. One line of thought is that "serial-lesion" findings with animals (preparations with multiple successive lesions; Finger, Walbran, and Stein, 1973) and human case reports of "momentum of lesion" are reflecting identical processes.

Two paradigms are basic to the animal-research literature on fast-

and slow-growing lesions, and in their simplest form (two-stage lesions) these designs are illustrated in Figure 7-1. In the first case (Row 1), a unilateral lesion is made in the first of two serial surgeries. As can be seen, the homologous area on the opposite side of the midline is subjected to an identical lesion at a later time. Alternatively, as is shown at the bottom of the figure (Row 5), the experimenter can make incomplete bilateral lesions which can be enlarged in the serial preparation. In either paradigm, the performance scores of animals with serial

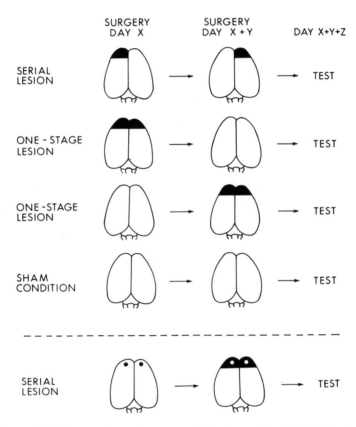

Figure 7-1.   The basic paradigms for many serial-lesion studies. Each design includes a group with sequential unilateral lesions, a group without ablations, and two groups with one-stage bilateral lesions; one matched in time to the first operation sustained by the serial group, and the other matched to that group's second operation. Modifications of this design may include elimination of the latter group (see text), the addition of lesion "control" groups, and preoperative and/or interoperative testing for some or all of the animals in each group. The time period between the lesions is usually referred to as the interlesion interval (ILI).

lesions can be compared to those of subjects with anatomically matched lesions produced in a single operation (Rows 2 and 3) as well as to animals without insult in this part of the brain (e.g., sham operations: Row 4). When the animals with successive lesions do better than those with simultaneous lesions, it may be designated the "serial-lesion effect" (Finger *et al.*, 1973). This can refer either to faster recovery after a deficit or to no apparent loss (sparing) in the serial preparation.

The large majority of experimenters who have explored serial-lesion effects have chosen the sequential unilateral lesion design (Row 1), although the bilateral lesion paradigm has been utilized in a few instances (Barbas and Spear, 1976; Finger, Marshak, Cohen, Scheff, Trace, and Neimand, 1971; Treichler, 1975). In addition, more complex designs derived from these two basic paradigms have been described (see review by Stein and Lewis, 1975). In one such study, Rosen, Stein, and Butters (1971) subjected monkeys to four surgeries spaced 3 weeks apart. Each operation involved removal of one bank of sulcus principalis (e.g., left hemisphere, lower bank), and on each succeeding operation the hemisphere and bank were changed (e.g., operation 2: right hemisphere, upper bank). They reported that monkeys with serial lesions made significantly fewer errors on a battery of spatial discriminations than did one-stage animals. This was the case in spite of the complication that the four surgical entries resulted in adhesions and unexpectedly larger lesions in the multistage lesion group.

One problem confronting experimenters doing this type of research is that of equating the postoperative recovery periods for the various lesion groups. Take as representative a study in which the two-stage animals experience successive unilateral lesions spaced 30 days apart, with testing on a discrimination problem starting 20 days after the last surgery. If the one-stage animals also have a 20-day postoperative recovery period, it can be claimed that the serial subjects are at a distinct advantage since one side of the brain in that group has 30 additional days for recovery. In contrast, if the one-stage animals are given 50 days for recovery, this being equal to recovery time from the first lesion of the two-stage animals, the one-stage subjects will have the advantage since the two-stage group will have some target tissue damaged with considerably less time for recovery. This confounding is particularly troublesome in studies in which the interlesion interval is very long while the recovery from the second operation is short and in experiments in which lesion effects are short lived.

When laboratory animals cannot be examined repeatedly over time, a strong case for less severe impairments with multistage lesions can be made if the experimenter measures the recovery period for the one-stage animals from the time of the first surgery in the two-stage condition. In this instance if the multistage animals still perform better than the one-stage animals, the power of the effect can be emphasized since, if anything, the bias is in favor of the opposite result.

Alternatively, the experimenter might choose to have some one-stage animals operated upon when the serial subjects have their first surgery and other one-stage animals operated upon when the serial subjects have their second surgery (see Figure 1). In this case the serial-lesion effect can be evaluated in the light of the significance of the post-operative recovery period for the one-stage animals if all of the groups begin testing at the same time. Furthermore, by subjecting the one-stage animals to sham operations at the time of the other surgery of the two-stage squad, anesthetic and drug effects can be equalized among the lesion groups.

Scanning the serial-lesion literature will reveal that experimenters typically have used only a single one-stage lesion group in their serial-lesion studies and that the designs are approximately equally split in terms of whether the one-stage subjects were operated upon at the time of the first or the second surgery of the serial animals. Nevertheless, the one-stage animals were not found to be better than the serial animals in any of these investigations, and in all but a handful of cases, in which all lesion groups performed poorly, the serial subjects performed better than the one-stage animals on the tasks. These data, and findings in experiments with two or more one-stage lesion groups, argue strongly against the notion that staged-lesion phenomena typically reflect temporal artifacts, although one cannot dismiss the possibility that differential recovery periods may have affected the findings in some of the experiments surveyed.

In this context it might be pointed out that the first serial-lesion study from this laboratory was one in which the one-stage animals had recovery periods timed from the second surgery of the two-stage rats (Finger, *et al.*, 1971). The multistage animals performed much better than the single-stage rats and resembled control animals in this experiment. When it was realized that the two-stage operates had 65 days to recover from their first surgery, while the one-stage operates had 30 days to recover from their only surgery, additional groups of one-stage animals were tested (Finger and Reyes, 1975). Some of the new rats were given months and some were given years to recover from one-stage somatosensory cortex lesions. In no instance, however, did any of the one-stage groups perform well on the series of two-choice tactile discriminations. Thus, in this case at least, the differential recovery times that were given to the one-stage and two-stage animals did not underlie the serial-lesion effect that appeared in a paradigm that might have favored the two-stage subjects (see also discussion by Spear and Barbas, 1975).

3. THE RANGE OF SERIAL-LESION EFFECTS

In the nineteenth century many researchers (e.g., Flourens, 1824) who had been investigating the effects of extensive brain lesions on animals found that survival of their subjects depended on the use of serial-lesion techniques. That is, large bilateral lesions made in one operation were found to be associated with lower survival rates than equivalent-sized lesions produced more slowly over time.

In the present century, Lashley (1929) also performed staged ablations, but only when more than 50% of the neocortex was to be extirpated. Since his rats with smaller lesions received one-stage extirpations, the details of some of his frequently cited behavioral findings (i.e., the slopes of graphs relating lesion size and performance) may reflect in varying degrees this methodological confounding. Kleitman and Camille (1932), in their experiments on sleep and wakefulness in dogs, also relied on staged extirpations of the cortex because of the high mortality rate that was associated with decortication in a single operation.

Perhaps the most striking example of mortality differences with fast- and slow-growing lesions is described in an experiment primarily involving the reticular formation (Adametz, 1959). In this investigation some 80 adult cats were subjected to extensive mesial tegmental lesions of the rostral midbrain. When large bilateral lesions were made in one operation, the inevitable result was coma and, with one exception, death, in spite of tube feeding, antibiotics, and special care to maximize survival. These same lesions placed in two or more sittings spaced 1–2 weeks apart resulted in wakefulness shortly after each operation. Furthermore, motor functions such as standing and walking and other behaviors such as self-feeding and grooming returned relatively rapidly to the serial cats:

> After the 2nd operation the animals again were able to eat unaided upon the 1st postoperative day, despite the fact that they now had an aggregate of lesions approximating those described above for the 1-stage comatose animals. From that time on their recovery progressed somewhat more slowly, but beyond comparison with the recovery rate of any animal in which bilateral lesions had been made at one sitting. Two months postoperatively several of these animals nearly approached normal except for movements upon horizontal ladders. Their inadequate placing reactions made them somewhat unsteady. They pursued mice, could jump a distance of several

feet, and groomed themselves regularly. All were alert and constantly interested in their surroundings. At no time after the first few days was a significant disturbance of the normal sleep–waking cycle observed: the animals
slept at night and remained awake much of the day (Adametz, 1959,
pp. 88–89).

Results such as these have been confirmed in related experiments
(e.g., Kesner, Fiedler, and Thomas, 1967; Lourie, Vanasupa, and
O'Leary, 1960) and constitute one aspect of the serial-lesion literature.
Experiments involving locomotion and motor abilities and those utilizing sensory learning paradigms represent other areas in which equally
dramatic effects have been reported.

Prior to a report by Travis and Woolsey (1956), it had been believed that bilateral removal of Brodmann areas 4 and 6 in adult monkeys inevitably led to a permanent loss of all useful motor function.
These animals could not walk, stand, or even right themselves as a
result of the muscular contractures that resulted from the lesions.

The monkeys in the Travis and Woolsey (1956) study underwent a
variety of sequential motor cortex ablations spaced over a number of
months. The adult animals that experienced these gradual lesions
never lost the ability to right themselves, walk, or feed, although constant care and special attention had to be given to some of them immediately after the ablations. Two of the monkeys then were subjected to
additional lesions which rendered them totally decorticate. One of
these animals showed "a remarkable preservation of motor abilities,"
and could sit up, right itself, and walk shortly after all of the surgeries
had been completed. Hopping and grasping reflexes also remained intact. The other monkey, while still exhibiting motor abilities far exceeding those previously reported for decorticate monkeys, was able to walk
with assistance, although it was less impressive than the first subject in
its retained abilities.

In contrast to this work, early evidence that serial lesions might be
less disruptive than one-stage lesions on a perceptual task resulted
somewhat by accident. Ades (1946) planned to ablate Brodmann areas
18 and 19 bilaterally in a group of monkeys in a single operation with
the hope of assessing the functions of the parastriate cortex. However, the condition of one of his animals necessitated the termination of
surgery after a unilateral lesion. Following a short recovery period this
monkey was retested, and the preoperatively acquired size, shape, and
color discriminations were found to be perfectly retained. Following a
second operation 18 days after the first, the habits still remained intact.
In contrast, the one-stage animals exhibited poor retention on all of the
discriminations.

Ades and Raab (1949) later reported a comparable finding when

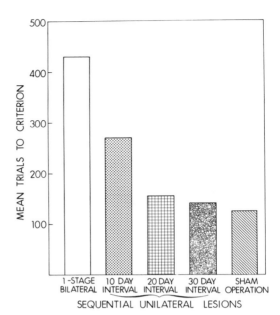

Figure 7-3. Performance of rats with simultaneous or sequential lesions of the frontal cortex or sham operations on a spatial-alternation problem (after Patrissi and Stein, 1975).

4.3. Ordering of the Lesions

There are related data which indicate that the ordering and configuration of damage produced in each operation may also be of some importance under certain conditions. Isseroff, Leveton, Freeman, Lewis, and Stein (1976) subjected rats to bilateral hippocampal lesions in stages. Some animals first had unilateral, dorsal–ventral hippocampal damage and then were given a matched lesion on the other side some 4 weeks later. Other rats had nonhomologous bilateral lesions of the dorsal or ventral hippocampi in the first operation, and remaining target tissue in each hemisphere was electrocoagulated after an equivalent recovery period. The results of this experiment showed that the ordering of surgery played an important role in recovery of a series of spatial-reversal tasks. Thus, even though there was extensive bilateral damage, recovery was dependent not as much on the amount of tissue removed as on the order in which hippocampal areas were damaged.

Barbas and Spear (1976), in contrast, could not find any differences which could be attributed to medial and then lateral versus lateral and then medial bilateral lesions of the visual cortex in rats. In their experiment these and other animals with serial lesions were examined on a preoperatively learned brightness discrimination. The one-stage animals had more difficulty relearning this problem than any of the lesion groups with successive unilateral or enlarged bilateral ablations. An informative discussion on how topographical organization within a target area could affect the results of an experiment on the ordering and configuration of serial lesions is provided by Barbas and Spear in their paper.

4.4. Interoperative Testing and Training

The role of interoperative testing appears to be important under some conditions, as has been discussed (see also Finger *et al.,* 1973). However, because one-stage animals and other two-stage animals rarely are given an equivalent amount of additional training, the significance of *interoperative* training (as opposed to *any* additional training) is not as clear as it sometimes is made out to be.

Glendenning (1972) is one of the few experimenters who has controlled for general "overtraining" effects. He demonstrated that interoperative training can be a significant determinant of behavior on a two-choice discrimination task after visual cortex lesions in rats. A recent experiment from the present author's laboratory, however, showed that formal interoperative training is not needed for good retention of a two-choice tactile discrimination after serial somatosensory cortical lesions in rats (Finger and Simons, 1976).

4.5. Environmental and Pharmacological Effects

The importance of the nature of the environment during the interlesion interval was first demonstrated by Meyer *et al.* (1958). In this study rats were subjected to sequential lesions of the visual cortex after they had learned a conditioned avoidance response to light onset. Some of the animals spent the 12-day interlesion interval in light, and the remaining rats were kept in the dark. It was found that the serial procedure was effective in sparing the habit when the animals were kept in the lighted environment, but that this was not the case when the rats were kept in the dark. These findings are summarized in Figure 7-4.

It is now known that stimulation in the auditory modality may compensate for the absence of visual stimulation in experiments such as the one conducted by Meyer and his colleagues. Isaac (1964), for example, reported that while retention of a visual-avoidance response is maximal with noise and light during the interlesion interval, noise

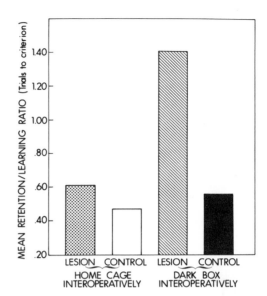

Figure 7-4. Performance of rats with serial lesions of the visual cortex or sham operations on a brightness-avoidance problem. Some animals were kept in darkness and others were kept in their home cages (light/dark) between surgeries (after Meyer *et al.*, 1958).

alone would facilitate performance above the level exhibited by animals kept in both dark and quiet conditions.

Issac's work (1964) suggests that nonspecific stimulation could also prevent the loss of a visual habit in animals kept in the dark condition. Experiments with stimulant drugs have lent some credence to this idea. In one such study, Cole *et al.* (1967) added small amounts of *d*-amphetamine or phenobarbital sodium to the drinking water of groups of rats between successive unilateral visual cortex ablations. Two groups showed good retention: those permitted light and noise but no drugs, and those kept in the dark and quiet environment but given amphetamine. Retention was impaired in the two remaining groups: rats kept in the dark and quiet condition without drugs, and animals housed with light and noise but given phenobarbital.

Isaac has postulated that these effects could be accounted for on the basis of the activity of the reticular formation. Whether his theory is correct or not, these experiments show that both environmental and pharmacological manipulations can affect performance in the serial-lesion paradigm.

4.6. Postoperative Recovery Period

The postoperative recovery interval has already been discussed in the context of the difficulties involved in matching one-stage and multistage animals in terms of recovery time. Surprisingly, the effects of giving serially operated animals different postoperative recovery periods has received little attention. In our laboratory, Reyes (1977) has examined the effects of sequential unilateral lesions of the somatosensory cortex in rats given one of three postoperative recovery intervals (7, 21, 49 days) and one of three interlesion intervals (7, 21, 49 days). His acquisition data indicate that recovery is best when a long recovery period is combined with a long interlesion interval. The 49-day postoperative recovery period did not seem to benefit animals with very short interlesion intervals, and, conversely, functional recovery was somewhat precluded when a short recovery period followed the 49-day interoperative period. These results are consistent with those presented in an earlier report (Finger *et al.*, 1971).

4.7. Age at Time of Surgery

In 1973, when serial-lesion experiments were last reviewed, it was stated that with the exception of some early observations by Kennard (1942), published reports on the significance of age at the time of surgery had not appeared in the serial-lesion literature.

Two recent reports now show that age can be an extremely important variable in staged-lesion studies. In the first case (Stein and Firl, 1976), serial or one-stage frontal cortex ablations were made in young mature laboratory rats and in animals that were approximately 2 years old. These lesions were spaced 30 or more days apart and recovery periods were equated among the groups. As expected, young adult animals with serial lesions showed sparing of function on a delayed spatial-alternation task, while those with one-stage lesions performed poorly. In contrast, both one-stage and two-stage old rats showed no impairments in comparisons with aged-matched control animals on the same problem when surgery was performed late in life, although they were disrupted on an active-avoidance problem.

Somewhat different findings were reported in an acquisition study dealing with lesions of the somatosensory cortex in prepubescent, mature, and old rats (Walbran, 1976). In this case the middle group showed a serial-lesion effect on the first of two tactile tasks, but both the 30-day-old operates and the old animals performed poorly regardless of whether the lesions were made in one or in two operations. These data strongly suggest that at least some serial-lesion effects may be age dependent.

4.8. Task Difficulty

Task difficulty is another variable that has received little systematic attention in the serial-lesion literature and one which could also account for the negative findings obtained in some experiments (e.g., Isaacson and Schmaltz, 1968).

Two recent studies from this laboratory have examined this factor in detail. Each experiment assessed retention of a tactile discrimination after large lesions of the somatosensory cortex in rats. The methods, the lesions, and the experimental designs were the same, but in one case the tactile problem was one which took naive rats more than 40 days to master (Simons, Puretz, and Finger, 1975), while in the other case most naive animals were able to meet criterion within 15 days (Finger and Simons, 1976).

The serial-lesion effect did not appear on the difficult tactile problem. Both one-stage and two-stage animals showed severe retention deficits on this task and there was no evidence for any one lesion group performing any better than any other lesion group. On the easier problem, the one-stage animals (without overtraining) again were markedly impaired relative to the sham-operated animals. However, in this case the rats with sequential lesions performed better than the animals with one-stage lesions and were statistically indistinguishable from the control group.

Task difficulty, of course, can be manipulated by varying the physical characteristics of the stimuli, as was done above, or by varying the nature and amount of training prior to exposure to the discrimination task in question. The latter possibility can be exemplified by looking at the "difficult" ridge–smooth discrimination used by Simons *et al.* (1975) under two conditions. When Simons *et al.* put rats with somatosensory cortical lesions directly onto this problem, their subjects performed very poorly regardless of whether they had one-stage or two-stage surgery. In contrast, when rats were exposed postoperatively to a series of easier but related tactile discriminations prior to encountering this problem, the operated rats with serial ablations (but not simultaneous lesions) were able to master it as rapidly as the sham-operated animals (Finger *et al.*, 1971).

4.9. Cortical versus Subcortical Structures

Serial-lesion effects have been reported at all levels of the central nervous system. Thus, these phenomena do not appear to be limited to the cerebral cortex or limbic system. However, because different questions have been asked with lesions placed at different levels, it is not possible to state with any certainty that the type of sparing seen at one level of the nervous system would be seen in other places as well. For example, acquisition and retention paradigms with specific sensory stimuli have been used in the large majority of cortical ablation studies but appear in very few experiments assessing the effects of subcortical lesions (e.g., Reyes *et al.*, 1973). Thus, although eating, drinking, and sleeping may be spared with some subcortical serial lesions, it is not known whether perceptual-learning effects like those found at the level of the cortex would appear with thalamic or tectal lesions.

4.10. Species Differences

While the factors necessary for obtaining a serial-lesion effect in one species may eventually be found to differ from the conditions that must be met for an analogous effect to be demonstrated in another species, there is no evidence to support the position that these effects are strictly limited to some mammals and not to others. If anything, the data currently available strongly indicate that a general rule is involved, although interspecies differences might be expected to appear on selected functions (e.g., mating behavior after olfactory system lesions; Macrides, Firl, Schneider, Bartke, and Stein, 1976; Rowe and Smith, 1973; Winans and Powers, 1974). Evidence that the speed of lesion development is important in man already has been discussed (e.g., Riese, 1948). In addition, as has been mentioned, numerous studies on laboratory animals have demonstrated serial-lesion effects in one form or another. These studies have been conducted on rodents such as mice and rats, on carnivores including cats and dogs, and on primates.

5. NEURAL BASIS OF SPARING AND RECOVERY

Little is known about the neural bases of functional recovery in man and animals, and although there has been considerable debate on the relevant issues (cf. Laurence and Stein, this volume), there now seems to be a slight trend in the serial-lesion literature away from arguing for one of many theories and toward presenting alternative models or even hedging on the issue entirely.

A number of reasons can be advanced to explain the paucity of material that deals directly with the mechanisms underlying these effects. For example, one key factor would have to be that neurophysiologists and neuroanatomists have rarely been involved with these preparations. In addition, there is a belief among some investigators that the mechanisms underlying sparing and recovery of function cannot be approached adequately until the specific and unique contributions of particular structures can be ascertained. A third limiting factor may be that most behavioral tests used in serial-lesion experiments permit the use of a wide variety of maneuvers and strategies. In short, most dependent measures may not have the sensitivity required to detect subtle changes in behavior that might help to differentiate among the possible neural models.

Notwithstanding these criticisms, some of the major theories that have been put forth to account for differences between fast- and slow-growing lesion effects deserve mention. One frequently cited hypothesis holds that large, acute lesions result in greater and more prolonged neural and/or general shock than multiple small lesions distributed over time (cf. Lewis and Lancione, 1976). On the basis of this schema, recovery and sparing would represent the diminution of shock in parts of the system that were not destroyed by the lesion. Riese (1948), for example, wrote that:

> According to this author's experiences (1947) signs of neural shock cannot only be seen in such sudden lesions as brain injuries or apopletic insults, but also in rapidly growing brain tumors, whereas they are absent in slowly growing neoplasms involving the same regions . . . Thus, the doctrine of neural shock has its far reaching practical implications, since a number of so-called negative cases of cerebral localization (frequently misleading the physician), can be explained in a satisfactory manner, by the time factor implied in Diaschisis (p. 66).

And the high survival rates of cats with multiple-stage lesions of the reticular formation was explained in this way by Adametz (1959):

> While presumably destruction of the reticular activating system is a primary factor in the production of coma by mesial tegmental lesions, other considerations have importance also. The experiments herein establish a shock factor (diaschisis), more enduring in the instance of bilateral lesions produced in 1 sitting than in corresponding lesions produced in 2 stages (p. 95).

Evidence that tissue surrounding small cortical lesions may suffer temporary loss of function immediately after surgery is best seen in a behavioral and electrophysiological investigation involving multiple small lesions of the cat's sensorimotor cortex (Glassman, 1971; see also Kempinsky, 1958). One might postulate that because of differential shock effects animals with staged lesions may make better use of spared fragments of target tissue than subjects with one-stage lesions. In addition, shock and metabolic theories might also be considered in those cases in which both one-stage and multistage subjects show some recovery relatively soon after surgery, and perhaps in some instances in which performance deficits appear to reflect impaired "access to engrams" (cf. Meyer, 1972).

Nevertheless, the phenomena of neural and general shock are not easily evaluated, and few if any investigators would claim that these factors could account for all short- and long-lived staged-lesion effects. Blatt and Lyon (1968), for example, specifically argued against surgical trauma as a major variable when they evaluated the effects of simultaneous or successive mesencephalic lesions on feeding behavior. Their position was based primarily upon the fact that asymmetrical "control" lesions and large unilateral lesions produced minimal disruption relative to smaller, bilaterally symmetrical lesions. The theory also has difficulty in dealing with cases in which "successful" postoperative behaviors do not closely resemble preoperative behaviors. Considerable similarity would be predicted when this "reestablishment" model is employed *in isolation* from other theories since structures that were originally involved with the behavior should again be mediating the function as the shock subsides.

Brain lesions centered in one structure may trigger a state of supersensitivity in associated structures and such changes could represent another potential recovery mechanism (Sharpless, 1964). The "law" of denervation supersensitivity as defined by Cannon and Rosenblueth (1949) holds that:

> When in a functional chain of neurons one of the elements is severed, the ensuing total or partial denervation of some of the subsequent elements in the chain causes a supersensitivity of all of the distal elements, including those not denervated, and effectors if present, to the excitatory or inhibitory action of chemical agents and nerve impulses; the supersensitivity is greater for the links which immediately follow the cut neurons and decreases progressively for more distal elements (p. 186).

Thus, fragments and elements which may have played a minimal role in mediating certain behaviors prior to damage may acquire the sensitivity necessary to do this after a lesion. Cannon and Rosenblueth (1949) hypothesized that such connections, once used, could be maintained after the supersensitivity subsides, and that denervation supersensitivity could lead not only to the "opening" of preexisting pathways, but to "devious nervous connections" which would not be employed under normal circumstances (see p. 213).

The idea that increased postsynaptic sensitivity could negate decreased presynaptic input is used by both Glick and Zimmerberg (1972) and Walbran (1976) to explain serial-lesion data. One potential criticism of this model, however, is that the supersensitivity might be expected to be most pronounced with lesions of rapid onset; yet animals with slow-growing lesions typically show faster recovery. This issue is critically evaluated in at least one paper (Glick and Zimmerberg, 1972).

The concept of functional reorganization is found throughout the serial-lesion literature (e.g., Bekoff, Lockwood, and Meikle, 1973; Dru, Walker, and Walker, 1975; Greene, Stauff and Walters, 1972; Meyer *et al.*, 1958; Stein *et al.*, 1969), although mechanisms such as supersensitivity are rarely specified and although it is not always clear whether "functional reorganization" is meant to imply functional switching within established circuitry, dynamic changes in anatomy, or something else. In fact, it is not always claimed that "recovered" and unoperated animals are identical (cf. Stein and Lewis, 1975). In general, the point is only that tissue spared after the first of multiple surgeries serves as a stimulus or template for change.

Ades and Raab (1946) first argued for what they called "some undetermined sort of reorganization" on the basis of additional lesions made after apparent recovery from serial lesions. Their additional lesions were placed in loci where ablations had no discernable effects on the task, given that the rest of the cortex was intact. Animals, that "recovered" from serial lesions, however, showed marked deficits when subjected to this additional surgery (see also Ades and Raab, 1949; Finger and Simons, 1976; Simons, *et al.*, 1975).

Another case for reorganization of function comes from an experiment by Scheff and Wright (1977) in which only rats that "recovered" from serial lesions of the visual cortex exhibited visual evoked potentials in adjacent cortex. On logical grounds neither this experiment nor that of Ades and Raab (1946) can be considered hard evidence for anatomical change or for one structure taking over another's function (see Dawson, 1973; LeVere, 1975). Nevertheless, it is not difficult to imagine how the potential for functional reorganization could differ with fast and slow-growing lesions. Jackson's (1881) analogy to governmental function in his treatise on postepileptic conditions bears on this issue, although it could relate to cue and strategy-selection models (see below) as well:

> Were the highest governing people in this country suddenly destroyed, we should have to lament the loss of their offices. . . . We should also have to lament the now permitted anarchy of the now ungoverned people consequent on that loss . . . But . . . if, in this country, the highest governing peoples were slowly removed . . . the rest of the country would not be, or would be only slightly anarchial [*sic*]. The lower governing bodies would, being then highest, gradually become efficient substitutes for general purposes. (pp. 399–400)

The search for mechanisms which might underlie reorganization of function may have been slowed by the strong belief that changes other than perhaps increased synaptic contracts would not be found in the mature mammalian nervous system. This type of thinking now has been tempered by a rapidly growing number of recent experiments on new connections ("sprouts") which may appear after brain damage (e.g., Goodman and Horel, 1966; Raisman, 1969). Moore and his colleagues (e.g., Moore, Björklund, and Stenevi, 1971), for example, have stated that axonal sprouting is observable within a period of days after surgery and that these new connections can be physiologically active. As regards one-stage and serial lesions, one thought is that target tissue spared after the first surgery may serve as an added stimulus for sprouting, or that greater shock resulting from simultaneous bilateral lesions could suppress the formation of new connections more effectively than would the slower-growing lesions.

Many questions remain unanswered with regard to sprouting, especially as it relates to behavior. This, of course, is understandable given the recent emergence of these findings and the fact that few anatomists have attempted to assess behavioral correlates of these changes (cf. Kerr, 1975). Among the possibilities that still must be considered are (1) the chance that these new aberrant connections may introduce "noise" into the system (Raisman, 1969); (2) the possibility that responses diametrically opposed to those which were lost might emerge, these maladaptive behaviors being both specific and stable (see Schneider, 1970); and (3) the idea that these new connections generally have a limited distribution and may even prevent the original pathways from reestablishing themselves by occupying vacated synaptic sites. In addition, the fact that the sprouting literature is essentially (but not entirely) a rodent literature with relatively young subjects has bothered some investigators, especially in the face of Wall and Egger's (1971) warning that the rat is "an animal which continues to grow throughout adult life perhaps therefore retaining certain embryological characteristics" (p. 545).

In the light of the current interest in some of the aforementioned models, it may be sobering to consider the concept of stability in mature biological systems (LeVere, 1975) and the idea that some staged-lesion effects might be due to changes in cue selection and strategy formation. A distinct possibility is that the initial damage causes a partial loss of an important capacity and that as a result of this the subject begins to explore and attend to other relevant cues which may vary concomitantly with those originally selected (see Morgan, 1951). Following additional insult, the subject might still be able to solve the problem, but this time by relying on the *new* cues, whereas animals with more acute lesions may never have learned that these other (somtimes subtle) cues are available in the testing situation. (In that this theory does not require a structure to assume a new, unusual function, it shares at least some common ground with shock theories.)

New strategies and compensatory actions may signify underlying functional deficits even though a problem may be mastered in a short amount of time. Nevertheless, one must consider the possibility that only the hierarchy of preferred responses could have changed as a result of insult and that with a change in conditions it might be possible to demonstrate that nothing is in fact lost. That is, while a subject may still be capable of solving the problem in the same way, it may now choose to do so with a new solution or strategy even though the new approach may not always equal the one used previously in terms of efficiency. If one defines recovery in terms of "goals" rather than by "means to an end" (see discussion by Laurence and Stein, this volume) the question of deficits versus preferences might not seem very important. The issue of whether something is indeed lost, however, must be addressed when recovery is evaluated on the basis of *how* the subject reaches the goal.

When means to a goal are considered, behaviors that appear to be only slightly different from those observed preoperatively can be especially perplexing and difficult to judge. Is recovery really present when one now observes a rat rubbing a tactile stimulus a bit harder than it did before somatosensory cortex surgery, or when a cat switches from a go–no go strategy to a simultaneous-sampling procedure while successfully confronting two visual stimuli at a choice point in a maze? Like an ape who must now use a healthy right paw to guide a deafferented left paw to a food cup, these changes may be demanded by the injury. Notably, in every case the animal would be considered "recovered" if testing had taken place in a black box (goals analysis).

Cue and strategy-selection theories usually are associated with lesion studies in which learning paradigms are used since, as mentioned, different means could be used to pursue the same ends in many such experiments (see Goldberger, 1972). It is more difficult to apply these concepts to studies on sleep and wakefulness, or to specific experiments on eating and drinking (Blatt and Lyon, 1968) and mating behaviors (Rowe and Smith, 1973) after certain lesions. In addition, these models hardly seem applicable to much of the vast clinical literature on aphasias after fast- and slow-growing lesions. Thus, the behavioral-substitution theories may also have limited applicability, although they could be very informative in some situations. This, of course, might mean that many mechanisms working separately or together could underlie the broad spectrum of serial-lesion effects, a possibility that was raised previously (Finger *et al.*, 1973). At the present time one might be

hard pressed to argue against such a notion, although some investigators have postulated that radical reorganizational models might not
be critical to a viable multifaceted formulation (Dawson, 1973; LeVere,
1975).

Although the basis of the serial-lesion effect is obviously both speculative and complex, experiments on seemingly recovered animals with
one-stage and multistage lesions do seem to indicate that the substrates
underlying recovery might not be the same in two instances. One supporting observation is that the two groups of "recovered" animals respond differently to drugs, although it is possible to argue that this
could reflect other things as well (Glick and Zimmerberg, 1972). However, a related observation is that "recovered" one-stage and multistage
subjects also appear to be affected in different ways by additional lesions. Finger and Simons (1976) and Simons et al., (1975) noted this
when lesions of frontal and occipital cortex were made after one-stage
or two-stage lesions of the somatosensory cortex in rats that had just
relearned a tactile task. In both studies the animals that originally had

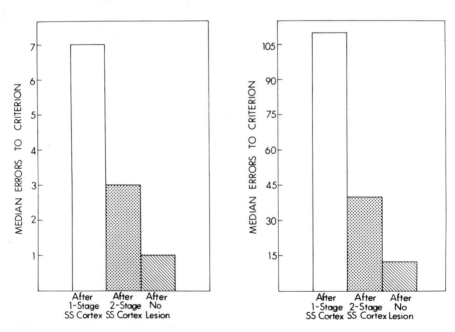

Figure 7-5.   Performance of animals on an easy (graph on left) or a difficult (graph on
right) tactile discrimination following large lesions of the cortex anterior and posterior to
the somatosensory areas. All animals previously had relearned the identical discrimination after (1) one-stage lesions of the somatosensory cortex, (2) two-stage lesions of the
somatosensory cortex, or (3) sham operations (after Finger and Simons, 1976, and
Simons et al., 1976, respectively).

one-stage lesions were more impaired by the additional ablations than were the rats that previously experienced the multistage operations (see, however, Scheff *et al.*, 1977). These data are summarized in Figure 7-5 and at least indirectly argue against identical neural substrates in the two conditions.

6. PRESENT AND FUTURE

Because the experimental investigation of lesion-momentum effects is relatively new, it is difficult to say which studies were most influential in attracting attention to these phenomena. The pioneering efforts of Ades and his co-workers, and the experiments of Travis and Woolsey (1956), Meyer, *et al.*, (1958), and Adametz (1959), however, may be among the most significant in this regard. These studies not only showed the range and complexity of serial-lesion effects, but did so in a manner such that more researchers were persuaded to explore these phenomena in greater detail.

In spite of its short history, the animal-research literature appears to be continuously undergoing change. One noticeable trend may be in the increased sophistication of the investigations. It is also interesting to consider the fact that negative data (no differences between the scores of animals with simultaneous and successive lesions) did not appear in print until relatively recently (e.g., Dawson, *et al.*, 1973; Isaacson and Schmaltz, 1968; LeVere, 1969; LeVere and Weiss, 1973).

The potential for new and significant research on lesion-momentum phenomena is great, and a number of voids are readily apparent in this field. For example, there have been almost no systematic analyses with mechanical compression (Tarlov, 1954), and fast- and slow-growing tumor substances have yet to be used. Both approaches would appear to be more representative of human clinical material than the ablation and electrolytic techniques that are currently employed.

In addition, much still remains to be learned about the conditions that must be met for serial-lesion effects to be observed and about animals that appear to have recovered from one-stage and multistage operations. Subjecting "recovered" animals to additional lesions (Finger and Simons, 1976; Simons *et al.*, 1975; Scheff *et al.*, 1977) and to drugs (Glick and Zimmerberg, 1972) is already proving informative. Cinematographic records of the animals also could be valuable, especially in terms of assessing behavioral strategies and maneuvers after insult (see Gentile, Nieburgs, Schmeltzer, and Stein, 1975).

The greatest need for systematic study has been and continues to be in delineating the anatomical and physiological correlates of these lesion effects. This is best exemplified by the fact that investigators have just started to examine multiple-unit characteristics in tissue adjacent to the lesions (Scheff and Wright, 1977), while attempts to assess single-unit properties in one- and two-stage animals have yet to appear. At the same time very little attention has been devoted to assessing how primary and secondary anatomical effects of rapid- and slow-growing lesions compare to each other or change over time (see Wolf and Di-Cara, 1969). Some behavioral scientists seem willing to assume that the secondary effects are the same in the two instances, but the current absence of published data to the contrary hardly provides strong support for this position. In fact, in a recent abstract some intriguing structural differences between the two preparations have been described (Scheff, Bernardo, Cotman, and Lynch, 1976). An ideal place in which to begin detailed anatomical and physiological analyses of fast- and slow-growing lesion-induced changes might be in a well-defined minisystem, such as the barrel fields of the rat or mouse somatosensory cortex. These regions have been described by Woolsey and van der Loos (1970) and Welker and Woolsey (1974) in recent publications.

Additional empirical research on factors such as these should help to resolve some of the controversy surrounding serial-lesion effects. A theoretical predisposition to view the nervous system as a system and not just as a collection of discrete parts (cf. Benton, 1976) may enhance one's perspective of both old and new findings pertaining to these generally neglected but important phenomena.

ACKNOWLEDGMENT

The preparation of this chapter was supported in part by NINCDS Grant NS-11002.

7. REFERENCES

Adametz, J. H. Rate of recovery of functioning in cats with rostal recticular lesions. *Journal of Neurosurgery*, 1959, *16*, 85–98.

Ades, H. W. Effects of extirpation of parastriate cortex on learned visual discriminations in monkeys. *Journal of Neuropathology and Experimental Neurology*, 1946, *5*, 60–66.

Ades, H. W., and Raab, D. H. Recovery of motor function after two stage extirpation of area 4 in monkeys (*Macaca mulatta*). *Journal of Neurophysiology*, 1946, *9*, 55–60.

Ades, H. W., and Raab, D. H. Effects of preoccipital and temporal decortication on learned visual discrimination in monkeys. *Journal of Neurophysiology*, 1949, *12*, 101–108.

Barbas, H., and Spear, P. D. Effects of serial unilateral and serial bilateral visual cortex lesions on brightness discrimination relearning in rats. *Journal of Comparative and Physiological Psychology*, 1976, *90*, 279–292.

Bekoff, M., Lockwood, A., and Meikle, T. H., Jr. Effects of serial lesions in cat visual cortex on a brightness discrimination. *Brain Research*, 1973, *49*, 190–193.

Benton, A. L. Hemispheric development of the concept of hemispheric cerebral dominance. In S. F. Spiker and H. T. Engelhardt, Jr. (Eds.), *Philosophical dimensions of the neuro-medical sciences*. Dordrecht, Holland: D. Reidel Publishing Co., 1976.

Blatt, B., and Lyon, M. The interrelationship of forebrain and midbrain structures involved in feeding behavior. *Acta Neurologica Scandinavica*, 1968, *44*, 576–595.

Broca, P. Remarques sur la siège de la faculté du langage articulé; suivies d'une observation d'aphemie. *Bulletin de la Societé Anatomique de Paris*, 1861, *6*, 330–357.

Broca, P. Localisation des fonctions cérébrales. Siège du langage articulé. *Bulletin de la Societé Anthropologique de Paris*, 1863, *4*, 200–203.

Broca, P. Sur la siège de la faculté du langage articulé. *Bulletin de la Societé Anthropologique de Paris*, 1865, *6*, 377–393.

Butters, N., Butter, C., Rosen, J., and Stein, D. G. Behavioral effects of sequential and one-stage ablations of orbital prefrontal cortex in the monkey. *Experimental Neurology*, 1973, *39*, 204–214.

Cannon, W. F., and Rosenblueth, A. *The supersensitivity of denervated structures*. New York: Macmillan, 1949.

Chow, K. L., and Survis, J. Retention of overlearned visual habit after temporal cortical ablation in monkey. *Archives of Neurology and Psychiatry* (Chicago), 1958, *79*, 640–646.

Cole, D. D., Sullins, W. R., and Isaac, W. Pharmacological modification of the effects of spaced occipital ablations. *Psychopharmacologia* (Berlin), 1967, *11*, 311–316.

Dawson, R. G., Recovery of function: Implications for theories of brain function. *Behavioral Biology*, 1973, *8*, 439–460.

Dawson, R. G., Conrad, L., and Lynch, G. Single and two-stage hippocampal lesions: A similar syndrome. *Experimental Neurology*, 1973, *40*, 263–277.

Dax, G. Notes sur le même sujet. *Gazette Hebdomadaire de Médecine et de Chirurgie* (Paris), 1865, *2*, 262.

Dax, M. Lesions de la moitié gauche de l'encéphale coincidant avec l'oublie des signes de la pensée. *Gazette Hebdomadaire de Médecine et de Chirurgie* (Paris), 1865, *2*, 259–262.

Dru, D., Walker, J. P., and Walker, J. B. Self-produced locomotion restores visual capacity after striate lesions. *Science*, 1975, *187*, 265–266.

Fass, B., Jordan, H., Rubman, A., Seibel, S., and Stein, D. Recovery of function after serial or one-stage lesions of the lateral hypothalamic area in rats. *Behavioral Biology*, 1975, *14*, 283–294.

Finger, S., and Reyes, R. Long-term deficits after somatosensory cortical lesions in rats. *Physiology and Behavior*, 1975, *15*, 289–293.

Finger, S., and Simons, D. Effects of serial lesions of somatosensory cortex and further neodecortication on retention of a rough-smooth discrimination in rats. *Experimental Brain Research*, 1976, *25*, 183–197.

Finger, S., Marshak, R. A., Cohen, M., Scheff, S., Trace, R., and Neimand, D. Effects of successive and simultaneous lesions of somatosensory cortex on tactile discrimination in the rat. *Journal of Comparative and Physiological Psychology*, 1971, *77*, 221–227.

Finger, S., Walbran, B., and Stein, D. G. Brain damage and behavioral recovery: Serial lesion phenomena. *Brain Research*, 1973, *63*, 1–18.

Flourens, P. *Investigations of the properties and the functions of the various parts which compose the cerebral mass*. Paris; Crevot, 1824, pp. 85–122. Reprinted in G. von Bonin (trans.), *Some papers on the cerebral cortex*. Springfield, Ill.: Charles C. Thomas, 1960.

Gentile, A., Nieburgs, A., Schmeltzer, W., and Stein, D. G. Recovery of locomotion following cortical lesions in rats. Paper presented at the 5th Annual Meeting of the Society for Neuroscience, New York City, November 2–6, 1975.

Glassman, R. B. Recovery following sensorimotor cortical damage: Evoked potentials, brain stimulation and motor control. *Experimental Neurology,* 1971, *33,* 16–29.

Glendenning, R. L. Effects of training between two unilateral lesions of visual cortex upon ultimate retention of black-white discrimination habits in rats. *Journal of Comparative Physiological Psychology,* 1972, *80,* 216–229.

Glick, S. D., and Zimmerberg, B. Comparative recovery following simultaneous- and successive-stage frontal brain damage in mice. *Journal of Comparative and Physiological Psychology,* 1972, *79,* 481–487.

Goldberger, M. E. Restitution of function in the CNS: The pathologic grasp in *Macaca mulatta. Experimental Brain Research,* 1972, *15,* 79–96.

Goodman, D. C., and Horel, J. A. Sprouting of optic tract projections in the brain stem of the rat. *Journal of Comparative Neurology,* 1966, *127,* 71–88.

Greene, E., Stauff, C., and Walters, J. Recovery of function with two-stage lesions of the fornix. *Experimental Neurology,* 1972, *37,* 14–22.

Head, H. *Aphasia and kindred disorders of speech.* Cambridge, Mass.: Cambridge University Press, 1926.

Isaac, W. Role of stimulation and time in the effects of spaced occipital ablations. *Psychological Reports,* 1964, *14,* 151–154.

Issacson, R. L., and Schmaltz, L. W., Failure to find savings from spaced, two-stage destruction of hippocampus. *Cummunications in Behavioral Biology,* 1968, *1,* 353–359.

Isseroff, A., Leveton, L., Freeman, G., Lewis, M. E., and Stein, D. G. The limits of behavioral recovery from serial lesions of the hipppocampus. *Experimental Neurology,* 1976, *53,* 339–354.

Jackson, J. H. On affections of speech from disease of the brain. *Brain,* 1879, *2,* 323–356.

Jackson, J. H. Remarks on the dissolution of the nervous system as exemplified by certain post-epileptic conditions. *Medical Press and Circular,* 1881, *1,* 329ff.

Jackson, J. H. The factors of insanities. *Medical Press and Circular,* 1894, *2,* 615–619.

Joynt, R. J. Presentation 5: Anatomical determinants of behavioral change. In A. L. Benton (Ed.), *Behavioral changes in cerebrovascular disease.* New York: Harper and Row, 1970, pp. 37–39.

Joynt, R. J., and Benton, A. L. The memoir of Marc Dax on aphasia. *Neurology* (Minneapolis), 1964, *14,* 851–154.

Kempinsky, W. H. Experimental study of distant effects of acute focal brain injury—a study of diaschisis. *Archives of Neurology and Psychiatry,* 1958, *79,* 376–389.

Kennard, M. A. Cortical reorganization of motor functions. *Archives of Neurology and Psychiatry* (Chicago), 1942, *48,* 227–240.

Kerr, F. W. L. Structural and functional evidence for plasticity in the central nervous system. *Experimental Neurology,* 1975, *48,* 16–31.

Kesner, R. P., Fiedler, P., and Thomas, G. J. Function of the mid-brain reticular formation in regulating level of activity and learning in rats. *Journal of Comparative and Physiological Psychology,* 1967, *63,* 452–457.

Kircher, K. A., Braun, J. J., Meyer, D. R., and Meyer, P. M. Equivalence of simultaneous and successive neocortical ablations in production of impairments of retention of black-white habits in rats. *Journal of Comparative and Physiological Psychology,* 1970, *71,* 420–425.

Kleitman, N., and Camille, N. Studies on the physiology of sleep. VI. The behavior of decorticated dogs. *American Journal of Physiology,* 1932, *100,* 474–480.

Lashley, K. S. *Brain mechanisms and intelligence.* Chicago: University of Chicago Press, 1929.

LeVere, T. E. Recovery of function after brainstem lesions in the rat. *Journal of Comparative and Physiological Psychology*, 1969, *69*, 339–344.

LeVere, T. E. Neural stability, sparing, and behavioral recovery following brain damage. *Psychological Review*, 1975, *82*, 344–358.

LeVere, T. E., and Weiss, J. Failure of seriatim dorsal hippocampal lesions to spare spatial reversal behavior in rats. *Journal of Comparative and Physiological Psychology*, 1973, *82*, 205–210.

Lewis, M. E., and Lancione, R. L. A mathematical model of recovery from brain damage. *Brain Theory Newsletter*, 1976, *1*, 65–66.

Lourie, H., Vanasupa, P., and O'Leary, J. Experimental observations upon chronic progressive lesions of the brain stem tegmentum and midline thalamus. *Surgical Forum*, 1960, *10*, 756–760.

Macrides, F., Firl, A. C., Schneider, S. P., Bartke, A., and Stein, D. G. Effects of one-stage or serial transections of the lateral olfactory tracts on behavior and plasma testosterone levels in male hamsters. *Brain Research*, 1976, *109*, 97–109.

Meyer, D. R. Access to engrams. *American Psychologist*, 1972, *27*, 124–133.

Meyer, D. R., Isaac, W., and Maher, B. The role of stimulation in spontaneous reorganization of visual habits. *Journal of Comparative and Physiological Psychology*, 1958, *51*, 546–548.

Moore, R. Y., Björklund, A., and Stenevi, U. Plastic changes in the adrenergic innervation of the rat septal area in response to denervation. *Brain Research*, 1971, *33*, 13–35.

Morgan, C. T. Some structural factors in perception. In R. R. Blake and G. V. Ramsey (Eds.), *Perception: An approach to personality.* New York: Ronald Press, 1951, pp. 25–55.

Patrissi, G., and Stein, D. G. Temporal factors in recovery of function after brain damage. *Experimental Neurology*, 1975, *47*, 470–480.

Petrinovich, L., and Carew, T. J. Interaction of neocortical lesion size and interoperative experience in retention of a learned brightness discrimination. *Journal of Comparative and Physiological Psychology*, 1969, *68*, 451–454.

Raisman, G. Neuronal plasticity in the septal nuclei of the adult rat. *Brain Research*, 1969, *14*, 25–48.

Reyes, R. Effects of interlesion interval and postoperative recovery period on recovery of function following serial lesions of somatic cortex in rats. Unpublished doctoral dissertation, Washington University, 1977.

Reyes, R., Finger, S., and Frye, J. Serial thalamic lesions and tactile discrimination in the rat. *Behavioral Biology*, 1973, *8*, 807–813.

Riese, W. Aphasia in brain tumors. *Confinia Neurologica*, 1948, *9*, 64–79.

Riese, W., *Principles of neurology in the light of history and their present use.* New York: Nervous and Mental Disease Monographs, 1950.

Rosen, J., Stein, D., and Butters, N. Recovery of function after serial ablation of prefrontal cortex in the rhesus monkey. *Science*, 1971, *173*, 353–356.

Rowe, F. A., and Smith, W. E. Simultaneous and successive olfactory bulb removal: Influences on the mating behavior of male mice. *Physiology and Behavior*, 1973, *10*, 443–449.

Scheff, S., Bernardo, L., Cotman, C., and Lynch, G. Cumulative effects of sequential lesions on axon sprouting in the hippocampus. Paper presented at the 6th Annual Meeting of the Society for Neuroscience, Toronto, November 7–11, 1976.

Scheff, S. W., and Wright, D. C. Behavioral and electrophysiological evidence for cortical reorganization of function with serial lesions of the visual cortex. *Physiological Psychology*, 1977, *5*, 103–107.

Scheff, S. W., Wright, D. C., Morgan W. K., and Bowers, R. P. The different effects of additional cortical lesions in rats with single or multiple stage lesions of the visual cortex. *Physiological Psychology*, 1977 *5*, 97–102.

Schneider, G. E. Mechanisms of functional recovery following lesions of visual cortex or superior colliculus in neonate and adult hamsters. *Brain Behavior and Evolution*, 1970, *3*, 295–323.

Schultze, M. J., and Stein, D. G. Recovery of function in the albino rat following either simultaneous or seriatim lesions of the caudate nucleus. *Experimental Neurology*, 1975, *46*, 291–301.

Sharpless, S. K. Reorganization of function in the nervous system—use and disuse. *Annual Review of Physiology*, 1964, *26*, 357–388.

Simons, D., Puretz, J., and Finger, S. Effects of serial lesions of somatosensory cortex and further neodecortication on tactile retention in rats. *Experimental Brain Research*, 1975, *23*, 353–366.

Spear, P. D., and Barbas, H. Recovery of pattern discrimination ability in rats receiving serial or one-stage visual cortex lesions. *Brain Research*, 1975, *94*, 337–346.

Stein, D. G., and Firl, A. Brain damage and reorganization of function in old age. *Experimental Neurology*, 1976, *52*, 157–167.

Stein, D. G., and Lewis, M. E. Functional recovery after brain damage in adult organisms. *INSERM*, 1975, *43*, 203–228.

Stein, D. G., Rosen, J. J., Graziadei, J., Mishkin, D., and Brink, J. J. Central nervous system: Recovery of function. *Science*, 1969, *166*, 528–530.

Stein, D. G., Butters, N., and Rosen, J. A comparison of two and four-stage ablations of sulcus principalis on recovery of spatial performance in the rhesus monkey. *Neuropsychologia*, 1977, *15*, 179–182.

Stewart, J. W., and Ades, H. W. The time factor in reintegration of a learned habit after temporal lobe lesions in the monkey (*Macaca mulatta*). *Journal of Comparative and Physiological Psychology*, 1951, *44*, 479–486.

Tarlov, I. M. Spinal cord compression studies: III. Time limits for recovery after gradual compression in dogs. *Archives of Neurology and Psychiatry*, 1954, *71*, 588–597.

Thompson, R. Retention of a brightness discrimination following neocortical damage in the rat. *Journal of Comparative and Physiological Psychology*, 1960, *53*, 212–215.

Travis, A. M., and Woolsey, C. N. Motor performance of monkeys after bilateral partial and total cerebral decortications. *American Journal of Physical Medicine*, 1956, *35*, 273–310.

Treichler, F. R. Two-stage frontal lesion influences upon severity of delayed response deficit. *Behavioral Biology*, 1975, *13*, 35–48.

von Monakow, C. *Gehirnpathologie*. Vienna: Hölder, 1897.

von Monakow, C. *Die Lokalisation im grosshirn und der Abbau der Funktion durch kortikale Herde*. Wiesbaden: J. F. Bergmann, 1914.

Walbran, B. B. Age and serial ablations of somatosensory cortex in the rat. *Physiology and Behavior*, 1976, *17*, 13–17.

Wall, P. D., and Egger, M. D. Formation of new connexions in adult rat brains after partial deafferentation. *Nature*, 1971, *232*, 542–545.

Welker, C., and Woolsey, T. A. Structure of layer IV in the somatosensory neocortex of the rat: Description and comparison with the mouse. *Journal of Comparative Neurology*, 1974, *158*, 437–454.

Winans, S. S., and Powers, J. B. Neonatal and two-stage olfactory bulbectomy: Effects on male hamster sexual behavior. *Behavioral Biology*, 1974, *10*, 461–471.

Wolf, G., and DiCara, L. V. Progressive morphologic changes in electrolytic brain lesions. *Experimental Neurology*, 1969, *23*, 529–536.

Woolsey, T. A., and van der Loos, H. The structural organization of layer IV in the somatosensory region (SI) of the mouse cerebral cortex: The description of a cortical field composed of discrete cytoarchitectonic units. *Brain Research*, 1970, *17*, 205–242.

8

Time and Recovery from Brain Damage

J. JAY BRAUN

1. INTRODUCTION

The time course of behavioral recovery following brain trauma varies substantially from the few minutes or hours of disorientation that occur following a mild concussion (Russel and Nathan, 1946) to the years required for any recovery following a left temporal lobectomy in humans (e.g., Blakemore and Falconer, 1967). The amount of time over which recovery will be observed, as well as the extent of ultimate recovery as assessed by some measure of asymptotic performance of affected behaviors, is determined by many factors: the nature, extent, and level of nervous system damage, the rate of onset of the damage (e.g., degenerative disease versus acute trauma), age at time of trauma, and the extent and permanence of indirect trauma produced by accessory complications such as edema and hypoxia. In addition, the particular choice of measures used to assess recovery can affect markedly an experimenter's judgment of when or whether or how abruptly recovery has occurred. These factors suggest events which underlie and ultimately determine the time course of recovery.

Two broad classes of factors enter into accounts of the recovery process: psychological and physiological. Examples of psychological factors are those related to generalized arousal, stimulation, and special training procedures which have been found to encourage recovery of function. Physiological factors include biochemical, regenerative, ho-

J. JAY BRAUN • Department of Psychology, Arizona State University, Tempe, Arizona 85281

meostatic, and developmental variables which are hypothesized to underlie behavioral recovery following brain damage.

These two classes of factors, of course, are not mutually exclusive. This becomes apparent by conceptually partitioning them in a fashion that relates to empirical considerations. Again, they fall into two broad categories of variables: those which are directly manipulable (independent variables) and those which are potentially measurable as outcomes (dependent variables) along a frame of reference provided by the ubiquitous "time" variable. Independent variables include such things as special training and surgical procedures, various pharmacological manipulations, and "time" from a developmental perspective. Dependent variables include time-related measures of electrophysiological, biochemical, and morphological changes in the nervous system. These two sets of variables represent potential "causes" and "correlates," respectively, of *behavioral* recovery following brain damage. One research challenge is to relate these two classes of variables to each other and to the outcome of behavioral recovery.

The following section discusses relationships of behavioral recovery to endogenous correlates of the recovery process. It emphasizes potential contributions of a trauma factor to both losses and sparing of neurological function and to defining the time course over which recovery may be observed to occur.

2. CORRELATES OF RECOVERY

"Time," in various guises (e.g., "spontaneous recovery" from diachisis: von Monakow, 1914), has had the role of an intervening variable in accounts of recovery following brain damage. In such a role, it has served mainly to identify a lack of understanding of the factors that actually are responsible for recovery. However, although time *per se* may not heal any wounds, various time-related processes appear to be important. Methodological considerations involving the control and selective manipulation of the time variable help to identify and partition the existence and role of such processes in recovery. An analysis presented by Meyer in 1958 illustrates this point.

2.1. Time and Stimulation

Meyer began by discussing the results and conclusions of Stewart and Ades' (1951) study of recovery following sequential, unilateral ablations of temporal neocortex in monkeys. Steward and Ades had noted that a preoperatively instated auditory habit was lost following simultaneous bilateral ablations, but that it was retained following successive unilateral ablations which ultimately included the same total amount of tissue as had the simultaneous bilateral procedure. However, using the successive–unilateral procedure, retention of the habit was observed only when a time interval of at least 7 days intervened between the two unilateral operations. This suggested to Steward and Ades that endogenous factors operated in this recovery, which they described as being due to a process of "spontaneous reorganization." Such an identification implied some underlying but unspecified fundamental physiological process that depended on the presence of relevant intact cortical tissue for a certain critical period of time between successive operations.

It is worthwhile to point out at this juncture that a conclusion relevant to recovery of function would not have been reached by Steward and Ades if they had not systematically varied the interoperative time period. If they had used only a short time interval (less than 7 days), for example, the previous functional localization conclusion would have been supported. A time-correlated process was clearly indicated, however, but beyond this there were no clues from the study concerning the specific nature of the process. The words "spontaneous reorganization" simply identified the observation of an interaction between the surgical procedure and a measure of time.

Addressing the concept of "spontaneous reorganization," Meyer, Isaac, and Maher (1958) conducted a study which was the first demonstration of the importance of exogenous stimulation during the interoperative interval for retention of a learned habit following sequential, unilateral lesions. They used a light-avoidance habit in a shuttle box to train normal rats to jump from one compartment to another within 2 seconds of light onset. In pilot work, they had established that simultaneous bilateral removals of visual neocortex resulted in a loss of the habit, as did successive unilateral ablations using a 6-day interoperative interval. However, when the interoperative interval was extended to 12 days during which the rats resided in their home cages in the normally lighted laboratory environment, a significant number of the operated rats retained the light-avoidance habit according to a savings measure. Up to this point, then, the experiment is exactly analogous to the Stewart and Ades study: Simultaneous bilateral lesions resulted in a loss of the preoperatively instated habit, but successive, unilateral lesions with an interoperative time period beyond a certain critical time duration resulted in retention of the habit.

Some time-correlated process essential for retention was identified in the Meyer *et al.* study, as it had been in the Stewart and Ades (1951) study. However, a new perspective was added by the observation that significant retention of the brightness habit following successive unilateral ablations separated by 12 days was *not* observed in a group of rats that were kept in the *dark* during the interoperative interval. Therefore, retention of the habit was not only "time correlated," but it appeared to be stimulation dependent as well. Hence, the role of time *per se* was substantially diminished in explanations of this recovery effect. Although diminished, however, it naggingly persists to this day as a reminder of the fact that the critical-period aspect of this form of recovery remains unexplained. Progress toward a solution to this problem might come from studies designed to relate a quantitative measure of endogenous factors, such as neural sprouting or various biochemical changes, with behavioral recovery, using the time variable as a common measure. The promise of this possibility is suggested by the increasing expression of both clinical and experimental interest in it over the past decade (e.g., Brodal, 1973; Stein, Rosen, and Butters, 1974).

2.2. Time as a Correlative Frame of Reference

The establishment of relationships following brain trauma between behavioral recovery and its physiological foundations requires a correlative approach by which separately derived measures of behavioral changes and morphological or biochemical changes in the brain are each related to a measure of time and then, through time, to each other. First, relationships must be established between a measure of time and measurements of post-trauma biochemical and/or morphological changes in the brain. Second, time-based measures of possible relevant behavioral changes must be established. Third, the degree of correspondence between the two sets of measures must be determined. Fourth, the interdependency of any promising relationships indicated in the third step must be tested by asking whether manipulations of one set of measures result in concomitant and predicted changes in the other.

Some of the most promising potential behavioral–physiological relationships have been indicated in studies which measure unusual behavioral changes following brain damage. The word "change" is used here instead of "recovery" in order to include instances of unusual behaviors which appear to be maladaptive but which nonetheless might be induced by measurable, concomitant processes of physiological reorganization. They include such changes as the inappropriate visually guided head turning responses in hamsters with damaged visual systems: This aberrant behavior appears to be related to the development of anomalous retinotectal projections (see Schneider and Jhaveri, 1974). Other examples include the development of spasticity, which might be due to collateral sprouting following dorsal root sectioning (McCouch, Austin, Liu, and Liu, 1958), and the possibility that anomalous sprouting might underlie the unusual impairments of mating behavior in hamsters with partial olfactory tract lesions in infancy (Devor, 1975).

The development of these unusual behavioral changes coincident with sprouting supports the hypothesis that the phenomenon of sprouting might underlie the observed changes. However, most behavioral changes over time following brain damage are in a direction that can be characterized as adaptive rather than as maladaptive. These adaptive-appearing changes include instances of exaggerated behavioral tendencies which clearly diminish over time in a constant setting (e.g., the septal hyperemotionality syndrome, Brady and Nauta, 1953), and they include behaviors which are greatly diminished, or initially eliminated, but which eventually tend to reappear over time (e.g., feeding behavior following lateral hypothalamic lesions, Teitelbaum and Epstein, 1962). Behavioral recovery in appropriate directions is evident in these cases. But to what degree might processes like sprouting underlie these kinds of adaptive-appearing behavior changes?

Loesche and Steward (1977) have recently published a compelling experiment attesting to the possibility of clearly defined central reinnervation following brain damage serving as a foundation for behavioral recovery. Previous work by Lynch and colleagues had established the development of reinnervation of the dentate gyrus of the hippocampus following unilateral lesions of the entorhinal cortex (Lynch, Matthews, Mosko, Parks, and Cotman, 1972) and had established the source of the reinnervation to be surviving afferents from the contralateral hippocampus (Lynch, Stanfield, and Cotman, 1973) and contralateral entorhinal cortex (Steward, Cotman, and Lynch, 1976). Loesche and Steward pointed out that the surviving afferents appeared to reinnervate the granule cells of the dentate gyrus in an apparently normal fashion, and that electrophysiological and autoradiographic studies had revealed reinnervation to occur predominantly between 8 and 12 days following unilateral entorhinal lesions. Their experiment established that marked deficits in reinforced alternation behavior occur following unilateral entorhinal cortex lesions and that the behavior appeared to recover to normal levels in about 10 days. A group of rats which received continuous training throughout the 10 days did not recover any faster than a group for which training was not begun for 10 days. Furthermore, subsequent lesions of the surviving entorhinal cortex and lesions of the dorsal psalterium, through which passes crossed projections from entorhinal cortex to the dentate gyrus, severely disrupted the recovered alternation behavior. However, in trained animals without unilateral entorhinal lesions, damage to the psalterium had negligible effects on alternation performance. Hence, Loesche and Steward were able to suggest that recovery of normal alternation behavior in rats with unilateral entorhinal lesions depends on reinnervation of the ipsilateral dentate gyrus via axons from contralateral entorhinal cortex which pass through the dorsal psalterium. Their study therefore strongly indicates that collateral sprouting underlies at least one instance of adaptive behavioral recovery following brain damage.

The discussion thus far has assumed that dynamic physiological processes of regrowth or reorganization may typically underlie behavioral recovery. But there is reason to suspect that many cases of such recovery may simply reflect the functioning of spared, but not necessarily reorganized, neural tissue. The following section addresses this less dramatic but very important possibility.

2.3. Recoveries, Deficits, and Diaschisis

Accounting for behavioral recovery over time and accounting for initial post-trauma deficits are conjoint problems in recovery research. Initial deficits represent a baseline from which recovery is measured, and an explanation of the deficit implies an explanation of the recovery. Consider, for example, the theoretical accounts of aphagia following lateral hypothalamic lesions in rats (Anand and Brobeck, 1951). Interpreting aphagia as representing a loss of motivation for food (Teitelbaum and Epstein, 1962), the reappearance of feeding behavior as displayed in "stage II" (anorexia) of recovery could be viewed as activation of a feeding response by the extreme deprivational state that eventually occurs as aphagia persists. When interpreted as an inability to eat produced by a disruption of sensorimotor coordination (Marshall and Teitelbaum, 1974), the reappearance of feeding behavior implies some sort of reacquisition of the coordination necessary to eat. Viewed as caused by a disruption of visceral activity which rapidly produces gastric ulcers, the reappearance of feeding can be interpreted as being based on the recovery of balanced visceral activity and the healing of the stomach ulcers (Grijalva, Lindholm, Schallert, and Bicknell, 1976). When the marked depletion of brain catecholamines following lateral hypothalamic lesions is suggested as a foundation for aphagia, the reappearance of feeding can be interpreted as due to compensatory changes in remaining catecholaminergic neurons and their postsynaptic receptors (Stricker and Zigmond, 1976). Finally, if the initial aphagia is interpreted as representing temporary lack of motivation to eat produced by a lowering of body weight set point (Powley and Keesey, 1970), and if a measure of body weight is used to assess recovery, then it can be suggested that the apparent recovery of feeding behavior is an epiphenomenon: that it occurs when body weight is reduced to a new regulatory set point. The observation by Powley and Keesey that body-weight reduction prior to surgery can eliminate a period of postoperative aphagia supports this interpretation.

These various interpretations of the aphagia produced by lateral hypothalamic lesions are not mutually exclusive, and they are listed here, in a greatly simplified form, merely to point out the interdependency between interpretations of losses and interpretations of recoveries that follow a specific brain lesion. A particularly broad range of potential foundations for recovery is implied in these examples, from the view that it is based on residual hypothalamic tissue or on reorganization of remaining extrahypothalamic parts of the feeding system (see Teitelbaum, 1971), to a view emphasizing the role of visceral or biochemical factors. In addition, on the basis of Powley and Keesey's work the view can be offered that the return of feeding following lateral hypothalamic lesions may not reflect a fundamental underlying process of recovery at all (see LeVere, 1975).

2.3.1. Reversible Brain Trauma

Regardless of the specific interpretation emphasized, however, a general statement at a more fundamental level can be made regarding the causes of initially apparent behavioral deficits following any kind of brain damage. They can be caused by reversible brain trauma, such as that produced by a temporary reduction of the oxygen supply to parts of the brain, and by more permanent types of brain damage. It is the latter cause that occupies most attention in recovery of function research because it provides the particularly interesting problem of accounting for behavioral recovery when an apparently crucial integrative system for the behavior in question has been removed or irrevocably damaged. However, the present discussion will emphasize the former cause, reversible brain trauma, for several reasons. First, reversible physiological processes are interesting substrates of recovery in their own right; they probably underlie much of the recovery observed after human brain trauma (e.g., Luria, Naydin, Tsvetkova, and Vinarskaya, 1969), and they have not received a great deal of attention in brain–behavior studies. Second, behavioral deficits measured immediately after brain damage inevitably will reflect confounding of the permanent effects with the reversible traumatic effects that probably always accompany the instrumentation of permanent damage. Ideally, in order to assess accurately the portion of observed behavioral recovery that might be attributable to some sort of neural reorganization or functional reinstatement, one must estimate and subtract that portion of the losses due to reversible indirect physiological consequences of brain damage. Third, transient brain trauma becomes permanent when the conditions producing it are prolonged beyond a critical time. For example, it is believed that permanent brain injury due to ischemia "accounts for more of the nonprogressive neurological deficits seen in children than any other type [of brain injury]" (Volpe, 1976). For these reasons, greater attention to both *reversible* and *irreversible* long-term consequences of ischemia is deemed especially important.

2.3.2. Ischemia and Permanent Brain Damage

Persistent brain ischemia can result in irreversible damage to parts of the nervous system surrounding, and sometimes distant from, the intended area of focal damage. This means that measured behavioral debilities can reflect diffuse damage extending beyond, and confounded with, the damage of intent in brain-lesion experiments. This problem was brought out in a study of the role of neocortex in feeding behavior (Braun, 1975). In this experiment, clear evidence of subcortical focal necrosis, which was produced, presumably, by ischemia, was observed. The degree of necrosis was highly variable, which is a characteristic of ischemic damage (Levine, 1960), and dense concentrations of calcium salts were observed in the necrotic areas; this condition can be produced by degenerating vascular tissue. In addition, the damage extended through a route similar to that described for the lenticulostriate arteries in human brains, which includes the striatum and medial thalamus. Striatal lesions produce profound disruption of feeding behavior (Sorenson and Ellison, 1970; Levine and Schwartzbaum, 1973). Therefore, it was not possible in Braun's study to attribute the disruptions of consummatory behavior observed after the neocortical ablations to neocortical processes alone.

In addition to illustrating the potential permanence of ischemic damage, the observations outlined above lead to the sugestion that ischemia is not necessarily "nonspecific." Its pattern of representation in the brain probably varies widely with the location and extent of the specific injury that produced it.

2.3.3. Transient Ischemia

Recent evidence suggests that the brains of animals (dogs and monkeys) can recover remarkably, at least according to bioelectrical and biochemical indices of metabolic recovery, following prolonged periods of complete ischemia (1 hour) and subsequent postischemic recirculation (e.g., Kleihues, Hossmann, Pegg, Kobayashi, and Zimmerman, 1975; Sobotka, Jirasek, and Gebert, 1974). The significance of these findings in terms of behavioral recovery is not known, but they provide a foundation for behavioral assessments.

Sobotka *et al.* (1974) briefly discussed the complication of post-ischemic edema as a source of considerable variance in their physiological measures of recovery. Post-traumatic edema is one of the major causes of restricted blood flow in the brain, and it is likely that this condition can endure for prolonged periods of time, at levels sufficient to maintain fundamental vitality of brain tissue but insufficient to maintain the contribution of restricted tissue to the integrative activity of the brain. The progressive diminution of this pathological state could underlie some kinds of relatively long-term behavioral recovery. Luria *et al.* (1969) have emphasized the potential role of such factors in clinical cases and discuss the effects of procedures designed to overcome them.

2.3.4. Electrophysiological Studies

Glassman (1971) found that behavioral recovery following damage to part of the somatosensory neocortex in cats occurred concomitantly with electrophysiological signs of recovery in spared tissue adjacent to a lesion. Recovery was correlated also with a return of excitability of the adjacent tissue as determined by evoked movements produced by direct electrical stimulation. In a more recent article, Glassman and Malamut (1976) describe a finding that is especially relevant to the possibility of relatively long-term influence of nonspecific factors on measures of behavioral recovery. In this study, a number of cats with frontal damage displayed delayed onset (about 1 week following surgery) of abnormal electrophysiological responses accompanied by the development of behavioral deficits more severe than those which immediately followed surgery. Glassman and Malamut expressed the possibility that the cause of this was "indirect, via some metabolic alteration, and not relevant to any neural recovery process specifically concerned with the function of the damaged area" (p. 352).

2.3.5. Explant Cultures

Studies of explant cultures of neural cells have shown that changes in the environment surrounding the cells can lead to reversible degenerative changes. Varon (1970) describes the course of degenerative changes of cells in such cultures from the time of explantation. During the first week, the cell bodies of many surviving neurons increasingly display signs of chromatolysis similar to those displayed by damaged neural cells *in vivo*. Over the ensuing *weeks,* the chromatolytic pattern can be observed to reverse with gradual enlargement of the cell body and centralization of the nucleus to the point where the configuration of a normal, healthy neural cell is observed. These kinds of dynamic cytological observations suggest a straightforward foundation for many instances of behavioral recovery following brain damage.

2.3.6. Spinal Trauma

The potential importance of greater attention to physiological events and manipulations which occur immediately following nervous system trauma can be illustrated by the results of a study by Parker and Smith (1974). These investigators studied functional recovery following spinal cord trauma in dogs. The "trauma" was produced in a highly consistent manner by dropping a sterilized 20 g weight down fixed lengths of plastic cylinder onto the exposed spinal cords of the anesthetized subjects. The dogs had been prepared with a dorsal laminectomy which uncovered the cord segments underlying the top two lumbar vertebrae and the bottom thoracic vertebra, but the meninges were left intact during application of the trauma. This procedure had been shown to result in various degrees of paralysis of the hindlimbs as indicated by comprehensive assessments of spinal reflexes using a carefully calibrated nine-point scale, from "normal" to complete "flaccid or spastic paralysis." The critical independent variable was the presence or absence of a post-trauma longitudinal incision in the spinal meninges; half of the dogs received such an incision and the other half (the control group) did not. This simple manipulation reduced recovery time by about 50% (see Figure 8-1).

It was suggested that the immediate meningeal incision reduced the intradural pressure caused by post-traumatic edema. The incision thus averted some of the ischemia and was followed by complete reflex recovery in a median of 9 days. Interestingly, two dogs did not appear to recover at all over 27 days of testing and both were in the nonincised control group. In addition, they were the only dogs that had evidenced complete loss of reflex function on the first postoperative testing day. Potentially transient trauma apparently became permanent in these dogs, at least according to the behavioral measures. Unfortunately, this study did not include a correlational assessment of the relationship between the amount of damage ultimately sustained by the spinal cord and the degree of observed behavioral recovery.

2.3.7. Diaschisis: Recovery as Sparing

It is suggested that many instances of behavioral recovery following brain damage simply reflect the physiological recovery of spared

lations and methods of behavioral analysis used in a particular study can substantially influence the degree to which one or the other of these perspectives is supported. This is most clearly illustrated by the results of brain-lesion studies which were responses to suggestions that certain areas of the brain are either necessary for, or, conversely, are not involved in, particular behavior functions.

Early work Smith (1937a) indicated that the visual neocortex of the cat was not involved in horizontal optokinetic nystagmus responses. Cats lacking visual neocortex displayed normal bidirectional tracking movements of the head when placed in a revolving drum with stripes on the inside. This result was consistent with the idea that a simple reflex response like nystagmus was principally integrated at the brain stem level: The function of generating optokinetic nystagmus appeared to be spared completely according to these results. Smith and Bridgeman (1943) and others (see Braun and Gault, 1969) had shown that afoveate species with near-complete decussation of the optic tracts (guinea pigs, rabbits, pigeons), while clearly displaying nystagmus, were deficient in monocular tests when the visual field was revolved in a nasal-to-temporal direction with respect to the viewing eye. Several lines of evidence suggested to Wood, Spear, and Braun (1973) that cats lacking visual neocortex might likewise display deficient optokinetic nystagmus in this monocular viewing condition. A test of this hypothesis revealed the following results (see Figure 8-2): Consistent with Smith's observations, Wood et al. found cats lacking visual neocortex to display normal bidirectional optokinetic nystagmus responses when both eyes viewed the moving field. The responses also appeared normal under monocular conditions when the field was moving in a temporal-to-nasal direction with respect to the viewing eye. However, the responses resembled those of afoveate species when, under monocular viewing conditions, the field rotated in a nasal-to-temporal direction. An interesting contribution of visual neocortex to optokinetic nystagmus was clearly indicated by these results. With regard to the present discussion, the outcome of the Wood et al. study provides a case in which a brain area classically interpreted as *not* involved in a particular behavior was found to be deeply involved in a certain aspect of it: The function was thus both spared *and* deficient following the neocortical ablation. Smith missed this because he did not systematically test his brain-damaged cats under monocular viewing conditions.

A study by Braun, Lundy, and McCarthy (1970) illustrates the transformation of a tentative functional localization conclusion into a sparing of function conclusion by a procedural manipulation. Meyer, Anderson, and Braun (1966) had found that the visual cliff performances of hooded rats lacking visual neocortex were no different from

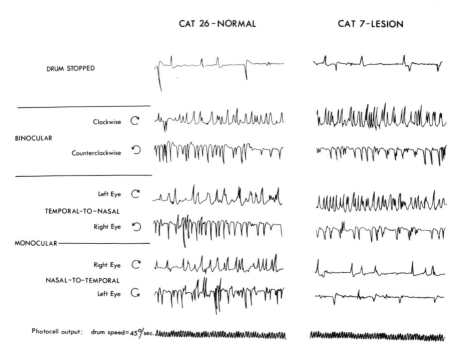

Figure 8-2.　Representative differential recordings of horizontal eye movements of two cats in an optokinetic nystagmus (OKN) testing situation. The cats were in a drum with vertical stripes on the inside, and the drum could be revolved in either direction. OKN was recorded under both monocular and binocular viewing conditions. The arrows preceding each record indicate the direction of drum rotation. The sample records are 30 seconds long. The abrupt shifts from baseline represent the fast component of the nystagmus response; the change in polarity with the change in direction of drum rotation reflects a shift in the direction of the fast component. A photocell (see bottom of figure) was used to monitor drum rotation. The figure compares the OKN records of a cat with a large posterior neocortex lesion to those of a normal cat. Note the weak OKN responses of the brain-damaged cat when the drum was rotated in a nasal-to-temporal direction with respect to the viewing eye. This selective deficiency was a reliable feature of cats with posterior neocortex lesions in a study by Wood *et al.* (1973), from which this figure is taken.

those of blinded rats. It appeared that the normal rat's ability to avoid the deeper of two alternatives in this situation depended upon the integrity of area striata. Using a shock-motivated discrimination situation and a miniature version of a visual cliff lying on its side for "deep" and "shallow" discriminada, Braun *et al.* found that rats lacking visual neocortex could learn a depth discrimination even when differential luminous flux, linear perspective, and localized luminosity cues were eliminated or greatly reduced. But it was noted that the performances of operated rats were deficient relative to those of normal rats (see Figure 8-3).

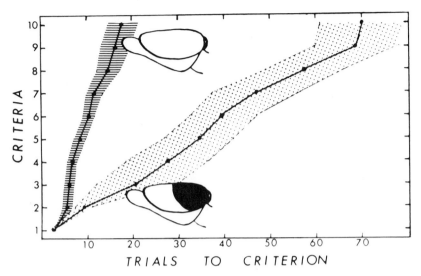

Figure 8-3. Mean trials to successive criteria on a depth-discrimination problem. The figure compares the acquisition performance of a group of 9 rats lacking visual neocortex to that of 12 normal rats. The "successive criteria" represent runs of consecutive correct responses; each point portrays the mean trial upon which a particular criterion was achieved for the first time, minus the criterion trials. The shading represents the standard error of the mean. The figure is based on data collected, but not presented in detail, by Braun *et al.* (1970).

3.3. Confounding Time and Experience

The inevitable confounding of experiential factors with time is a special problem in experiments concerned with partitioning the relative roles of exogenous and endogenous factors in recovery and in studies which use learning or relearning measures of recovery. One way to approach this problem is to use control groups which begin training or testing after an experimental group has displayed recovery. If the control group requires the same number of trials to recover as the experimental group, then recovery can be considered as a function of specific experience with the task. However, if the control group recovers in fewer trials, an explanation of recovery in terms of endogenous growth or neural reorganization as opposed to experiential factors is not clearly indicated because the extended recovery period represents both an unusual period of postoperative experience with the recovery environment and an extended opportunity for endogenous readjustments.

Finger and Reyes (1975) pointed this out in a learning experiment devoted to testing whether increased recovery time is associated with greater recovery. Rats were trained on five graded tactile discrimination problems after receiving simultaneous bilateral lesions of somatosensory neocortex. Training began after 14, 35, 180, 365, or 730 days of recovery for independent groups of rats, and performances were compared to those of sham-operated control groups which had the same recovery times. Although there was evidence of sparing in this experiment (20 of the 37 rats with somatosensory neocortex lesions learned at least one of the discrimination problems), the rats with cortical lesions were deficient relative to controls at each of the recovery intervals and there was no evidence of recovery defined as a diminishing degree of deficit with time. Although Finger and Reyes interpreted their results to suggest that there was no evidence of an influence of time-related factors on recovery after somatosensory cortical ablations, they also acknowledged that evidence of recovery as a function of time could not have been interpreted as being due to the time factor: The rats with longer recovery times also had more experience with whatever tactile stimuli were produced by moving about in their cages during the recovery period.

Given that one cannot create the pure conditions of time-without-experience and experience-without-time to which to assign experimental groups of subjects, differentiating between the effects of experience and of time requires holding one constant while systematically varying the other. However, since additional time inevitably implies additional experience, one is left with the control manipulation of varying experience while holding time constant.

Braun (1966) used this procedure in a study of the recovery of visual placing behavior in rats following ablations of neocortex. The number of animals and time available for the study were limited. Given some uncertainty concerning the ultimate amount of time the recovery phase of the experiment would take, and given the threat of an additional group being required as a control for aging factors if a group of operated rats were not permitted postoperative experience with the behavior until after the other groups had completed postoperative testing, a compromise strategy was necessary. The recovery period was held constant and one group of rats was given a crash program of rehabilitation by administering three times more testing (practice) trials for placing behavior than were given to the other groups in the experiment. Recovery of visual placing was found to be a function of practice and not a simple function of time: It was significantly enhanced by increasing the number of practice trials without increasing the period of time within which they were given, and the group receiving the extra experience achieved in only 4 days of testing the modest level of performance exhibited by the comparison group in 18 days. Massed practice had a definite facilitory effect on the recovery of this simple behavior, as did amphetamine treatment and the sequential, unilateral lesioning procedure (see Figure 8-4).

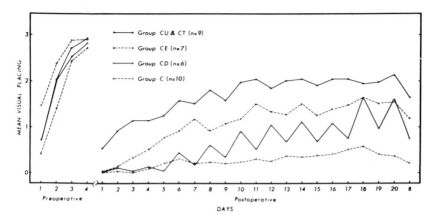

Figure 8-4. Visual placing performances of four groups of rats before and after complete ablations of neocortex separated by a 3-week recovery period. The consistent high level performances of normal rats (not displayed) indicated that the postoperative loss of visual placing was due to the cortical lesion. The visual placing scale is ordinal and represents increasing degrees of alacrity and accuracy on controlled tests for visual placing. Head orientation to the edge of a visual placing platform was scored 0.5, while accurate and immediate placing of the front feet on the platform was scored 3. Groups CU and CT had received two-stage ablations of neocortex and extensive interoperative practice. Group CE was postoperatively given 9 test trials per day instead of the usual 3. Group CD was injected with amphetamine on even-numbered days. Group C was given 3 test trials a day; this group never progressed beyond the recovery of head-orientation responses. The recovery of visual placing responses was reliably evident for each of the three experimental groups, but these responses tended to be sluggish and sometimes inaccurate. This figure is taken from Braun (1966).

3.4. Crowding the Limits: Long-Term Experiments

An extreme functional localization perspective is difficult to support because it demands a persistent loss over an extended time period and under conditions known to facilitate recovery. But behavioral capacities which appear to be lost following specific brain lesion and after a generous postoperative recovery period provide a convincing baseline against which to discern the exent of recovery produced by various independent manipulations. This was the strategy adopted in the Braun (1966) study of visual placing in brain-damaged rats described above. The results of several long-term studies have challenged extreme functional localization positions and provide convincing estimates of the limits within which recovery can be expected to occur. Experiments by Spear and Braun (1969b) and Wood, Spear, and Braun (1974) on the abilities of cats lacking visual neocortex to discriminate two-dimensional patterns are relevant here. Earlier research had suggested, on the one hand, that visual neocortex was necessary for pattern discrimination ability, and, on the other hand, that it was not (see Spear and Braun, 1969*b*, for a detailed analysis of the previous studies).

A number of features distinguished the two sets of earlier studies. Especially pertinent were the following three distinctive features of those which reported sparing of pattern (or form) discrimination: The stimuli were transilluminated, as opposed to being illuminated by reflected light. The stimuli were not equated for local luminosity cues; cats lacking visual neocortex readily learn to discriminate luminosity differences as shown by Smith (1937*b*), Urbaitis and Meikle (1968), and others. Finally, a greater number of postoperative training trials were used.

Accordingly, Spear and Braun's experiment was intended to resolve the ambiguities concerning the pattern discrimination abilities of cats lacking neocortex by (1) using pattern (rather than form) stimuli that were carefully equated for local luminosity differences and for total amount of contour (horizontal versus vertical stripes), (2) transilluminating the stimuli so as to produce marked contrast between the black and white stripes, and (3) using an automated training situation and being prepared to continue postoperative retraining (the cats had been trained prior to surgery) until obtaining convincing evidence that pattern discrimination ability was either present or absent. The cortical ablations included areas 17, 18, and most or all of 19.

In both the Spear and Braun (1969*b*) experiment and its more comprehensive follow-up (Wood *et al.*, 1974), the operated cats generally began with initial performances indistinguishable from chance and then advanced to a period of hundreds of trials during which performance was only marginally, but consistently, above chance. In the Spear and Braun study, for example, one of the cats (cat No. 3) performed at levels barely above chance (about 60% correct) for over 1300 trials, then appeared to reach an asymptote for an additional 2400 trials at about 75% correct. Only after 3760 trials did it reach the arbitrary criterion of at least 90% correct responding in two consecutive 40-trial training sessions. Preoperatively, this cat had mastered the pattern discrimination problem in about one-tenth this number of trials (see Figure 8-5).

Throughout these exeriments it was difficult to decide when to terminate training. In the Spear and Braun study, for example, conclusions concerning the ultimate capacity of cats lacking visual neocortex to perform the pattern habit would have been influenced by earlier, justifiable decisions to conclude the experiment. With regard to the measure employed (percent correct responding in blocks of 40 trials), the recovery of cat No. 3, for example, could have been judged as

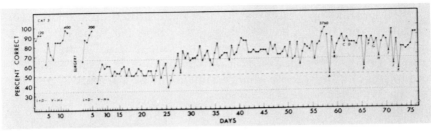

Figure 8-5.   The preoperative and postoperative performance of cat No. 3, from a study by Spear and Braun (1969b) on brightness and pattern discrimination tasks. Each point on the figure represents a session of 40 trials; two sessions were run on some days. The first function to the left represents the original acquisition of a brightness habit in three blocks of trials; the second function represents acquisition of a pattern habit in 10 blocks of trials. After surgery and a month of recovery, the cat was retrained on these two tasks, requiring 5 blocks of trials to relearn the brightness habit and 94 blocks of trials to relearn the pattern discrimination to a terminal criterion. Test trials were conducted over days 58 through 76 in order to determine that the cat was discriminating the patterns and not some other feature of the testing situation; the performance disruptions portrayed occurred when either the bottom halves of the stimulus panels (closest to the reward cup) were covered or when transmission intensity of the stimulus light was markedly reduced using neutral density filters. The dashed line represents chance performance, and the two dotted lines represent the 95% confidence interval.

"minimal," "moderate," or "complete" depending upon whether we had stopped after 30, 60, or 94 blocks of trials (the "minimal" judgment would have been based on evidence of significant sparing relative to chance). The first two potential stopping points had been preceded by long runs of asymptotic-appearing performance which had provoked a rather pessimistic view of the chances for further recovery. But each of these runs was followed by a relatively abrupt transition to a consistently higher level of performance.

The Wood et al. (1974) study assessed pattern discrimination abilities of cats lacking suprasylvian gyri in addition to areas 17, 18, and 19. Here, the problem of deciding when to stop the assessment required a somewhat different approach. The performances of three cats with the most extensive lesions did not extend beyond "marginal" or "moderate" recovery after more than 7000 training trials. However, it was noted that all three of the cats with the most extensive lesions displayed highly significant sparing of pattern discrimination ability relative to chance performance, after having remained at chance for over 1400 trials. In addition, all cats with lesions restricted to areas 17, 18, and 19 eventually reached the terminal criterion. Upon completion of the histology, it was evident that the experiment provided a convincing demonstration of the abilities of cats with complete removal of areas 17, 18, and 19, plus all of the middle and posterior suprasylvian gyri (including the Clare-Bishop area) to perform reliably a discrimination between horizontal and vertical stripes, despite the fact that none of the cats with the most extensive lesions rereached the original training criterion. A tendency to display an inordinate number of errors while performing significantly above chance appears to be a feature of the discrimination performances of animals with posterior neocortex lesions. This observation is addressed in the following subsection of this chapter.

It should be mentioned that other investigators have since challenged the conclusion of the original Spear and Braun study. Doty (1971) presented evidence suggesting that ablation of the visual areas eliminated a capacity for pattern vision in cats. This conclusion was based on a performance deficiency that was exhibited by a cat lacking areas 17, 18, and 19. Wood *et al.* (1974) subsequently noted that Doty's cat, while not reaching the normal performance criterion, nonetheless had performed significantly above chance after extensive retraining (mean = 68% correct).

Recently, Ritchie *et al.* (1976) suggested that the Spear and Braun cats may have used differential flicker cues produced by horizontally scanning the stimulus panels. Wood *et al.*, (1974) had acknowledged this possibility, but a study by Bauman (1975) indicates that performances of recovered cats with visual neocortex lesions are not severely disrupted when transilluminated pattern stimuli are rapidly flashed on and off at various rates of flicker, singly and in combination. Such a manipulation should disrupt discriminations based on self-generated flicker cues. However, using a pattern problem involving "numerosity cues," cats with large posterior ablations in the Ritchie *et al.* study failed to perform consistently above chance in approximately 4000 trials; yet these cats displayed a clear relearning capacity when checkered stimuli were used. The old question concerning the pattern-discrimination capacity of cats lacking visual neocortex apparently has become a question of the properties of pattern stimuli which are associated with evidence of sparing or loss of a pattern habit when visual neocortex is ablated. The problems mentioned here concerning the relationship between neocortex and pattern discrimination ability are discussed more thoroughly by Spear (in press).

3.5. Criterial and Continuous Performance Measures

Restricted criterial measures of performance can confuse interpretations of recovery either by supporting an overstatement of its extent, as when the criteria are overly generous, or by indicating that recovery does not occur, as is sometimes the case when the criteria are very stringent. Spear and Braun (1969*b*) provided an example, based on an earlier analysis by Horel, Bettinger, Royce, and Meyer (1966), of the way in which the selection of different specific criterion levels could lead to a wide range of different conclusions concerning the performances of brain-damaged as compared to those of normal rats. Using different criteria, one could suggest that rats lacking visual neocortex were significantly superior, equivalent, or significantly inferior to unoperated rats on either of two brightness-discrimination problems (see Figure 8-6).

When performances over a range of criteria from 1 to 20 consecutive correct responses were graphed by Spear and Braun, the normal rats appeared "inferior" at low performance criterion levels; this was attributed to their greater aversion to light (Krechevsky, 1936). It was also apparent from the relative slopes of the learning functions that the performances of the operated rats became progressively retarded as more stringent criterion levels of performance were demanded: This reflected the cost, to the rat, of not having a visual neocortex. The criterial point of equivalent-appearing performances of the two groups reflected the crossover point of the two learning functions. This point

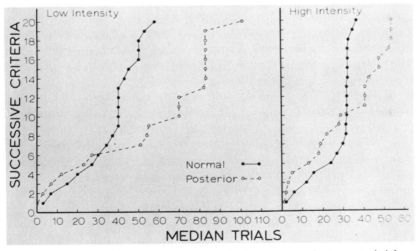

Figure 8-6.   Median trials to successive criteria by four groups of rats on two brightness-discrimination habits in which the brighter alternative was always positive. On one problem the brightness difference between the two stimuli was relatively low while on the other the difference was relatively high. The "successive criteria" represent runs of consecutive correct responses minus the criterion trials. Note the relative inefficiency of rats with posterior neocortex lesions at the higher criterion levels. This figure was taken from Spear and Braun (1969*a*).

appeared to vary as a direct function of the intensity difference between the two discriminative stimuli. Lashley's (1935) conclusion concerning the equivalence of learning performances of rats lacking visual neocortex and normal rats on a brightness-discrimination problem had been based on a measure of trials to a single, very stringent, criterion level, and he used a learning situation in which the brighter of the two alternative stimuli was always positive and was apparently quite intense relative to the darker alternative. Spear and Braun suggested that this outcome might have been a coincidental reflection of a special relationship between the stimulus parameters, the demands of the training situation, and the arbitrary criterion level that had been used by Lashley.

A tendency to exhibit inefficient discrimination performances while displaying consistent sparing of a learned habit appears to be a characteristic of animals with posterior neocortex lesions. This was shown in the studies of pattern discrimination in cats lacking visual neocortex (e.g., Spear and Braun, 1969a) and in the Braun et al., (1970) study of depth discrimination in which a disparity between normal and operated rats became more pronounced as a function of increasingly stringent criteria. To the degree these observations imply the possibility that this is a general feature of animals with any kind of neocortex lesion, decisions concerning the performance abilities (sparing) of such animals probably should not be based on measures of performance to a single criterion level. The Spear and Braun (1969b) analysis suggests that when criterial measures are used they should reflect a comprehensively broad range of performance levels. A characterization of performances of normal versus operated animals is probably more accurate and fine-grained when based on a description of their differences over such a range. This consideration is especially important in studies designed to relate performance changes to physiological changes or to various independent manipulations: In most experiments, one would have to be inordinately lucky to have a specific criterion level of performance correspond in time to some related underlying physiological change.

Selected criterial measures are useful for describing noteworthy inflections and other statistically interesting reference points in continuous data and for helping to decide when to stop an experiment. But it is suggested that such measures have only limited value when they constitute the principle or sole inferential data in brain–behavior experiments. Some ambiguities in the brain–behavior literature probably could be circumvented by the general use of measures reflecting continuity of performance over time.

3.6. Time-Defined Sequelae of Recovery

It is evident that specific kinds of brain trauma have broader effects on behavioral performances than are implied by the set of behavioral observations upon which a case study or an experiment chooses to focus. Highly specific dependent measures of loss and subsequent recovery tend to tap just a few of these effects. For example, in the visual placing study previously mentioned (Braun, 1966), rats lacking neocortex were noted to display recoverable deficits in feeding behavior and permanent-appearing deficits in tactual placing in addition to the visual placing deficits, but these additional observations were not elaborated.

Brain damage tends to produce syndromes which are defined by a profile of losses and recoveries over time. In short-term studies the specific nature of the losses can be obscured by a host of general, but transient, debilitating effects. Long-term studies are necessary to partition such effects and define accompanying losses. For example, the initially complete loss of consummatory behavior following lateral hypothalamic lesions, originally described by Anand and Brobeck (1951), overshadows the more subtle and permanent-appearing deficits and changes in such things as drinking behavior, responsiveness to flavor stimuli, set-point for body-weight regulation, salt appetite, meal patterns, and so on (see Epstein, 1971, for a comprehensive review). These persistent deficits give profound clues to the functioning of a neurological feeding system, and they can be observed clearly only after consummatory behavior and weight-regulation capacity have recovered.

From a recovery-of-function perspective, long-term studies provide the opportunity to characterize recovery as a sequence of changes over time to emphasize, where appropriate, the continuous and invariant nature of a particular recovery process (e.g., Teitelbaum, 1971). Such characterizations of recovery in terms of sequences of stages using a multivariate approach contribute to recovery research in two important ways: They provide a comprehensive basis for comparing separate studies of the consequences of damage to specific brain areas. In addition, a time-based measure of progression from one stage of recovery to another facilitates the assessment of the specific consequences of various rehabilitating manipulations. Both of these advantages were apparent in a recent long-term study concerning the effects of neocortex removal on feeding behavior in rats (Braun, 1975).

Braun's study was based on the comprehensive analysis of consummatory behavior pioneered by Teitelbaum and Epstein (1962) in their studies of the "lateral hypothalamic syndrome." Special attention was paid to the "invariant sequence" of recovery stages which Epstein

(1971) considers especially definitive of this syndrome. The most striking result of the study was the degree of correspondence between the "lateral hypothalamic syndrome" and the "neocortical feeding syndrome" according to these measures. Rats lacking neocortex were initially aphagic and adipsic (stage I, according to Teitelbaum and Epstein, 1962). This was followed by a period of anorexia and adipsia during which only highly palatable wet foods were eaten, but not in amounts sufficient to maintain a constant level of body-weight (stage II). Next, the rats recovered the capacity to regulate body weight on wet foods, and nibbled the dry food that was continuously available, but did not drink water (stage III, adipsia). This was followed by a return of water-drinking and the ability to regulate body weight on dry food alone, indicating that the final recovery stage had been reached (stage IV). This pattern and sequence of recovery was as characteristic of rats that sustained lesions restricted to anterolateral neocortex as it was of rats completely lacking neocortex. However, the group with the more restricted lesion progressed through the stages in 7 days as opposed to the 17 days that were required for the group with larger lesions, suggesting a mass action effect. The pattern of distinct recovery stages over time was *not* observed following large posterior or unilateral cortical ablations. From this it was inferred that disruption of intrinsic cortical systems related to feeding, rather than nonspecific trauma, was responsible for the feeding deficits observed in the anterior and complete preparations, and that such systems were focused in anterior neocortex (this is supported by the observations of Kolb and Nonneman, 1975, in a study which was published shortly before Braun's study appeared).

The study was continued for 4 months beyond the initial observation of stage IV recovery, during which time body weight was monitored and tests of finickiness and prandial drinking were conducted. Again, as previously observed in rats with lateral hypothalamic lesions (see Epstein, 1971), rats with near-complete ablations of neocortex were found to be abnormally finicky when their drinking water was adulterated with quinine, and they displayed prandial drinking by showing an abnormal reduction of fluid intake when their dry food was withdrawn for a day. They also displayed what appeared to be a permanent reduction of their set-point for body-weight regulation as described by Powley and Keesey (1970) for rats with lateral hypothalamic lesions.

The effects of neocortical ablation and the effects of lateral hypothalamic lesions show striking parallels in both the sequencing of recovery stages and the nature of the apparently permanent deficits. Qualitatively, the two quite different lesions appear to have the same kinds of effects. Quantitatively, however, there are differences: Rats with lateral hypothalamic lesions appear to remain longer in each stage of recovery, so that overall recovery takes longer. The similarities strongly suggest that neocortical and hypothalamic contributions to feeding behavior are interdependent, rather than unique. The differences suggest a more modest contribution to feeding behavior by neocortical systems.

Braun's (1975) experiment also contained a group of rats that were subjected to sequential unilateral ablations of neocortex. This was done because it had been noted in passing, but not quantified (Braun, 1966), that rats subjected to this procedure did not require the degree of postoperative care and special feeding that had been necessary for a group receiving simultaneous bilateral ablations. The comprehensive analysis of feeding behavior in the 1975 study provided a solid foundation for examining some of the details of recovery that might be facilitated by the sequential unilateral procedure. The results were as follows: After the second ablation, rats with sequential unilateral ablations displayed a foreshortened stage I of recovery (they began to eat wet foods significantly faster than the single-stage group), and they by-passed stage III altogether by drinking their first water on the same day that they ate dry food for the first time. However, their consummatory behavior was not sufficient to arrest a sharp decline in weight to levels equivalent to those reached by the simultaneous bilateral group. They did not begin to regulate body weight any sooner than the bilateral group, and their body weight remained significantly lower than normal throughout the duration of the experiment (120 days following the second-stage ablation). Like the bilateral groups, they displayed finickiness and prandial drinking.

Appropriate feeding and drinking behaviors appeared much earlier for the sequentially lesioned group, but this did not have significant effects on their level of body-weight regulation. In other words, behaviors that would be expected to recover anyway recovered earlier following the sequential procedure whereas deficiencies that appeared to be relatively permanent were not obviously affected by the sequential lesioning procedure. Thus, the comprehensive analysis of consummatory behavior used in this study allowed an interesting distinction to be made between the effects of simultaneous bilateral and sequential unilateral ablations of neocortex.

The continuous nature of many instances of recovery following brain trauma, as defined by a sequence of changes occurring over time, is also reflected in clinical observations. Those by Gershuni (described by Luria et al., 1969, page 370) regarding the loss and subsequent recovery of hearing following concussions induced by blast injuries pro-

vide a particularly interesting example. The gradual progression of recovery in moderately severe cases begins with an initial stage of total
unresponsiveness to auditory stimulation. This is followed by a stage of
high thresholds for the elicitation of certain physiological responses to
sound (e.g., the "cochleopupillar reflex" which is dilation of the pupil
to sudden intense sounds) without concomitant evidence of auditory
perception—the brain responds to the sound without the person whose
brain it is appearing able to report hearing the sound. The next stage
of recovery is characterized by a gradual diminution of the threshold
for the elicitation of the cochleopupillary reflex; this is followed by evidence of auditory perception of only very intense stimuli. Finally, there
is a progressive lowering of the threshold for auditory perception to a
point below the intensity necessary to elicit the cochleopupillary reflex.
This represents the restoration of approximately normal auditory perception.

These kinds of analyses obviously provide a much more compelling and meaningful frame of reference for evaluating the extent of a
brain injury as it concerns behavior in the first place, and they provide
a more sensitive perspective from which to evaluate the effectiveness of
any therapeutic procedures that might be attempted.

4. SUMMARY AND CONCLUDING REMARKS

This chapter addressed two related problems in brain lesion research: (1) the problem of accounting for the physiological foundations
of apparent behavioral recovery following brain trauma and (2) the an-
alytical problem of characterizing the behavioral consequences, the
losses as well as the recoveries, of brain damage. The specification of
relevant physiological processes and their relationships to recovery obviously depends to a great degree on the adequacy, comprehensiveness,
and sensitivity of the behavioral measures by which their influences are
inferred. However, unique physiological events probably will not be
found to underlie all instances of behavioral recovery; indeed, such
events may be very limited. Various psychological processes related to
learning, perception, motivation, generalized arousal, and so on must
be taken into account as adjunctive and perhaps sometimes even superordinate to physiological factors. Psychological processes will be "adjunctive" to the extent that they possibly contribute to the activation of
crucial physiological processes. In many instances of facilitated behavioral recovery following sequential unilateral lesions, for example, interoperative experience or stimulation appears to be necessary (Meyer,
1958; see also Finger, this volume); these experiential and stimulation

factors may induce and/or guide crucial physiological processes in some cases. Psychological factors will be "superordinate" to the extent that special training and stimulation factors are observed to promote recovery of a behavioral capacity that was not observed over prolonged periods of postoperative recovery time. Such behavioral capacities often can be interpreted as representing reinstitution of function (see Goldberger, 1974; LeVere, 1975) insofar as they are based on the development of new ways of adaptively responding to old environmental contingencies by using either different stimuli or new response strategies.

The chapter began by denying time *per se* as important to recovery while acknowledging events which are confounded with measures of time as the foundation for rational theoretical accounts of the recovery process. Although the expression *time-dependent events* may be useful for describing empirical observations of endogenous processes with which behavioral recovery may be thought to concur, *event-dependent time* is viewed as a more accurate theoretical expression of the relationship between time and such processes. The utility of this point of view should become apparent when sequences of endogenous processes relevant to recovery are ultimately described and the biophysical foundations of these processes are determined. For the present purposes, "time" was viewed simply as providing a framework within which to specify and analyze endogenous events and as a convenient umbrella under which to integrate the broad range of topics covered in the chapter.

Within this framework, time can play several kinds of roles in recovery-of-function experiments. As elaborated under Correlates of Recovery (section 2), time can be used as a relatively neutral intervening variable which implies endogenous processes which themselves define the course of recovery. The time variable is also useful empirically as a correlative frame of reference within which to determine relationships between measures of endogenous processes and measures of behavioral recovery following brain damage. In this regard, the discussion emphasized reversible endogenous processes which normally accompany brain trauma as probably accounting for a substantial portion of the temporal course of both short-term and long-term recovery following brain damage. Thus, the first substantive section of the chapter ended by making a case for a diaschisis hypothesis as a most parsimonious theoretical explanation of recovery in view of available data.

The second major section of this chapter, "The Limits of Recovery: Methodological Considerations," began by defining the expressions *behavioral recovery, sparing,* and *deficiency* as they relate to behavioral assessments in brain–behavior studies. This was followed by a discussion of how interpretations of brain function and recovery based on such assessments can vary substantially as a function of simple procedural variables. Special problems encountered with the inevitable confounding of time and experience during recovery were discussed, as were the value and some of the difficulties of long-term experiments as they relate to both recovery of function and functional localization concerns. In addition, restricted criterial measures of performance were described as having limited utility in brain–behavior experiments. Finally, the role of time in defining comprehensive sequelae of recovery and losses following brain damage and the value of characterizing the effects of brain damage in these terms were discussed.

Thus, two important factors in accounts of the temporal course of recovery following brain damage have been reviewed with the following general conclusions: Reversible endogenous brain processes probably underlie a substantial portion of the behavioral recovery that occurs following brain damage. The comprehensiveness and grain of behavioral analyses applied to assessing the limits of recovery underlies the degree to which (1) the limits of recovery are accurately estimated and (2) the behavioral consequences of brain damage are appropriately characterized.

5. REFERENCES

Anand, B. K., and Brobeck, J. R. Hypothalamic control of food intake in rats and cats. *Yale Journal of Biology and Medicine,* 1951, *24,* 123–140.

Bauman, T. P. Behavioral cues and brain areas involved in functional recovery after removal of visual cortex in the cat. Master's Thesis, 1975, Kansas State University.

Beach, F. A., Hebb, D. O., Morgan, C. T., and Nissen, H. W. *The neuropsychology of Lashley.* New York: McGraw-Hill, 1960.

Blakemore, C. B., and Falconer, M. A. Long-term effects of anterior temporal lobectomy on certain cognitive functions. *Journal of Neurology, Neuro-Surgery, and Psychiatry,* 1967, *30,* 364–367.

Brady, J. V., and Nauta, W. J. H. Subcortical mechanisms in emotional behavior: Affective changes following septal forebrain lesions in the albino rat. *Journal of Comparative and Physiological Psychology,* 1953, *46,* 339–346.

Braun, J. J. The neocortex and visual placing in rats. *Brain Research,* 1966, *1,* 381–394.

Braun, J. J. Neocortex and feeding behavior in the rat. *Journal of Comparative and Physiological Psychology,* 1975, *89,* 507–522.

Braun, J. J., and Gault, F. P. Monocular and binocular control of horizontal optokinetic nystagmus in cats and rabbits. *Journal of Comparative and Physiological Psychology,* 1969, *69,* 12–16.

Braun, J. J., Meyer, P. M., and Meyer, D. R. Sparing of a brightness habit in rats following visual decortication. *Journal of Comparative and Physiological Psychology,* 1966, *61,* 79–82.

Braun, J. J., Lundy, E. G., and McCarthy, F. Depth discrimination in rats following removal of visual neocortex. *Brain Research,* 1970, *20,* 283–291.

Brodal, A. Self-observations and neuro-anatomical considerations after a stroke. *Brain*, 1973, *96* (Pt. IV), 675–694.

Devor, M. Neuroplasticity in the sparing or deterioration of function and early olfactory tract lesions. *Science*, 1975, *190*, 998–1000.

Doty, R. W. Survival of pattern vision after removal of striate cortex in the adult cat. *Journal of Comparative Neurology*, 1971, *143*, 341–370.

Epstein, A. N. The lateral hypothalamic syndrome: Its implications for the physiological psychology of hunger and thirst. In E. Stellar and J. M. Sprague (Eds.), *Progress in physiological psychology*. Vol. 4. New York: Academic Press, 1971.

Finger, S., and Reyes, R. Long-term deficits after somatosensory cortical lesions in rats. *Physiology and Behavior*, 1975, *15*, 289–293.

Glassman, R. B. Recovery following sensorimotor cortical damage: Evoked potentials, brain stimulation, and motor control. *Experimental Neurology*, 1971, *33*, 16–29.

Glassman, R. B., and Malamut, B. L. Recovery from electroencephalographic slowing and reduced evoked potentials after somatosensory cortical damage in cats. *Behavioral Biology*, 1976, *17*, 333–354.

Goldberger, M. E. Recovery of Movement after CNS lesions in monkeys. In D. G. Stein, J. J. Rosen, and N. Butters (Eds.), *Plasticity and recovery of function in the central nervous system*. New York: Academic Press, 1974.

Goldman, P. S. An alternative to developmental plasticity: Heterology of CNS structures in infants and adults. In D. G. Stein, J. J. Rosen, and N. Butters (Eds.), *Plasticity and recovery of function in the central nervous system*. New York: Academic Press, 1974.

Grijalva, C. V., Lindholm, E., Schallert, T., and Bicknell, E. J. Gastric pathology and aphagia following lateral hypothalamic lesions in rats: Effects of preoperative weight reduction. *Journal of Comparative and Physiological Psychology*, 1976, *90*, 505–519.

Horel, J. A., Bettinger, L. A., Royce, G. J., and Meyer, D. R. Role of neocortex in the learning and relearning of two visual habits by the rat. *Journal of Comparative and Physiological Psychology*, 1966, *61*, 66–78.

Kerr, F. W. L. Structural and functional evidence of plasticity in the central nervous system. *Experimental Neurology*, 1975, *48*, 16–31.

Kleihues, P., Hossmann, K. A., Pegg, A. E., Kobayashi, K., and Zimmermann V. Resuscitation of the monkey brain after one hour complete ischemia: III. Indications of metabolic recovery. *Brain Research*, 1975, *95*, 61–73.

Kolb, B., and Nonneman, A. Prefrontal cortex and the regulation of food intake in the rat. *Journal of Comparative and Physiological Psychology*, 1975, *88*, 806–815.

Kreschevsky, I. Brain mechanisms and brightness discrimination learning. *Journal of Comparative Psychology*, 1936, *21*, 404–445.

Lashley, K. S. The mechanism of vision: XII. Nervous structures concerned in habits based on reactions to light. *Comparative Psychology Monograph*, 1935, *11*, 43–79.

Lashley, K. S. In search of the engram. *Society of Experimental Biology Symposium No. 4: Physiological Mechanisms in Animal Behavior*. Cambridge, England: Cambridge University Press, 1950, pp. 454–482. (Reprinted in Beach, Hebb, Morgan, and Nissen, 1960).

Lennenberg, E. H. The effect of age on the outcome of cortical nervous system disease in children. In R. L. Isaacson (Ed.), *The neuropsychology of development*. New York: John Wiley and Sons, 1968.

LeVere, T. E. Neural stability, sparing, and behavioral recovery following brain damage. *Psychological Review*, 1975, *82*, 344–358.

Levine, M. S., and Schwartzbaum, J. S. Sensorimotor functions of the striatopallidal system and lateral hypothalamus and consummatory behavior in rats. *Journal of Comparative and Physiological Psychology*, 1973, *85*, 615–635.

Levine, S. Anoxic-ischemic encephalopathy in rats. *The American Journal of Pathology,* 1960, *36,* 1–17.

Loesche, J., and Steward, O. Behavioral correlates of denervation and reinnervation of the hippocampal formation of the rat: Recovery of alternation performance following unilateral entorhinal cortex lesions. *Brain Research Bulletin,* 1977, *2,* 31–39.

Luria, A. R., Naydin, V. L., Tsvetkova, L. S., and Vinarskaya, E. N. Restoration of higher cortical function following local brain damage. In P. J. Vinken and G. W. Brugh (Eds.), *Handbook of clinical neurology.* New York: John Wiley and Sons, 1969.

Lynch, G., Matthews, D. A., Mosko, S., Parks, T., and Cotman, C. Induced AChE-rich layer in rat dentate gyrus following entorhinal lesions. *Brain Research,* 1972, *42,* 311–319.

Lynch, G., Stanfield, B., and Cotman, C. Developmental differences in postlesion axonal growth in the hippocampus. *Brain Research,* 1973, *59,* 155–168.

Macht, M. B. Effects of d-amphetamine on hemidecorticate, decorticate, and decerebrate cats. *American Journal of Physiology,* 1950, *163,* 731–732.

Maling, H. M., and Acheson, G. H. Righting and other postural activity in low decerebrate and in spinal cats after d-amphetamine. *Journal of Neurophysiology,* 1946, *9,* 379–386.

Marshall, J. F., and Teitelbaum, P. Further analysis of sensory inattention following lateral hypothalamic damage in rats. *Journal of Comparative and Physiological Psychology,* 1974, *86,* 375–395.

McCouch, G. P., Austin, G. M., Liu, C. N., and Liu, C. Y. Sprouting as a cause of spasticity. *Journal of Neurophysiology,* 1958, *21,* 205–216.

Meyer, D. R. Some psychological determinants of sparing and loss following damage to the brain. In H. F. Harlow and C. N. Woolsey (Eds.), *Biological and biochemical bases of behavior.* Madison, Wis.: The University of Wisconsin Press, 1958.

Meyer, D. R. Access to engrams. *American Psychologist,* 1972, *27,* 124–133.

Meyer, D. R., and Meyer, P. M. Dynamics and bases of recoveries of functions after injuries to the cerebral cortex. *Physiological Psychology,* 1977, *5,* 133–165.

Meyer, D. R., Isaac, W., and Maher, B. The role of stimulation in spontaneous reorganization of visual habits. *Journal of Comparative and Physiological Psychology,* 1958, *51,* 546–548.

Meyer, P. M., Horel, J. A., and Meyer, D. R. Effects of dl-amphetamine upon placing responses in neodecorticate cats. *Journal of Comparative and Physiological Psychology,* 1963, *56,* 402– 405.

Meyer, P. M., Anderson, R. A., and Braun, M. G. Visual cliff preferences following lesions of the visual neocortex in cats and rats. *Psychonomic Science,* 1966, *4,* 269–270.

Parker, A. J., and Smith, C. W. Functional recovery from spinal cord trauma following incision of spinal meninges in dogs. *Research in Veterinary Science,* 1974, *16,* 276–279.

Powley, T. L., and Keesey, R. E. Relationship of body weight to the lateral hypothalamic feeding syndrome. *Journal of Comparative and Physiological Psychology,* 1970, 25–36.

Ritchie, G. D., Meyer, P. M., and Meyer, D. R. Residual spatial vision of cats with lesions of the visual cortex. *Experimental Neurology,* 1976, *53,* 227–254.

Rosner, B. S. Recovery of function and localization of function in historical perspective. In D. G. Stein, J. J. Rosen, and N. Butters (Eds.), *Plasticity and recovery of function in the central nervous system.* New York: Academic Press, 1974.

Russell, W. R., and Nathan, P. W. Traumatic amnesia. *Brain,* 1946, *69,* 280–300.

Schneider, G. E., and Jhaveri, S. R. Neuroanatomical correlates of spared or altered function after brain lesions in the newborn hamster. In D. G. Stein, J. J. Rosen, and N. Butters (Eds.), *Plasticity and recovery of function in the central nervous system.* New York: Academic Press, 1974.

Smith, K. U. The postoperative effects of removal of the striate cortex upon certain unlearned visually controlled reactions in the cat. *Journal of Genetic Psychology,* 1937*a,* *50,* 137–156.

Smith, K. U. Visual discrimination in the cat: V. The postoperative effects of removal of striate cortex upon intensity discrimination. *Journal of Genetic Psychology,* 1937*b, 51,* 329–370.

Smith, K. U., and Bridgeman, M. The neural mechanisms of movement vision and optic nystagmus. *Journal of Experimental Psychology,* 1943, *33,* 165–187.

Sobotka, P., Jirasek, A., and Gebert, T. Morphological consequences of prolonged complete brain ischemia. *Brain Research,* 1974, *79,* 111–118.

Sorenson, C. A., and Ellison, G. D. Striatal organization of feeding behavior in the decorticate rat. *Experimental Neurology,* 1970, *29,* 162–174.

Spear, P. D. Behavioral and neurophysiological mechanisms of recovery from visual cortex damage. In J. M. Sprague and A. N. Epstein (Eds.), *Progress in psychobiology and physiological psychology.* Vol. 7. New York: Academic Press, in press.

Spear, P. D., and Braun, J. J. Non-equivalence of normal and posteriorly neodecorticated rats on two brightness discrimination problems. *Journal of Comparative and Physiological Psychology,* 1969*a, 67,* 235–239.

Spear, P. D., and Braun, J. J. Pattern discrimination following removal of visual neocortex in the cat. *Experimental Neurology,* 1969*b, 25,* 331–347.

Stein, D. G., Rosen, J. J., and Butters, N. (Eds.), *Plasticity and recovery of function in the central nervous system.* New York: Academic Press, 1974.

Steward, O., Cotman, C., and Lynch, G. A quantitative autoradiographic and electrophysiological study of the reinnervation of the dentate gyrus by the contralateral entorhinal cortex following ipsilateral entorhinal lesions. *Brain Research,* 1976, *114,* 181–200.

Stewart, J. W., and Ades, H. W. The time factor in reintegration of a learned habit lost after temporal lobe lesions in monkeys. *Journal of Comparative and Physiological Psychology,* 1951, *44,* 479–486.

Stricker, E. M., and Zigmond, M. J. Recovery of function after damage to central catecholamine-containing neurons: A neurochemical model for the lateral hypothalamic syndrome. In J. M. Sprague and A. N. Epstein (Eds.), *Progress in psychobiology and physiological psychology.* Vol. 6. New York: Academic Press, 1976.

Teitelbaum, P. The encephalization of hunger. In E. Stellar and J. M. Sprague (Eds.), *Progress in physiological psychology.* Vol. 4. New York: Academic Press, 1971.

Teitelbaum, P., and Epstein, A. The lateral hypothalamic syndrome: Recovery of feeding and drinking after lateral hypothalamic lesions. *Psychological Review,* 1962, *69,* 74–90.

Urbaitis, J. C., and Meikle, T. H., Jr. Relearning a dark-light discrimination by cats after cortical and collicular lesions. *Experimental Neurology,* 1968, *20,* 295–311.

Varon, S. S. In vitro study of developing neural tissue and cells: Past and prospective contributions. In F. O. Schmitt (Ed.), *The neurosciences, second study program.* New York: Rockefeller University Press, 1970.

Volpe, J. J. Perinatal hypoxic-ischemic brain injury. *Pediatric Clinics of North America,* 1976, *23,* 383–397.

Von Monakow, C. "Die Lokalisation im Grosshirnrinde und der Abban der Funktion durch korticale Herde," 1914, Wiesbaden: J. F. Bergmann.

Wood, C. C., Spear, P. D., and Braun, J. J. Direction-specific deficits in horizontal optokinetic nystagmus following removal of visual cortex in the cat. *Brain Research,* 1973, *60,* 231–237.

Wood, C. C., Spear, P. D., and Braun, J. J. Effects of sequential lesions of suprasylvian gyri and visual cortex on pattern discrimination in the cat. *Brain Research,* 1974, *66,* 443–466.

9

Testing Procedures and the Interpretation of Behavioral Data

ULF NORRSELL

1. INTRODUCTION

The most common experimental approach in studies of the various functional assignments of different parts of the central nervous system has been studies of the behavioral effects of localized lesions of that system. A given type of behavior has been compared either in the same individual before and after the lesion, or between individuals some of which have suffered the lesion and others not. The theory behind this approach is attractive for its simplicity; if a structure is necessary for a function, then that function should become altered or disappear following its removal. The application of that theory is, unfortunately, less simple. The functions which are compared before and after the lesions are rarely if ever isolated and static phenomena, but more or less integrated with other processes which belong to everyday life. For that reason defects can often be masked by compensatory behavior. Alternatively, changes may occur between the preoperative and postoperative periods or between animals even without any lesions. Of the many problems concerning lesion experiments, some of those regarding the actual testing will be discussed below.

The behavioral functions which are investigated can usually (with some exceptions like sleep studies) be characterized as stimulus–response events. The use of this type of behavior has the advantage of

ULF NORRSELL • Department of Physiology, University of Göteborg, Göteborg, Sweden

providing quantifiable data by being divisionable into discrete "trials" in relation to the presentation of stimuli or the occurrence of responses. The experimental situation can be designed so as to permit selective evaluation of stimulus reception (i.e., afferent systems) or response characteristics (i.e., efferent systems) or superimposed functions (structures concerned with motivation or learning, etc.).

Stimulus—response events often refer to variations of classical conditioned reflexes (e.g., a dog salivating at the ticking of a metronome, which is followed by the serving of food; see Pavlov, 1927) or to discriminative operant behavior (e.g., a pigeon pecking a button which has become illuminated, thereby leading to the appearance of grains; see Honig, 1966). A definition characterizing the experimental environment as a stimulus (Konorski, 1948) leads to the inclusion of, for example, rats pressing levers in constant surroundings. The types of tests which are commonly used for examining motor functions can also be regarded as stimulus–response events. Functional aspects of the cortico-spinal tract in the monkey have been evaluated in lesion experiments with studies of "relatively independent finger movements" (Lawrence and Hopkins, 1976). This behavior is a motor response involving the grasping of small pieces of food between thumb and index finger, but it is elicited by a specific stimulus, the presence of "morsels of food in small food wells." Simple tests for locomotor precision like a cat's walk along a narrow bar (Lindström and Norrsell, 1971) are also stimulus dependent. The probability is very low for cats to walk on bars placed on the floor. The height from the floor to the bar provides a stimulus (or incentive) for the cat to produce the desired response.

The tests for motor function which have been described differ from tests involving conditioning with regard to learning. The difference may be quantitative rather than qualitative, however, since it is notoriously difficult to exclude learning from any behavioral performance (see, e.g., Barnett, 1973). It is probably safest to assume that learning is involved to a certain extent in all tests, and that the closer the testing situation lies to the common behavior of the species in question the less time will have to be spent on the training of the experimental subjects. It follows that tests demanding formal training, although they may appear to be cumbersome, actually have the advantage of involving quantifiable and thus controlled learning.

A single test and its results will provide a set of experimental data, but at the same time it is part of a behavioral continuum and thus also a precept for subsequent tests. A test can be designed for establishing the presence of a function. The same test may, on the other hand, be unsuitable for studying its absence. It is, for example, simple to study the normal behavior of a cat walking on a bar. Cats with serious motor defects, however, do not walk on bars, but tend to cling desperately to the part where they are placed, especially after having fallen down once or twice. Thus, in the context of lesion experiments, bar-walking is suitable for showing an absence of defects after some lesions, but not the type of defects caused by others.

A behavioral defect which appears after a lesion can emanate from a disturbance in any part of the set of functions which constitutes the tested behavior: signal reception, motivation, memory, response, or reinforcement mechanisms. The traditional way to circumvent this problem of interpretation is to perform several different tests which emphasize different functions, and thus to single out common denominators. It is sometimes possible to utilize the bilaterality of most nervous structures for this type of control. The afferent and/or efferent functions, whichever will be studied, are in this case restricted to and tested in one body half at a time. It then becomes possible to show after unilateral lesions that a given function is defective unilaterally, the experimental subject serving as its own control for the soundness of all other functions.

A very large number of different training and testing techniques have been used in lesion experiments. A general survey of such techniques is therefore not within the scope of this chapter, and the reader wanting details of special techniques is directed to handbooks of neurology (e.g., Vinken and Bruyn, 1969–1976) or animal learning (e.g., Kimble, 1961; Mackintosh, 1974). Two techniques which we have used extensively in our laboratory (type II conditioning in dogs, and T-maze discrimination in cats), however, can be used to illustrate some general problems.

I. *Definitions of Stimulus and Response.* A negative finding, i.e., the lack of postoperative defects, is valid only if (1) it can be shown that the behavior is still being generated by the same stimulus and (2) that the response is unchanged, not only the behavioral results, but also the behavioral performance and stategy.

II. *Level of Training.* Behavior generally changes with either repetition or nonrepetition. Postoperative effects for that reason can be different depending on the amount of preoperative training.

III. *Level of Performance.* It is necessary to work with comparable levels of performance of a given behavior if a comparison is to be made between different periods of time or different subjects. For that reason it is often desirable to establish the optimal performance (e.g., the threshold of a stimulus discrimination) in each case. Testing of the optimal performance, on the other hand, is very straining to the experimental subject.

2. METHODS

Figure 9-1 illustrates a type II conditioned reflex which we have been using. The dog in the picture had not been fed for 24 hours and had learned that a push on the button in front of its nose with the nose would result in food being served from a rotating food tray in the hole beneath its head. The dog had learned also that the response is effective only when it is receiving light tactile stimulation of one hindlimb.

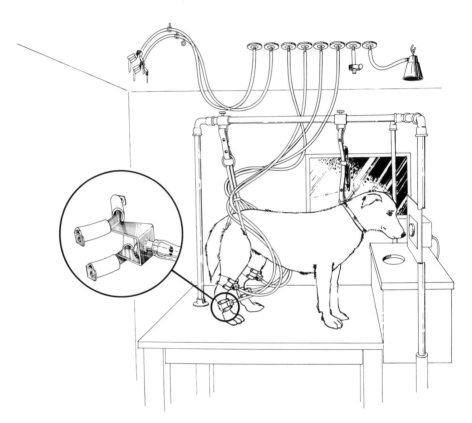

Figure 9-1.   Dog being tested for light tactile sensitivity with a type II conditioned reflex. The dog had learned to push the button in front of its nose when being stimulated by puffs of air through one of the nozzles attached to the hindlimbs. Pushing the button interrupted the stimulation and caused food to be served in the hole below the head. The dog was alone in a semisoundproof chamber and was watched through the oneway window seen behind the head. A white noise was used to mask acoustic accessory cues, and the bell-shaped instrument in the ceiling produced its supersonic components with compressed air. Reproduced after Norrsell (1975) with the permission of *Acta Neurobioliae Experimentalis*.

The stimulus was puffs of air (3/sec) through one of the four nozzles which were attached to the hindlimbs. The stimulation was interrupted when the dog pushed the button (and got food) or after 10 sec in the absence of response.

The training of this behavior was made in several steps. The dogs were first taught that a button push led to food being served. The food was then withheld intermittently in order to make the dogs push several times for each portion. The number of pushes for each reinforcement was increased gradually on a temporal basis until an interval between reinforcements was reached which was suitable for the presentation of stimuli. The stimuli were then introduced as prerequisites for reinforcement. Under these circumstances some of the responses happened to coincide with the stimulation and food was served. With repetition the dogs began to respond regularly at the onset of stimulation with a fairly constant latency. The number of button pushes in absence of stimulation decreased in parallel, albeit more slowly. The ideal testing situation was reached when the animal responded to every stimulation with optimal speed and refrained from pushing the button during the intervals. Unfortunately, these two criteria are to a certain extent antagonistic (i.e., quiet dogs are sometimes inattentive). Depending on the dog the ideal situation could be difficult to reach when using light tactile stimulation. It was certainly easier with acoustic or visual stimuli, or stronger stimuli in Pavlov's (1927) terminology.

The dog of Figure 9-1 was secured by a leash and loops around the hindlimbs. It bears mentioning that this was done in order to prevent inadvertent displacement of the stimulating nozzles. There was no need to leash the animals in order to stop them from jumping down. Experimental situations where the animals have to be restrained by force, in our experience, tend to produce erratic behavior. For that reason dogs were used rather than cats when working with light tactile stimulation with attached stimulators (Norrsell, 1975). Cats are not so easily subdued but, on the other hand, have the advantage of a better-explored nervous system. There are other techniques, however, which are more suitable for cats.

The T-maze provides an experimental situation where cats perform reliably, even after large central nervous lesions. The technique is tractable after removal of the cerebral cortex of one hemisphere in adult cats (Norrsell, 1976) or bilaterally in newborn animals (Bjursten, Norrsell, and Norrsell, 1976). The traditional T-maze consists of three narrow alleys which are joined at right angles. One alley is used for starting the tests and leads to the junction where the two testing alleys branch off to the right and to the left. One of the testing alleys arbitrarily is attributed to be correct (i.e., leading to a reward), and the cat is provided with a stimulus acting as a cue for choosing the alley at the junction of the alleys or just after having entered one of the testing alleys. The correct alley is changed "at random" between trials, and the ability of the animal to collect the reward in more than 50% of the trials thus can be used as an indicator for its ability to receive and/or evaluate the stimulus. A given animal can be tested only a limited number of times under comparable conditions and for that reason so-called pseudo-random series are used for changing the stimuli between the testing alleys. A commonly used series is one published by Gellerman (1933). There are other sets of pseudo-random series, and Durup (1967) has published a cyclic series which has the advantage of being more easily used with programming equipment.

Figure 9-2 shows from above a modified T-maze which is suitable for cats. The maze does not look like a T but is technically comparable with the animal waiting in a starting "alley" (Figure 9-2, 1) before the trial. The trial begins when a door (Figure 9-2, hatched, inverted, and slanted T in the left upper corner) slides upward and gives access to two testing alleys branching at equal angles to the right (Figure 9-2, 2) and to the left (Figure 9-2, 3). The stimulation occurs when the cat enters the narrow parts of the testing alleys. The stimulus can be either the floor of that part of the alley (e.g., texture or temperature) or a visual stimulus which is presented at the moment when the cat touches that floor (e.g., by being projected onto the wall at the end of the alley). Alternatively, acoustic stimuli can be presented at that moment. The cat can walk back and forth between the testing alleys and compare the stimuli *ad libitum* before making the decision which terminates the trial. The response or decision consists of touching the floor beyond the narrow part of one of the testing alleys. The trial was started by a T-shaped sliding door opening and the decision makes that door close again behind the cat. At the same time another door slides open in the wall of the relevant testing alley (Figure 9-2, hatched lines in left, lower, and right upper corners) providing a way back to the starting "alley." When the cat leaves the testing alley, food is served from a food tray rotating one step below the aperture in the starting alley (Figure 9-2, right, lower corner) if the decision was correct. In all circumstances the second sliding door closes and the apparatus is set for the following trial when the cat leaves the testing alley.

The main difference between this technique and the traditional T-maze lies in the displacement of the food reward from the testing alleys to the starting alley. This change has the advantage of removing undesirable olfactory indicators of the correct solution. Another advan-

Figure 9-2. Modified T-maze for testing discriminative behavior of cats (seen from above). The maze consisted of three separate "alleys" when the three sliding doors indicated by the hatched lines were closed. The starting alley is indicated by the number 1, the right testing alley by 2, and the left testing alley by 3. A trial was started when the door shaped like a slanted, inverted T in the upper, left corner opened and gave the cat access to the two testing alleys. The cues were presented at the narrow parts of the testing alleys, and the cat finished a trial by passing through that part of one testing alley to its inner section. At that moment the T-shaped door closed behind the

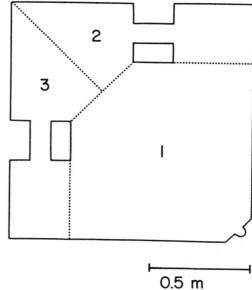

0.5 m

cat and the door opened in the side of the testing alley in which the cat was standing. The second door closed when the cat returned to the starting alley, and at that moment a food reinforcement was served, if applicable, in the aperture at the lower, right-hand corner.

tage is that the cat is returned to the pretesting conditions automatically without that handling by the experimenter which is unavoidable in a traditional T-maze. The shape of the maze does not appear to be critical as long as the animal is provided with sufficient space (see, e.g., Norrsell, 1974).

3. DEFINITIONS OF STIMULUS AND RESPONSE

3.1. The Stimulus

In lesion experiments regarding sensory systems it is obviously critical to establish the relevant stimulus parameters. The aim of the dog experiments which were described was to evaluate structures involved in tactile sensitivity (Norrsell, 1975). The standard stimulus was an air stream passing through nozzles (Figure 9-1) at 40 m/sec. This ostensibly high velocity is not very dramatic if a 3-mm internal diameter of the nozzle is considered, and the experience of a human observer getting the stimulus applied to the back of one hand was that of light tactile stimulation. The attentive observer would also notice faint swishes. The dogs, on the other hand, unless prevented would respond mainly to the acoustic components of the stimuli despite the nozzles being attached to their hindlimbs. For that reason a white noise covering the range 0.04–35 kHz was presented in the experimental chamber during all testing sessions.

The airstream causing the tactile stimulation could be deflected by the introduction of an obstacle in the path between the opening of the nozzle and the hairs of the hindlimb. This maneuver did not remove the acoustic components of the stimulus which thus could be tested in isolation in pre- and postoperative sample sessions and excluded as accessory cues. The lack of response to such "blind" stimuli also served as an extra control for temporal cues. Temporal cues (i.e., the subject's increasing expectations of a new test as time passed) are, on the other hand, quite easily avoided by making the intertrial intervals vary at random within a suitable range.

Undesirable accessory cues can be much less obvious and must always be avoided. It is, for example, not uncommon to use smooth paper versus sandpaper as stimuli in roughness-discrimination experiments. The two types of stimuli may smell different, however, at least to rats, as was found by Finger, Frommer, Carmon, and Inbal (1970). Needless to say, such accessory cues are easily overlooked and could lead to confusing results in a lesion experiment.

It is sometimes not only the quality of the stimulus which must be controlled but also the place of stimulation, as in experiments with subjects who will not accept attached stimulators. Cats were trained to discriminate differences of temperature in the T-maze shown in Figure 9-2. The aim was to locate spinal pathways for temperature sensitivity by making lesions of the cervical spinal cord, and receptive fields above that level thus had to be excluded. For that reason longitudinal barriers were placed above the temperature stimulators which were in the floor of the narrow section of the testing alleys (Figure 9-2, 2 and 3). In that way a cat would automatically touch a thermode with its feet when entering a testing alley but would be unable to reach it with its face because of the restricted space between the barrier and the walls.

Figure 9-3 shows a cat learning to perform that discrimination. The discriminanda (positive stimulus, 35°C; negative stimulus, 15°C) were introduced in the first session of the figure; the cat had been accustomed to the T-maze procedure before that time. The ambient temperature of the T-maze was 22°C during the period, and the cat was thus expected to distinguish between "warm" and "cold." The cat performed above chance after the fifth session, which indicates its having acquired the ability to discriminate between the stimuli (Figure 9-3,

indicate the percent initial entries into the right-hand-alley in each trial. At the initial $\Delta 10°$ level it was clear that the cat had a strong preference for the right-hand alley; i.e., expressed anthropomorphically, it considered how to proceed first after having entered the right-hand alley at the beginning of each trial. This behavior changed when the discrimination became more difficult because the cat then began to enter the left-hand alley at the beginning of the trials to an increasing extent. The change can be expressed anthropomorphically in this way: the cat had now started considering which alley was the correct one before encountering the cues. The curve marked with crosses in diagram B shows that there was no payoff for this change of behavior. This curve indicates the percentage of initial entries into the correct alley in each trial, which remained around 50% throughout the period. The only difference between the easier $\Delta 10°$ discrimination and the more difficult $\Delta 4°$ discrimination in this respect was a greater variability between the values from one daily session to the next.

The change between the two types of behavioral strategy which was seen in this cat has been observed in others, but not in all cats. There is no evidence that a shift from an easier to a more difficult discrimination is the only cause for the change. Different animals, in addition, appear to have a preference for one strategy or the other. It bears emphasizing, however, that the two strategies represent two different behaviors in the sense expressed in the citation from Skinner (1966) above. The two behaviors could be expected to have slightly different neural substrates, which might be critical in a lesion experiment.

4. LEVEL OF TRAINING

The testing of behavioral defects caused by lesions usually calls for a preoperative reference by either training or repetitive testing. The amount of preoperative training and/or testing may, on the other hand, influence the effect of a lesion. It has been found repeatedly that the more preoperative training used for a given behavior, the fewer the defects caused by a given lesion; a so-called overtraining effect (see Weese, Neimand, and Finger, 1973, for references). On that basis it has also been suggested that the lack of defects after some lesions could be due to the use of behavioral techniques which required a long series of preoperative testing (Orbach and Fantz, 1958).

cidence of the cat entering the right-hand testing alley (circles) and the correct testing alley (crosses) at the beginning of each trial. Diagram C shows the mean number of changes between the alleys per trial. The figure illustrates how the cat's initial preference for the right-hand alley diminished with the increasing complexity of the problem.

The reasons for the influence of overtraining on the defects caused by lesions is outside the scope of this chapter, but the definition of overtraining is not. "Overtraining" usually means further repetition of testing after the subject has reached an optimal level of performance (expressed in percent correct responses). This is an operative definition, and it has already been shown that behavioral success is not the only response parameter which may be studied. Perhaps our understanding of "overtraining" would be advanced if behavioral speed, "effort," strategy, etc., were studied as well. Nevertheless, it is critical to observe strict criteria with regard to the level of training in lesion experiments.

5. LEVEL OF PERFORMANCE

The level of the subject's optimal performance in a testing situation is decided by several factors. One factor is the biological bestowal, e.g., in a sensory test the resolution and/or threshold of the receptive system. Another factor is the testing situation. Miller and Murphy (1964) have shown that the rate of learning and level of performance of monkeys making a visual discrimination in a modified Wisconsin General Test Apparatus was different depending on the spatial relations of the cue, the response, and the reward. Figure 9-5 illustrates an experiment indicating similar factors to prevail with cats' discriminative behavior in a T-maze.

In the experiment of Figure 9-5 the cat was discriminating between two visual stimuli presented on the walls at the ends of the testing alleys of the maze described in Section 3 (positive stimulus: a 100-mm square formed by 16 weak electric bulbs of 10-mm diameter; negative stimulus: a single similar electric bulb). A secondary-reinforcement technique was used, namely, a tone was switched on when the cat made a correct decision by passing through the alley with the positive stimulus. The tone stopped when the cat returned to the starting alley and the reward was served; thus the tone constituted a link between response and reward in the capacity of conditioned stimulus of a classical conditioned reflex. Figure 9-5 shows a series of 33 consecutive daily sessions divided into three equal parts; the first 11 sessions with secondary reinforcement followed by 11 without, and at the end 11 sessions after the secondary reinforcement had been reintroduced. The upper curve (circles) shows the percentage of decisions following immediately after the cat had encountered the positive stimulus. The lower curve (crosses) shows the percentage of decisions made immediately after the cat had enountered the negative stimulus. The distance between the two curves indicates the cat's success in solving the problem, and the

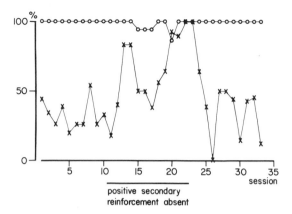

Figure 9-5. Cat performing a visual discrimination in a T-maze in the presence (Sessions 1–10, 23–33) and absence (Sessions 11–22) of an acoustic secondary reinforcement. Each point represents a daily session of 16 trials with 60 sec intertrial intervals. The upper curve (circles) shows the probability of the cat continuing to decision through the alley with the positive stimulus. The lower curve (crosses) shows the probability of the cat continuing to decision through the alley with the negative stimulus. The diagram illustrates how the cat originally had no doubt about the meaning of the positive stimulus and increased its success by turning back from the negative stimulus most of the time. Both types of behavior deteriorated after removal of the secondary reinforcement but were reinstated after its return.

levels of the curves indicate the method. During the initial 11 sessions the cat had an absolute propensity to continue to a (correct) decision whenever it enountered the positive stimulus. Its errors consisted of continuing to a decision in an average of 40% of the instances when it encountered the negative stimulus, and it solved the problem by turning back from the negative stimulus the rest of the time. The behavior changed drastically after the secondary reinforcement had been stopped. Not only did the cat start to turn back from the positive stimulus (sessions 15, 16, 17, and 20) but its tendency to turn back from the negative stimulus declined. The number of correct responses had dropped to chance level in the last session without secondary reinforcement (22) when the cat failed to turn back from either stimulus. It now continued to decision in whatever testing alley it first entered at the beginning of a trial. A reintroduction of the secondary reinforcement from the following session rapidly brought back the original behavior.

In the experiment of Figure 9-5 the level of the behavioral performance obviously was decided to a greater extent by the testing situation than by the stimulation parameters. In jest, it could be suggested that it might have become difficult to distinguish between visual and acoustic defects if that technique were used in a lesion experiment. In lesion experiments, however, the possibility of setting the level of performance by other than the stimulus parameters sometimes is useful. Cats who have been performing a discrimination at the 100% level in a T-maze sometimes stop working altogether after a few failures caused by the problem having become more complicated. The same cat, on the other hand, will accept a greater complexity of the problem without difficulty if the level of performance is first lowered by adjusting the relations between either the cue and the response or, as was seen above, the response and the reinforcement. By analogy the preoperative performance of an animal can be set at a suitable level depending on whether or not the lesion is expected to cause a defect and thus possible frustrations.

Questions are often asked in lesion experiments which involve very specific functions, e.g., with regard to particular receptive fields, submodalities, etc. For that reason it is often more difficult to obtain a sufficiently high level of performance than the opposite. It is sometimes possible, however, to make an animal produce better results than first appeared feasible with the use of shaping techniques. Finger and Norrsell (1974) found the cat's behavioral thresholds to be 1°C or less for both increases (warm) and decreases (cold) of temperature when using the paws. This finding was made despite the fact that the cats initially would learn to make only cold discriminations. Discrimination of warm temperatures were eventually obtained by starting the training with a combined warm–cold discrimination procedure. The cold temperature was then raised gradually and the cats worked into a true warm discrimination.

The shaping of a sensory performance does not have to be made within one sensory system. Miles and Jenkins (1973) have shown that rapid learning may be obtained by using two cues (in their case visual and acoustic) which summate. One of the cues can then be brought to control the behavior by diminishing the discriminability of the other.

6. FINAL COMMENTS

There are, to summarize, no general rules for the training/testing procedures of lesion experiments except that extreme caution must be observed at all times. The proper procedure will become evident only after having observed the results of the first lesions, and one should probably always be prepared to repeat an experiment with alternative techniques. This may appear self-evident if the time factor is forgotten. A lesion experiment with proper preoperative and postoperative controls may take up to a year or more. After that time a repetition of the experiment may appear less attractive in the advent of equivocal results. It may be concluded with regard to behavioral data that the recording of just the success or the failure of a test is probably too little. Again only the results can show what is relevant or not. Before that time it is probably safest to collect as much data as possible.

ACKNOWLEDGMENT

This work was supported by the Swedish Medical Research Council (Project No. 2857). Miss Eva-Britt Gordon and Miss Karin Göthner assisted in the experiments.

7. REFERENCES

Barnett, S. A. Animals to man: The epigenetics of behaviour. In S. A. Barnett (Ed.), *Ethology and Development. Clinics in Developmental Medicine,* 1973, *47,* 104–124.

Bjursten, L.-M., Norrsell, K., and Norrsell, U. Behavioural repertory of cats without cerebral cortex from infancy. *Experimental Brain Research,* 1976, *25,* 115–130.

Durup, H. Recherche de plans d'expériences temporels à transitions exhaustives simples ou multiples. *Bulletin du Centre d'Etudes et Recherches Psychologiques,* 1976, *16,* 21–39.

Finger, S., Frommer, G. P., Carmon, A., and Inbal, R. Roughness discrimination with sandpaper surface: An olfactory confounding. *Psychonomic Science,* 1970, *18,* 165–166.

Finger, S., and Norrsell, U. Temperature sensitivity of the paw of the cat: A behavioural study. *Journal of Physiology* (London), 1974, *239,* 631–646.

Gellerman, L. W. Chance orders of alternating stimuli in visual discrimination experiments. *Journal of Genetic Psychology,* 1933, *42,* 206–208.

Honig, W. K. Introductory remarks. In W. K. Honig (Ed.), *Operant behavior; Areas of research and application.* New York: Appleton-Century-Crofts, 1966, pp. 1–11.

Kimble, G. A. *Hilgard and Marquis: Conditioning and learning.* New York: Appleton-Century-Crofts, 1961.

Konorski, J. *Conditioned reflexes and neuron organization.* Cambridge: Cambridge University Press, 1948.

Lawrence, D. G., and Hopkins, D. A. The development of motor control in the rhesus monkey: Evidence concerning the role of corticomotoneuronal connections. *Brain,* 1976, *94,* 235–254.

Lindström, S., and Norrsell, U. A note on knee-joint denervation and postural reflexes in the cat. *Acta Physiologica Scandinavica,* 1971, *82,* 406–408.

Mackintosh, N. J. *The psychology of animal learning.* London: Academic Press, 1974.

Miles, C. G., and Jenkins, H. M. Overshadowing in operant conditioning as a function of discriminability. *Learning and Motivation,* 1973, *4,* 11–27.

Miller, R. E., and Murphy, J. V. Influence of the spatial relationships between the cue, reward, and response in discrimination learning. *Journal of Experimental Psychology,* 1964, *67,* 120–123.

Norrsell, K. Subcortical vision in cats. *Brain Research,* 1977, *127,* 357.

Norrsell, U. An automatic T-maze for temperature discrimination in the cat. *Physiology and Behavior,* 1974, *12,* 297–300.

Norrsell, U. Central nervous structures participating in the simple recognition of touch. *Acta Neurobiologiae Experimentalis,* 1975, *35,* 707–714.

Orbach, J., and Fantz, R. L. Differential effects of temporal neo-cortical resections on overtrained and non-overtrained visual habits in monkeys. *Journal of Comparative and Physiological Psychology*, 1958, *51*, 126–129.

Pavlov, I. P. *Conditioned reflexes. An investigation of the physiological activity of the cerebral cortex.* London: Oxford University Press, 1927.

Skinner, B. F. Operant behavior. In W. K. Honig (Ed.), *Operant behavior; Areas of research and application.* New York: Appleton-Century-Crofts, 1966, pp. 12–32.

Vinken, P. J., and Bruyn, G. W. *Handbook of clinical neurology.* Vol. 1–26. Amsterdam: North-Holland Publishing Co., 1969–1976.

Weese, G. D., Neimand, D., and Finger, S. Cortical lesions and somesthesis in rats: Effects of training and overtraining prior to surgery. *Experimental Brain Research*, 1973, *16*, 542–550.

10

Subtotal Lesions: Implications for Coding and Recovery of Function

GABRIEL P. FROMMER

1. INTRODUCTION

In introducing her chapter on the lesion technique in somesthesis, Semmes (1973) has written:

> . . . the general method of behavioral analysis following ablations . . . should help to answer not only the question of "where?" (localization) but also the more interesting question of "how?" (neural coding). Full exploitation of the method in animal studies depends, on the one hand, upon relating behavioral results to anatomical and physiological properties of tracts and areas, and on the other, upon advancing behavioral techniques. Ideally, once it has been found that a selected lesion produces impairment on a test, the analytical task has only begun. It proceeds in two directions, toward identifying the critical features of the lesion and toward defining as precisely as possible the function impaired (p. 719–720).

Analysis of the effects of incomplete lesions can contribute to this effort. Far from being merely a technical embarrassment, such lesions result in preparations that can provide useful information relevant to the interrelated problems of coding, localization of function, and recovery of function. Animals with such lesions often exhibit performance capacities that seem incongruent with the known anatomical and physiological properties of the system under study and with the functions that are implicitly or explicitly inferred from those properties. The dis-

GABRIEL P. FROMMER • Department of Psychology, Indiana University, Bloomington, Indiana 47401
Preparation of this paper was supported in part by USPHS Postdoctoral Fellowship MH 55989 and Research Grant MH 29204.

crepancy is due to an incomplete understanding of that underlying anatomy and physiology, a less than thorough analysis of what to expect of lesions (complete as well as incomplete) on the basis of what is in fact known, insensitivity of the behavioral measure to the deficit, or, most likely, a combination of these. A careful analysis of the data on incomplete lesions therefore may suggest new questions to ask about the physiology and anatomy of the system under investigation, provide an interesting and useful preparation in which to ask them, compel a more careful examination of the known anatomy and physiology to interpret the data obtained from lesion experiments, and provide a more rational basis for making lesions and selecting behavioral tasks and stimuli used to assess the effects of the lesions.

The usefulness of data from incomplete lesions has been noted by several writers. Rosner (1970) and Zangwill (1961) have treated them in relation to problems of recovery of function and localization of function. Weiskrantz (1961) and Doty (1973) have paid particular attention to them in relation to the functional organization of the visual system. The purpose of this paper is to pick up these threads by reviewing some of the data on incomplete lesions with special emphasis on sensory systems, and by developing some of the points at which these data have been or can be useful in extending our understanding of questions of functional organization, recovery, and coding.

The definition of subtotal lesion requires comment. A whole system, a particular pathway within a system, or a subdivision of a particular pathway can be taken as the unit of analysis, and a particular lesion may be considered subtotal, total, or "supertotal" depending on the level of analysis. For example, damage to the geniculostriate system resulting in complete degeneration of the dorsal lateral geniculate (LGD) is subtotal with respect to the whole visual system because several other central connections of the retina remain intact. It is total with respect to the geniculocortical pathway. But this pathway is not homogeneous, so such a lesion would be "supertotal" with respect to any component. Perhaps rather than treating them in purely anatomical terms, it is more appropriate to think of subtotal lesions as a strategy which emphasizes the relation between anatomical and physiological organization of the damaged system and what that system can do as well as what it cannot. This is the strategy that will be attempted in the pages that follow.

2. SOME "NONSENSORY" EXAMPLES

Many studies have reported a relation between lesion size and magnitude of deficit in performance. In one recent example (Villablanca, Marcus, and Olmstead, 1976) cats were prepared with lesions that destroyed from 27% to 100% of the caudate nucleus with little damage to neighboring areas. A compulsory approaching syndrome persisted in marked form for their survival (at least 3 months) in the cats with lesions destroying more than 70% of the caudate. Smaller lesions resulted in a proportionally shorter-lasting and weaker expression of this syndrome. This study, like many others, used the relation between lesion size and behavioral change largely in a descriptive manner.

Of greater interest are those studies in which such a relation is used more analytically. Good examples can be found in recent work on the effects of lesions in the lateral hypothalamus (LH). In their classic review Teitelbaum and Epstein (1962) noted that the length and severity of aphagia and adipsia depended on the size of the LH lesion. Expanding the size of a lesion that produced only transient aphagia and adipsia reinstated the syndrome, and the same recovery sequence followed. On the basis of such data they concluded that the recovery of feeding and drinking depended on the tissue surrounding the lesion.

Keesey and his coworkers have pursued this phenomenon further. Powley and Keesey (1970) destroyed about 20–35%, 45–60%, or 80–90% of the LH tissue by passing 1 mA for 4, 7, or 10 sec. The sizes of the lesions correlated negatively with the body weights at which the rats stabilized (Powley, cited in Keesey and Boyle, 1973). These weights were defended in much the same manner as normal animals defend their body weights (Keesey, Boyle, Kemnitz, and Mitchel, 1976). These studies suggest that damage to LH lowers the "set point" at which body weight is regulated in proportion to the volume of the critical tissue destroyed. Keesey *et al.* (1976) were careful to note that LH lesions could have other important consequences, but they argued that these factors either had little influence on long-range regulation of body weight or could be experimentally controlled. They also noted that damage could easily extend beyond the anatomical area critical for producing the phenomena they described to involve systems mediating other functions (e.g., sensorimotor functions, ability to feed).

This point raises again the question of the definition of the completeness of a lesion. Keesey's lesions destroyed a specific part of LH, a structure which can be subdivided on anatomical, neurochemical, and functional grounds. Hence, variation in lesion size is likely to affect differentially the subdivisions involved as well as, or in addition to, the proportion of the target system. Schallert and co-workers (Schallert, Whishaw, and Flannigan, 1977; Schallert and Whishaw, unpublished data) have recently found just this sort of subdivision in the LH associated with several different types of hypophagia. These include (1) active food rejection; (2) passive food acceptance; (2) sensorimotor specific aphagia; (4) uncoordinated activity aphagia; (5) emotionally dependent aphagia; (6) hyperthermia-dependent aphagia. The effects that were observed depended most importantly on the location of the lesion, but on its size as well. Large lesions, therefore, often produced combinations of these aphagia types. Functional differences between parts of the structure damaged by a lesion can, therefore, account for the nonmonotonic relationship sometimes observed between lesion size and behavioral effect. Hamilton, Kelsey, and Grossman (1970) have reported such an effect for septal lesions on performance in a shuttlebox avoidance task, and Marshall (1951) has described this phenomenon in the perception of pain in humans after wounds in the brain involving somatosensory cortical areas.

Stricker and Zigmond (1976) have developed a neurochemical model to account for the apparent recovery of function following LH lesions. It is based on the residual sparing of catecholamine-containing neurons in highly redundant systems. These become more effective through known adaptive processes which increase the availability of catecholamines in the remaining neurons and the sensitivity of the postsynaptic receptors to them. Stricker and Zigmond showed that these systems have extensive recuperative powers and that the duration of subnormal sensitivity in them is correlated in a highly nonlinear manner with the proportion of fibers destroyed. The model can account for a number of features of the recovered lateral hypothalamic animal. Body weight falls in proportion to the magnitude of the lesion because mild homeostatic imbalances become progressively less effective as the system is truncated. Nonspecific stress, arousal, and amphetamine facilitate eating by anorexic animals because these interventions provide the extra stimulation the remaining neurons require to release enough catecholamine to induce consummatory behavior. Severe homeostatic challenges fail to induce consummatory behavior because the limited catecholamine reserves available in the truncated system are rapidly depleted by such intense activation.

This work illustrates the experimental and theoretical usefulness of thinking in terms of what parts of a system are spared. These examples stress the role of partial lesions in the interpretation of recovery of function. In the review of studies on sensory systems that follows, special attention is paid to the analysis of coding as well.

3. SENSORY SYSTEMS: VISION

The well-known spatial representation of sensory surfaces in the central nervous system has traditionally been held to have functional significance for sensory discrimination. The literature on the effects of lesions in sensory systems has amply demonstrated that what that functional significance might be is not necessarily clear (Diamond, 1967, 1976; Diamond and Hall, 1969; Doty, 1961). The visual system deserves particular attention because its anatomical and physiological organization is well investigated. Most is known about the geniculocortical projection, which has an exquisitely precise spatial organization. Therefore one expects that behavioral tests depending on spatial distribution of light will be sensitive to lesions in it. The scotomas in humans bear out this expectation (Koerner and Teuber, 1973; Teuber, 1960). But scotomas are often found not to be absolute (Perenin and Jeannerod, 1975; Weiskrantz, 1961, Weiskrantz, Warrington, Sanders, and Marshall, 1974). Patients soon fail to notice them and report they fill in (e.g., Pribram, 1971; Teuber, 1960, 1966), as do normal subjects with artificial "scotomas" produced by stopped images (Gerrits and Vendrick, 1970). Conversely, patients with rather extensive sparing of visual fields have a variety of rather subtle deficits in perception of stimuli that fall outside their perimetrically measured field defects (Teuber, 1960, 1966). These observations are particularly vivid examples of the apparent noncorrespondence between the effects of subtotal lesions and the intricate spatially organized functional anatomy of the sensory projections. Any theory of coding and of recovery of function in sensory systems must deal with these phenomena, as well as many other related findings from the neurobehavioral analysis of sensory function in animals. In the following discussions these findings are reviewed in the context of the rapidly evolving literature on the effects of "complete" lesions.

3.1. Afferent Pathways

In animals, localized damage in the retina produces the predicted permanent and stable scotoma (Weiskrantz and Cowey, 1970). Saggital section of the optic chiasm results in the expected bitemporal field defect (Berlucchi, Sprague, Levi, and DiBerardino, 1972). It produces in addition deficits on monocular tests of tracking stimuli that move toward the (blind) ipsilateral field (Berlucchi et al., 1972) and on discriminations based on asymmetries toward the ipsilateral field (Hamilton, Tieman, and Winter, 1973).

Further centrally, massive lesions in the optic tract do not prevent pattern* discrimination (Chow, 1968, 1970; Galambos, Norton, and

---

*"Pattern" is used here and throughout this paper only in a descriptive sense, meaning differential spatial distribution of light and dark. Determining just how animals use this distribution is a difficult task (Doty, 1973). Use of a battery of test stimuli that vary in spatial distribution (Lashley, 1939; Winans, 1971) and intensity (Doty, 1971, 1973) is

Frommer, 1967). As little as 2% of the optic tract could mediate recovery of a discrimination between a 6 and a 9, preservation of only 1% permitted intensity but not pattern discrimination, and complete transection produced total blindness (Norton, Galambos, and Frommer, 1967). Evoked potentials recorded in visual cortex from these and other similarly prepared cats showed only modest changes in amplitude and configuration, except in cats with the most severe lesions (Frommer, Galambos, and Norton, 1968). Chow (1968, 1970) observed sparing of visual discrimination after subtotal optic-tract lesions in combination with large but incomplete lesions of the visual cortex. The latter finding together with the electrophysiology and general behavior of the cats described by Galambos and coworkers suggests that the remaining tract fibers had access to a fairly wide area of the visual projections and that the lesions did not produce massive scotomas leaving residual islands of vision. A more appropriate explanation of the sparing may be in terms of the relatively diffuse organization of the optic tract (Doty, 1961; McIlwain, 1964).

Keating's recent findings (Keating, 1977, Keating and Horel, 1976) on combined retinal and cortical lesions in macaques can fit this interpretation. Destruction of the receptors or of the orderly arranged retinal output at the optic disc combined with removal of the striate projection of the spared portion of the retina resulted in severe visual deficits. A small area of overlap in the sparing produced only a transient deficit. This result makes problematical the functional significance of optic tract units that respond to appropriate stimulation far from the conventionally defined receptive field (e.g., Krüger, Fischer, and Barth, 1975).

3.2. Organization of Central Visual Pathways

The interpretation of the effects of lesions in the central visual projections is complicated by several factors. There are technical dif-

---

necessary. Even the traditional horizontal versus vertical stripe display might be detected on the basis of the difference in total flux at the bottom of the display (Spear and Braun, 1969; see also Dodwell and Freedman, 1968; Lashley, 1939; Winans, 1971) or on the basis of the flicker or nystagmus the vertical stripes could induce when the animal moved its head horizontally (Murphy and Chow, 1974). In this matter one should follow Klüver's (1941) admonition: "To say that a differential response, for instance, to a horizontal and a vertical bar, indicates rudimentary 'pattern vision' serves no purpose. The problem is not whether certain differential responses can be considered as evidence for 'pattern vision' (it may even be argued that the response to a single light . . . is not possible without patterning of the field), but to determine the properties of various configurations which are or are not effective in influencing the reactions of the animals" (p. 39).

ferences between laboratories in behavioral assessment techniques, modes of presenting stimuli, and criteria used to define the extent and completeness of lesions. More interesting are the sometimes dramatically different data from different species. Mammals vary significantly in the anatomy of the central visual pathways (e.g., Masterton, Skeen, and RoBards, 1974), but they have two basic pathways from the retina to diencephalic and telencephalic projection areas (Diamond, 1976; Diamond and Hall, 1969). One is by way of the dorsal lateral geniculate (LGD) to the "primary visual cortex," which corresponds to striate cortex in many species. The other projects by way of the superior colliculus and pulvinar (lateral posterior) nuclei of the thalamus to several neighboring cortical areas which Diamond and Hall (1969) call collectively "visual belt cortex." Elements of this pattern also exist in avian and reptilian species (Karten and Hodos, 1970; Karten, Hodos, Nauta, and Revzin, 1973). In primitive mammals such as hedgehog, these projections overlap, and recent investigations in cat have also revealed an overlap as well as a widespread projection of LGD well beyond striate cortex (cf. Sprague, Levy, DiBerardino, and Berlucchi, 1977). Nevertheless, the cat's visual cortical areas have a complex, highly differentiated organization and contain at least 13 different representations of the visual field, each with its unique characteristics (Tusa, Palmer, and Rosenquist, 1975). In addition, extensive interconnections exist between different components of these projection systems (Jones, 1974). Of particular importance in the neurobehavioral literature summarized later is the topographic projection of the striate cortex onto prestriate cortex, which in turn projects to inferotemporal cortex or its apparent homologous structures in nonprimates.

3.3. Geniculocortical System

3.3.1. Visuomotor and Visuospatial Behavior

The effects of lesions to the occipital lobe have been a subject of controversy since the beginnings of neurobehavioral analysis (Weiskrantz, 1961, 1972). The influential work of Klüver (1942) together with clinical observations seemed to establish the idea that striatectomy results in cortical blindness, leaving only the capacity to discriminate differences in overall flux. However, both he and Smith (1937, 1938) also noted that spatial distribution of flux might be a significant variable in guiding behavior, and Klüver described visuospatial behavior similar to the remarkable capacities Humphrey (1974) described in a destriate monkey he studied extensively. After signs of visual following were noted some 19 months after striate destruction, this animal was tested on a variety of formal and "naturalistic" visual tasks. She gradually developed the ability to follow her gaze and reach accurately for small visual stimuli placed randomly in her visual field. She was able to respond differentially between pairs of stimuli on the basis of their "salience" as determined empirically by a preference procedure. Dimensions such as size, form, or brightness were irrelevant independent of their contribution to salience. This monkey also gradually developed the ability to navigate accurately in an open field, skillfully avoiding obstacles on the basis of visual cues.

Anatomical reconstruction of her visual system revealed that the central retina (but not the peripheral) had lost most of its ganglion cells and that a small fragment of the striate cortex was spared on one side. Although it was not possible rigorously to rule out the role of this small fragment in the recovery of this animal's visually guided behavior, careful observation in the testing situation and cinematographic and oculographic recording techniques failed to detect preferential use of any part of the visual field (except for an early dependence on *central* vision).

Keating and Horel (1972) and Denny-Brown and Chambers (1976) reported somewhat similar abilities in their destriate monkeys. The latter workers found losses in binocular fixation, visual recognition of still objects, and visually mediated social behavior. On the other hand, visuospatial orientation, judgment of depth, and accurate reaching for moving targets in the peripheral field recovered. They suggested that some of the abilities Humphrey had described did result from a small spared portion of area 17, because in their hands sparing of small parts of LGD was associated with more rapid recovery of tracking moving objects and locating small particles of food visually.

Precise perimetric assessment of the visual fields of monkeys with striate lesions has been reported. Weiskrantz and Cowey (1970) plotted the scotoma by requiring the monkey to make an instrumental response when a small, brief flash of light appeared somewhere in the central 40° of the visual field. The position of the eyes was photographed in synchrony with the flash. Failures of detection were roughly predictable from the size and position of the lesion in relation to electrophysiological maps of the visual cortex, but there were important qualifications. The size and density of the scotoma decreased as the intensity of the flash was increased and as testing continued over several months. This effect was not an artifact, because retinally produced scotomas did not vary in this manner.

Mohler and Wurtz (1977) used a somewhat different technique to demonstrate even more complete recovery. Deficits in detecting flashes in the scotoma and in the accuracy of visual saccades directed toward them virtually disappeared 6 weeks after the lesion was made. Specific practice was necessary for recovery, as Weiskrantz and Cowey (1970) had suggested. After the extent of the deficit was initially mapped, only half the affected area was subjected to continued testing. When recovery was complete in this part, the untested half still exhibited the deficits. Human clinical cases rarely have the neat, well-localized surgical excisions that can be produced in experimental animals, but Weiskrantz et al. (1974) have reported a patient with such a lesion in visual cortex. He could detect and localize stimuli presented in his scotoma and could make crude discriminations between pairs of them even though he failed to "see" them.

Other species also show significant sparing or recovery of visual placing, localization, and tracking, but the amount appears to vary significantly between laboratories. By far the most data are available from the cat. Sprague and coworkers (Berlucchi et al., 1972; Sprague, 1966a; Sprague et al., 1977) have found no discernable deficits in visual placing in cats with lesions ranging from complete removal of area 17 to destruction of 17 and most of 18 and 19 (LGD in one cat was completely degenerated). Sherman (1974) confirmed this finding in a similar testing situation, Wetzel (1969) reported little deficit in his cats on this sort of measure, and Cornwell, Overman, Levitsky, Shipley, and Lezynski, (1976a) obtained placing responses on 90% of the test trials with cats having less than 10% of LGD spared.

On the other hand, many workers reported that placing becomes less reliable and cruder (e.g., Baden, Urbaitis, and Meikle, 1965; Doty, 1961, 1971; Murphy, Mize, and Schecter, 1975) after ablation of the visual cortex and requires a brightly illuminated surface that sharply contrasts with the background (e.g., Fischman and Meikle, 1965; Spear and Braun, 1969; Winans, 1971). The extent of the damage is an important variable. Wetzel (1969) found that only lesions that produced the most extensive degeneration in LGD produced deficits in visual placing, and Doty (1971) reported excellent placing if lesions were largely limited to area 17.

When the lesions involved other visual areas on the posterior neocortex in addition to areas 17, 18, and 19, all workers report severe and lasting deficits in the placing response (Baden et al., 1965; Meyer, 1963; Ritchie, Meyer, and Meyer, 1976; Sherman, 1974; Sprague, 1966a; Urbaitis and Meikle, 1968). This response can be largely reinstated by injections of amphetamine (Meyer, Horel, and Meyer, 1963; Ritchie et al., 1976) or by removing the input from the contralateral to the ipsilateral superior colliculus (Sherman, 1974; Sprague, 1966b). Ritchie et al. specifically excluded the hypothesis that the amphetamine's action was mediated by spared islands of the geniculocortical system. Doty's studies (1961, 1971) did not show a simple correspondence between sparing in the geniculocortical system and sparing visuomotor behaviors such as placing. Sparing a small portion of this system preserved such responses, but only if other areas of the cortex that receive visual input were largely spared. Interaction between subtotal damage to the two corticopetal visual pathways also appears in formal tests of pattern vision (see below).

Reports on the effects of visual cortical lesions on visual localization and tracking also vary between laboratories. Sprague (1966a), Sprague et al. (1977), and Sherman (1974) appear to have found the least deficit. Even after extensive lesions involving the middle and posterior suprasylvian as well as areas 17, 18, and 19 on the marginal and postlateral gyri, deficits in visual following contralateral to these unilateral lesions were barely discernable after the seventh week of recovery (Sprague, 1966a). Sherman (1974) found deficits in his bilaterally lesioned cats only when testing was carried out monocularly. They failed to attend to stimuli in the contralateral field and tracked only stimuli that moved laterally from the midline into the ipsilateral field. In contrast, Murphy et al. (1975) found that visual following was almost entirely absent in their brain-damaged cats. Most workers report that the ability to localize and track bright, large, slowly moving stimuli is preserved (Baden et al., 1965; Doty, 1971; Fischman and Meikle, 1965; Winans, 1971). Destruction restricted to area 17 results in little or no loss on this measure, and cats with lesions of the marginal gyrus intended to spare representation of the peripheral field showed a smaller deficit than did cats whose lesions completely destroyed visual cortex (Cornwell, Overman, and Campbell, unpublished).

Fewer data are available from other species. One of two bushbabies (Galago senegalensis, a prosimian) with complete removal of striate cortex was unable to reach accurately for food, but the other was largely normal on this measure (Atencio, Diamond, and Ward, 1975). Using a different testing regimen Caldwell and Ward (1976) found substantial recovery in this preparation. Rats largely failed to orient toward a white disc that moved into the visual field contralateral to a unilateral posterior neocortical lesion (Kirvel, 1975; Kirvel, Greenfield, and Meyer, 1974). However, Ferrier and Cooper (1976) elegantly demonstrated that rats with bilateral destruction of the visual cortex could still accurately localize a source of light. Normal and destriate rats learned to jump accurately at an illuminated opening. Although the destriate rats took longer to reach criterion and had a longer latency to respond, goggles bearing field displacing wedge prisms or translucent occluders equally affected the jumping accuracy of both groups of animals. Goodale and Murison (1975) reported that after posterior neocortical lesions rats showed a transitory decline in the percent of trials on which they correctly selected the illuminated door from among four other darkened ones and a more lasting decline in the directness of their approach to the correct door.

Depth perception as measured on a visual-cliff test is usually reported to fall to chance after complete or nearly complete destruction of the geniculocortical system. Cornwell *et al.* (1976a), who have summarized this literature, found that cats with more than 20% of LGD spared showed normal or near normal performance, but that cats with less than 10% spared, usually in the splenial projection of the peripheral field, performed at chance throughout testing. They suggested that reports of successful performance on this test by cats with damaged visual cortex (Dalby, Meyer, and Meyer, 1970; Wetzel, 1969) may have been due to similar sparing of the geniculocortical system as well as to certain procedural variables. Other less formal measures of visuospatial capacities have been obtained from animals with visual cortical lesions. Doty (1973) has summarized these data.

Some species appear to show no deficit on this sort of measure after visual cortical lesions. Hamsters prepared this way were able accurately to track sunflower seeds dangled in front of and above them (Schneider, 1969). Tree shrews were so normal that the experimenters fully expected to find that the lesions were grossly incomplete. Even when the lesions completely destroyed striate cortex and extensively damaged the adjacent visual belt cortex, the animals could quickly and accurately reach for stationary or moving bait (Snyder and Diamond, 1968). The only obvious deficit was found in animals with the most extensive destruction of the striate and belt areas. These animals tended to fall off edges or through gaps in the surface on which they were walking.

The data summarized in the preceding paragraphs show that, in all species tested, animals sustaining essentially complete destruction of the geniculocortical component of the visual system can exhibit capacities for visually guided behaviors that exceed the capacities traditionally ascribed to them. Such animals have been reported to orient toward or reach accurately for visual targets under appropriate test conditions. They can make visually guided placing responses though usually less readily, accurately, or reliably. Incomplete destruction has been found to permit higher levels of performance on some measures. Ability to detect stimuli in the visual field corresponding to the incomplete lesions also recovered extensively with practice.

3.3.2. Learning and Retention of Visual Pattern Discriminations

3.3.2a. Complete Lesions. Animals suffering apparently complete destruction of the geniculocortical projection are able to relearn visual discriminations on the basis of the spatial distribution of light. What the effective stimulus dimensions may be has been difficult to identify. Some investigators have found that differences in total contour are effective (Mize, Wetzel, and Thompson, 1971; Weiskrantz, 1972, 1974; Wetzel, 1969; Cornwell et al., unpublished) or necessary (Dalby et al., 1970; Ritchie et al., 1976). Others have been successful with stimuli that did not differ markedly or reliably overall on this dimension. Stripe orientation was most commonly used, but simple patterns have also been employed. However, Sprague et al. (1977) have found that lesions in the visual system affect discrimination of stripe orientation less than of outline patterns. Some workers have reported failure under these conditions (Braun, Lundy, and McCarthy, 1970; Dalby et al., 1970; Doty, 1971; Keating, 1975; Kicliter, Loop, and Jane, 1977; Ritchie et al., 1976), but many have reported reliable though usually severely retarded and restricted acquisition or reacquisition (Atencio, et al., 1975; Doty, 1961; Hall and Diamond, 1968; Keating and Horel, 1972; Moore and Murphy, 1976; Murphy and Chow, 1975; Murphy et al., 1975; Spear and Barbas, 1975, Weiskrantz and Passingham, 1975).

Pasik and Pasik (1971) found that destriate monkeys could relearn discriminations on the basis of brightness, color, and spatial distribution with negative saving. Gross, irrelevant variations of the stimuli did not prevent reliable discrimination after the basic pattern task was finally mastered. They suggested that Klüver's (1942) more severe deficits were due at least in part to lesions that encroached on large parts of areas 18 and 19. The particular method of testing (the monkey drew luminous stimuli toward itself in complete darkness) may have been critical for the levels of performance that were obtained (Schiller, Pasik, and Pasik, 1972). Caldwell and Ward (1976) showed that destriate bushbabies could be trained to master an orientation discrimination with stripes subtending an estimated 18′ angle.

Winans' (1967, 1971) cats learned to discriminate between a series of upright and inverted solid triangles, the smallest of which were 5.4 cm high and 2.8 cm wide. Her brain-damaged cats mastered the series almost as quickly as the normal animals but showed no savings on transoperative retention except for one cat with an incomplete lesion. These animals were also tested on transfer stimuli in which size, position, figure–ground relations, and completeness of the figures were varied. Both control and operated cats performed at chance when the figure and ground were reversed. Both groups also tended to use differences at the bottom of the stimulus cards when these were available, but could perform above chance on test stimuli that were outline figures of triangles with the bases removed. She attributed her success to careful restriction of the lesions to areas 17, 18, and 19, training for up to 3000 trials, and use of training stimuli and contingencies that minimized strategies that were incompatible with learning the discrimination.

Some species are less affected by destruction of the geniculocortical system than are others. Diamond and coworkers (Killackey, Snyder, and Diamond, 1971; Snyder and Diamond, 1968; Ware, Diamond, and Casagrande, 1974) found that such lesions did not prevent transoperative retention or rapid relearning of discriminations in tree shrews, though Ward and coworkers (Ward, Frank, and Moss, 1975; Ward and Masterton, 1970) have reported a significant acuity loss. Such preparations did show a deficit when irrelevant background features were added or when the test stimuli changed daily (Killackey *et al.*, 1971, Killackey, Wilson, and Diamond, 1972). Preliminary studies on the gray squirrel have provided similar results (Casagrande *et al.*, cited by Atencio *et al.*, 1975). In pigeons Hodos and coworkers (Hodos, 1976; Hodos and Bonbright, 1974; Hodos, Karten, and Bonbright, 1973) had to use sensitive measures to detect deficits on brightness or pattern discriminations after extensive damage to the principal optic nucleus of the thalamus or its telencephalic projection in the accessory hyperstriatum in the Wulst, structures that are apparently homologous to LGD and its cortical projection. They attributed the modest, transient deficit in pattern discrimination reported by Pritz, Mead, and Northcutt (1970) to task variables such as difficulty and the more severe deficits Ziegler (1963) found to the extension of destruction into the main hyperstriatal mass.

3.3.2b. Incomplete Lesions. In many studies lesions accidentally or intentionally spared some portion of the cortical projection of LGD. After such lesions brightness and flux discriminations, which in many species must be relearned after complete removal of visual cortex, are usually largely preserved (Baden *et al.*, 1965; Fischman and Meikle, 1965; Lashley, 1935; Levey and Jane, 1975; Smith, 1937; see however, Barbas and Spear, 1976; Braun, Meyer, and Meyer, 1966; Horel, Bettinger, Royce, and Meyer, 1966; Zangwill, 1961). When pattern discrimination was tested many workers obtained an inverse relation between the presence or amount of sparing in visual cortex and the magnitude of the deficit on the tasks (Dalby *et al.*, 1970; Doty, 1961, Hall and Diamond, 1968; Killackey *et al.*, 1972; Levey and Jane, 1975; Mize *et al.*, 1971; Moore and Murphy, 1976; Schneider, 1969; Snyder and Diamond, 1968; Wetzel, 1969; Winans, 1971; Cornwell, Overman, and Campbell, unpublished). Other studies did not (Cowey and Weiskrantz, 1971; Killackey *et al.*, 1971; Murphy and Chow, 1974; Ritchie *et al.*, 1976; Ware *et al.*, 1974; Weiskrantz and Passingham, 1975). Differences in procedure, species, or range of anatomical variation may account for these different outcomes.

Several studies specifically showed that complete lesions and lesions sparing small parts of the geniculocortical system have markedly different outcomes: e.g., no learning versus learning to a strict criterion, or relearning with large negative savings versus relearning with positive savings. Weiskrantz (1961) and Doty (1973) have reviewed an extensive earlier literature on this topic. Lashley (1939), in his frequently cited paper, showed that a rat with only $1/50$th of its LGD intact could be trained to discriminate correctly on 90% or more of the test trials between horizontal and vertical stripes and between upright and inverted triangles, tasks on which animals with more complete lesions failed. The difference in luminous flux from the bottom of the stimulus cards, which has been proposed as the basis of this sort of discrimination (Dodwell and Freedman, 1968), was unlikely to have contributed to the rat's successful performance, because it performed at chance on a test between horizontal lines located at the top of one card and the bottom of the other. However, all animals in the series, even those with half of one LGD intact, were markedly deficient compared to control rats on the battery of visual tasks used in this study.

Similar findings have been reported for several other species. Keating (1975) found a marked difference in visually guided behavior between two macaques with 100% loss of normal cells in LGD and three with 82–98% loss. The former acted blind for 4 months after surgery and failed to distinguish visually between a raisin and a steel machine nut in over 1300 trials, while the latter showed visually guided behavior the day after surgery and relearned this task to a stringent criterion in a maximum of 777 trials. An even more marked difference appeared on a task requiring the monkeys to select a vertically striped panel from among 23 other, blank ones. The monkeys with incomplete lesions relearned this task and showed almost perfect transfer when an incorrect panel with horizontal stripes was added to the display. The completely destriate animals were not tested on the latter because they failed to master the former. No comment was made about anisotropy in the visual field. Similarly, Glickstein, Barrow, and Luschei (1970) attributed their destriate monkeys' capacity to recover a pattern discrimination after appropriate fading techniques were introduced to a spared fragment in the geniculostriate system.

Lesions restricted to the representation of the central visual field on the lateral striate cortex produce transient and inconsequential deficits in neurologically assessed visual function (e.g., Anderson and Symmes, 1969). They do retard the acquisition of some simple pattern discriminations (Butter, 1969, 1972; Wilson and Mishkin, 1959), but by no means all (Butter, 1969, 1974a; Butter, Mishkin and Rosvold, 1965; Cowey and Weiskrantz, 1967). Such lesions result in a substantial deficit in performance compared to unoperated animals when irrelevant background features are added to the display (Butter, 1969, 1972).

Butter interpreted this finding in terms of an attention deficit because the acquisition curve was normal until the animals were correct about 75% of the time, after which the rise to criterion was retarded. Weiskrantz and Cowey (1970) showed that monkeys with lateral striate lesions could detect finer gratings than could monkeys with retinal lesions that destroyed the equivalent representation of the visual field. They interpreted these and other data (see above) in terms of "lateral shunting" by means of divergent projections from points on the retina, a principle for which some physiological evidence exists (e.g., Doty, 1961; Frommer *et al.*, 1968; Krüger *et al.*, 1975).

Bushbabies with lateral striate lesions successfully learned a variety of pattern discriminations that animals with complete lesions could not, though they were markedly retarded in comparison to animals with lesions in inferior temporal cortex (Atencio *et al.*, 1975). As in macaques, performance was further retarded by addition of irrelevant background visual "noise" and failed entirely when the position of the discriminative stimuli varied on the stimulus card.

Cats with about 5% of the geniculocortical projection spared were able to relearn a simple pattern discrimination transoperatively or learn it postoperatively (Chow, 1968, 1970; Cornwell, Warren, and Nonneman, 1976b, Cornwell *et al.*, unpublished), but addition of irrelevant brightness and size cues disrupted performance (Cornwell *et al.*, 1976b, unpublished). Cats with more sparing of the visual cortex showed little deficit on unmasked visual patterns, even when they were relatively difficult for normal cats to learn (Cornwell *et al.*, unpublished). Addition of irrelevant background stripes also severely disrupted the performance of these animals but had virtually no effect on the normal cats. The magnitude of the impairment was proportional to the severity of the visual cortical involvement. Cats with lesions restricted to area 17 (Doty, 1971) or areas 17 and 18 (Chow, 1968, 1970; Sprague *et al.*, 1977) showed relatively little or no deficit in acquisition or retention on a variety of pattern discriminations. Cat VDC3 of Sprague *et al.* quickly recovered the discrimination between upright and inverted outline triangles embedded in circles, a difficult one for normal animals. Damage to the projection of the central visual field decreased cats' ability to discriminate line tilt (Berkley, 1976), in accord with the physiological finding that orientation selective cortical cells are less sharply tuned in the representation of the peripheral visual field.

3.3.3. Summary

The preceding discussion started from the supposition that the geniculocortical system is necessary for pattern vision. Evidence was marshaled to show that in many species under at least some experimental conditions some level of pattern vision is possible in the absence of this system. However, the stimulus dimensions and experimental conditions that permit learning or relearning pattern discrimination and that facilitate high levels of performance remain unclear. Species differences observed in these studies may reflect differences in the organization of the visual system or simply difficulty in obtaining strictly comparable lesions, tasks, and stimuli across species. Differences found within the same species may be based on differences in the demands the various stimulus conditions made on visual information processing or on much less interesting differences in extravisual aspects of the experiments (comparability of lesions; length of training; presence or absence of procedures, such as punishment, correction, and gradual introduction of more difficult problems that prevent response strategies incompatible with learning the discrimination; random variation within and between the small samples used in most studies; etc.).

But it is clear that animals without "visual cortex" have a greater capacity to process visual information than has ordinarily been attributed to them. Total contour is an effective dimension on which stimuli can vary, but it is not the only one. Stimuli that differ only in the orientation of stripes or of geometric figures can be discriminated successfully, as can different geometric patterns that are equated for contour and flux. It is further evident that animals with a part of the geniculocortical system spared do better, sometimes strikingly so, on visually guided behaviors than do animals suffering essentially complete destruction of this portion of the visual system. Spared pattern vision is, however, vulnerable to the interference of irrelevant background "noise."

Sparing parts of the geniculocortical system is not necessarily sufficient to spare pattern vision. Doty (1961) described chance performance on the simplest discrimination in his series by a cat with a lesion in marginal, postlateral, and posterior suprasylvian gyri which spared a portion of area 17. Earlier, Lashley (1931) had found that lesions sparing large portions of the rat's striate cortex but encroaching on a neighboring lateral area disrupted pattern vision. These data may be examples of the crucial role of extrastriate areas in pattern vision or may reflect the synergistic effects of partial destruction of striate and extrastriate visual cortex. Data on the effects of lesions in the extrastriate visual projection system on pattern discrimination are considered in the following section.

3.4. Extrageniculostriate Visual System

3.4.1. Superior Colliculus and Related Structures

3.4.1a. Visual Discrimination Learning and Retention.   Severe deficits have been reported in learned pattern-discrimination tasks following lesions of optic tectum in cat (Blake, 1959), pigeon (Hodos, 1976; Hodos and Karten, 1974; Jarvis, 1974), and tree shrew (Casagrande and Diamond, 1974) (see Sprague, Berlucchi, and Rizzolatti, 1973, for a recent review). In monkeys neurologic testing following bilateral destruction of the superior colliculus and corticomesencephalic fibers revealed a persistent loss of vision for still objects and objects that moved into the central visual field (Denny-Brown and Fischer, 1976). Other workers have found only rather selective and often subtle losses on discrimination learning or retention in cat (Berlucchi *et al.*, 1972; Winterkorn, 1975), monkey (Anderson and Symmes, 1969; Butter, 1974*a*; Keating, 1976) and hamster (Schneider, 1969). For example, the only deficit Anderson and Symmes (1969) detected was on the discrimination between two rates of movement of a pattern. Berlucchi *et al.*, (1972) observed deficits on acqustion but not retention. Butter (1974*a*) obtained a deficit only when the discriminative stimuli (colors) were spatially separated from the response plaque in the Wisconsin General Test Apparatus (WGTA). Keating's (1976) monkeys were deficient only in selecting which of two panels (out of a total of 24) had briefly been illuminated with the dimmer of two lights. Other workers have reported no deficit or only brief, transient deficits in cat (Myers, 1964), rat (Dyer, Marino, Johnson, and Kruggel, 1976; Thompson, 1969), and monkey (Thompson and Myers, 1971), though lesions that extended into neighboring structures delayed recovery or prevented it entirely (Myers, 1964).

A number of variables may contribute to these differences. Species differences are likely to be the basis of the relatively severe deficits found in pigeons and tree shrews, because the mild effect of lesions in the geniculocortical system in these species suggests that they depend more on the tectofugal pathways for pattern vision (see above). Lesion size and location produced variation in deficits within some studies (Berlucchi *et al.*, 1972; Hodos and Karten, 1974; Keating, 1976; Schneider, 1969; Winterkorn, 1975). Denny-Brown and Fischer (1976) found that preservation of some bundles of corticomesencephalic fibers in an otherwise complete removal of the superior colliculi permitted recovery of pattern vision. This variable may have contributed to the difference between the marked deficit in Blake's (1959) cats and Denny-Brown and Fischer's (1976) monkeys and the milder losses found in these species by others.

3.4.1b. Visuomotor and Visuospatial Behavior. Procedural variables are important because tests must tap the processes that are disrupted by the lesion in order to show a deficit. Many workers adopt the hypothesis that the superior colliculus plays a role in some aspect of visuospatial information processing and/or guidance (e.g., Berlucchi *et al.*, 1972; Butter, 1974a; Keating, 1976; Schneider, 1969; see, however, Denny-Brown and Fischer, 1976). After lesions of the superior colliculus behaviors such as tracking of, approach to, or orienting toward visual stimuli show deficits that seem to fit this label with some consistency (Berlucchi *et al.*, 1972; Kirvel, 1975; Latto and Marzi, 1975; Myers, 1964; Schneider, 1969; Sprague, 1966a; Sprague and Meikle, 1965). The deficits can be powerful enough to reverse the hemianopia produced on these measures by visual cortical destruction in the opposite hemisphere (Kirvel *et al.*, 1974; Sherman, 1974; Sprague, 1966b). However, other studies have reported quite restricted deficits that depend on the particular response measured. Anderson and Symmes' (1969) monkeys had only slight alterations in neurologic tests once the operative trauma had passed. Rats showed a deficit in approaching the location of an illuminated door when they had to jump but not when they could walk (Barnes, Smith, and Latto, 1970). Rats also *improved* in accuracy of a similar approach task following collicular lesions, and were less distracted from this task by irrelevant stimuli than were normal animals (Goodale and Murison, 1975). An analogous sparing has been reported in pigeon after lesions of the optic lobe (including tectum) that had devastating effects on pattern vision (Jarvis, 1974). Sparing of localization associated with retarded acquisition in pattern discriminations has also been reported in cat with superior collicular lesions (Tunkl and Berkley, 1974).

The only deficit Mohler and Wurtz's (1977) monkeys showed after discrete lesions in the superior colliculus was a slight increase in the latency of saccadic eye movements and in the frequency of small secondary saccades to brief light flashes in the visual field corresponding to the location of the lesion. Detecting the flashes and accuracy of saccades was unaffected. However, Schiller (Schiller, 1972; Schiller and Koerner, 1971) found that ablation of the superior colliculi disrupted the ability in three of four monkeys to direct their eyes at visual targets by saccadic eye movements, even though orientation and accurate reaching could be learned. Myers (1964) also found a dissociation between measures in his cats. Visually guided head turning was abolished but reaching and batting objects was not.

3.4.2. Lateral Posterior-Pulvinar

Fewer studies have been performed on the lateral posterior-pulvinar relay in the tectofugal pathway to extrastriate cortex. In monkeys, size constancy was unaffected by subtotal pulvinar lesions (Ungeleider, Ganz, and Pribram, 1977). Mishkin (1972) found negligible effects of either partial or complete destruction of the pulvinar of monkeys tested in the WGTA, but Thompson and Myers (1971) did report modest retention deficits on pattern discriminations. Their monkeys were trained preoperatively to a less stringent criterion that Mishkin's, and the lesions involved structures outside the pulvinar as well. Retention of a discrimination in which the pattern stimuli were presented very briefly (a much more difficult task for normal monkeys than the WGTA presentation) was severely impaired by damage to the inferior pulvinar (Chapula, Coyle, and Lindsley, 1976). Performance of the experimental animals that did recover was futher impaired by adding irrelevant background patterns. Magnitude of the deficit was not related to the size or location of the damage in an obvious way. In pigeons, lesions in nucleus rotundus, which stands in the same relation to the optic tectum and its telencephalic projection as does the lateral posterior-pulvinar in mammals, severely disrupted pattern discrimination (Hodos and Fletcher, 1974; Jarvis, 1974). The extent of the damage was inversely related to the rate and extent of recovery (Jarvis, 1974).

3.4.3. Prestriate Cortex of Monkey

Early studies found little or no deficit in pattern vision following damage to the prestriate cortex of monkeys (Gross, 1973a,b). Some writers (Gross, 1973a,b; Mishkin, 1972) have proposed that this was the result of incomplete destruction of this area. Monkeys with striate cortex isolated from inferotemporal cortex by total resection of the prestriate area failed to relearn a pattern discrimination in 2000 trials, despite showing "adequate visually directed behavior during testing" (Mishkin, 1972, p. 201). Partial destruction of this area had no effect on this measure. Two of Keating's (1975) monkeys with prestriate lesions succeeded in relearning an object and a stripe-orientation discrimination. Two others that failed had more degeneration in the inferior pulvinar than did the ones that succeeded. In Keating and Horel's (1972) study the one experimental monkey that showed no deficit in object recognition or perimetry had sparing in the "foveal prestriate area." The monkeys that had complete destruction of this area were more deficient on these tasks than were the animals with ablations of striate cortex.

Denny-Brown and Chambers (1976), using neurologic testing procedures, described a somewhat different pattern of loss following destruction of areas 18 and 19, sparing area 17. Their monkeys lost visuospatial behavior but quickly recovered object discrimination and the ability to fixate and track slowly moving targets. Different and less extensive destruction appears to produce less complete but still severe deficits in pattern discrimination (e.g., Butter, 1974a; Cowey and Gross, 1970; Gross, Cowey, and Manning, 1971). Prestriate lesions added to previously ineffective pulvinar lesions disrupted size constancy by inducing the monkeys to respond on the basis of the size of the retinal images (Ungeleider *et al.*, 1977). A specific deficit on a "landmark reversal" task has been reported after destruction of posterior parietal cortex including the representation of the lower parafoveal visual field in the dorsal prestriate cortex (Mishkin, 1972). This deficit may simply reflect a field defect (as may the disruption of pattern discrimination by foveal prestriate lesions) or a disturbance in perception of spatial relations among objects (Weiskrantz, 1974).

Others have failed to find any loss after apparently complete prestriate lesions (Pribram, Spinelli, and Reitz, 1969). Pribram (1974) has proposed that the discrepancy may depend on differences in the way stimuli were presented, together with a field defect resulting from damage to the underlying optic radiations. Christensen and Pribram (1977) have suggested that prestriate ablations must encroach on the adjacent posterior inferotemporal cortex or on the underlying optic radiations to produce severe, lasting deficits on visual discrimination. Weiskrantz (1974) discussed several explanations including differences in the extent of the lesions and duration of recovery.

3.4.4. Inferotemporal Cortex of Monkey

Lesions of monkey's inferotemporal cortex produce what have been characterized as visual learning deficits (in contrast to deficits attributable to sensory dysfunction following ablation of striate cortex). The complex nature of the deficits and the way in which they can be distinguished from deficits that follow striate lesions are described by Dean (1976), Gross (1973a,b), and Weiskrantz (1974). The effects of location and size of lesions in this structure have been investigated. Selective ablation of 5-mm wide strips produced about the same amount of retardation in pattern-discrimination learning, regardless of the rostro-caudal location on the gyrus (Mishkin, 1972). Analysis of larger but still incomplete lesions did reveal differences. More rostral damage retarded concurrent learning of eight different object discriminations more severely than learning of a two-dimensional pattern discrimination, while more caudal damage produced the opposite relation between the magnitude of deficit in these two tasks (Mishkin, 1972). More recent data appear to confirm this difference. Monkeys with lesions on the inferotemporal gyrus similar to Mishkin's (1972) more rostral lesions had to relearn pattern discriminations after interpolated visual tasks. Monkeys with partial destruction of the prestriate area retained the discriminations virtually perfectly (Dean and Cowey, 1977). Damage in the posterior portion of the classical inferotemporal visual area produced more "perceptual" deficits (Iverson, 1973). Highly experienced monkeys performed nearly normally on a concurrent discrimination learning task consisting of six pairs of stimuli, each pair differing on a different dimension. They were marked retarded when the concurrent tasks were composed of stimulus pairs that all differed on the same relevant dimension and also differed on one or more irrelevant dimension. However, in an effort to test the "perceptual" interpretation, Dean (1974) found an increase in reaction time on a more difficult choice task only in a monkey whose lesion encroached upon foveal prestriate cortex. An additive effect of inferotemporal and prestriate lesions has also been found on a pattern discrimination (Ettlinger, Iwai, Mishkin, and Rosvold, 1968; see also Christensen and Pribram, 1977).

Damage to the outflow through the albal stalk from inferotemporal cortex to subcortical structures, anterior commissure, and frontal cortex resulted in an inability to relearn a simply pattern discrimination in up to 1300 trials. Sparing a small fragment of this pathway permitted relearning at a rate roughly proportional to the amount spared (Horel and Misantone, 1976).

3.4.5. Extrastriate Cortex in Other Species

The homologies of extrastriate visual structures between monkey and other mammals have only recently begun to be worked out (Diamond, 1976; Jones, 1974), so only limited data from other species are available that are directly comparable to the data in monkey. In bushbaby, lesions of the inferior temporal cortex retarded acquisition or disrupted retention of a variety of pattern-discrimination tasks, but the nature of the deficit could not easily be characterized. There were marked individual differences on discriminations with irrelevant background "noise" or with variation in the position of the stimuli on the card (variations that devastated the performance of animals with lateral striate lesions), but these could not be ascribed to detectable differences in the lesion (Atencio et al., 1975).

Tree shrews with lesions of the temporal cortical projection of the pulvinar relearned brightness and simple pattern discriminations with negative savings. Spatial reversal learning was unaffected, but visual reversal shifts, whether intradimensional or extradimensional, were relearned without improvement over successive reversals (Killackey *et al.*, 1971, 1972). Pigeons with damage to the telencephalic projection of the tectofugal pathway onto the ectostriatum had deficits in relearning pattern discriminations, the magnitude of which was highly correlated with the amount of destruction of the target plus the periectostriatal belt (Hodos and Karten, 1970).

Lesions of the middle and posterior suprasylvian gyrus in cats usually produce at most modest deficits in pattern discriminations (Cornwell *et al.*, 1976*b*; Doty, 1971; Hara, Cornwell, Warren, and Webster, 1974; Wood, Spear, and Braun, 1974), but under some conditions they can be more severe. Campbell (1977) found that damage in the cat's posterior temporal cortex, the apparent homologue of the primate inferotemporal gyrus, retarded the acquisition of a pattern discrimination and other more complex visually guided tasks, a result comparable to findings in monkey. Sprague *et al.* (1977) studied in detail a series of cats with lesions involving various combinations of areas 19, 20, 21, and lateral suprasylvian area (roughly equivalent to prestriate and temporal visual cortex of monkey). The most extensive lesions resulted in severe deficits on various pattern discriminations, though discrimination of stripe orientation was near normal. Less extensive damage in these extrastriate areas resulted in milder deficits. Cornwell and co-workers (Cornwell *et al.*, 1976*b*; Hara *et al.*, 1974) also found substantial deficits in pattern discrimination after their most extensive resections of extramarginal visual areas. However, the lesions in many of these animals also involved the geniculocortical radiations. The possible role of interaction or facilitation between partial lesions in the two corticopetal visual pathways is treated in the following section.

3.4.6. Effects of Lesions Involving Both Visual Projection Systems

Anderson and Symmes (1969) have reported striking augmentation of deficits after lesions involving both visual projection systems. Lateral striate lesions combined with lesions of the superior colliculi, which alone produced modest deficits, produced severe, lasting deficits. These monkeys showed reduced visual arousal, depth perception, and recognition of edibles and of social stimuli. Butter (1974*b*) obtained less severe combined effects which he attributed to less extensive destruction of the colliculi in his monkeys. Trachtenberg and Gower (1975) found that combined lateral striate and pulvinar lesions exacerbated visual deficits in their monkeys. Mohler and Wurtz (1977) found that

spared components of the visual system. Mishkin's (1966, 1972) neuro-behavioral analysis of the circuitry that appears to underlie the visual functions of the inferotemporal gyrus in monkeys suggests a hierarchical, sequential processing system. Recent data suggest a further stage of sequential processing (Horel and Misantone, 1976) and confirm the importance of the prestriate relay (Butter, 1971a; Gross, 1973a,b; Keating, 1975; see, however, Pribram, 1974; Pribram et al., 1969) for pattern vision. There are some parallel neurobehavioral data in cat (e.g., Campbell, 1977; Cornwell et al., 1976a; Sprague et al., 1977), but the full complement of anatomical and behavioral data from this species suggests an alternative (and therefore more interesting) interpretation.

Based on their finding in cats that extrastriate lesions appeared to disrupt pattern vision more severely than did striate lesions Sprague et al. (1977) argued that several extrastriate visual areas participate in pattern vision in some integrated fashion relatively independently of the striate cortex. Taken together with the disruptive effect that tectal and pulvinar lesions can have on pattern vision in many species, these data are consistent with the idea that the first stages of simple pattern vision can be mediated by the tectopulvinar projection system at least in many species. But both pattern and brightness discriminations must be relearned after destruction of the geniculocortical system, indicating that it normally participates in these functions. Other neurobehavioral data suggest that the two systems work in concert, as the complex anatomical interconnections suggest. Denny-Brown and Fischer (1976) adopted such a position on the basis of the similarity in the deficits they found in monkeys after complete destruction of the striate cortex or of the superior colliculus and corticomesencephalic fibers. The facilitatory influence of visual cortex on superior colliculus (Kirvel et al., 1974; Sherman, 1974; Sprague, 1966b) and the synergistic effect of damage in the two systems (e.g., Anderson and Symmes, 1969; Butter, 1974b; Hara et al., 1974) are also consistent with this view.

3.5.3. Incomplete Lesions and Models of Functional Organization

The phenomena associated with incomplete lesions provide the most interesting data because they appear at first glance not to be compatible with the complex spatially organized anatomy and physiology of the visual system as it is ordinarily regarded. These data have often been cited to illustrate the fact that we do not understand the functional organization of the visual system (e.g., Doty, 1973; Rosner, 1970; Sprague et al., 1973; Teuber, 1960, 1966), and Pribram (1971, 1974) has used them (together with other kinds of data) to support a model of visual-information processing in which encoding and processing are distributed throughout the striate cortex (and presumably other visual representations as well) by repeated replication of each piece of information. In essence, Pribram challenges the relevance of visual maps for pattern vision, because a piece of the map seems to work quite well, and because there is evidence that the map is not drawn the way it is usually assumed to be. His alternative is an organization modeled after physical holograms. It has several appealing features in addition to its ability to predict sparing of form discrimination after subtotal lesions. These include large capacity and ability to match inputs that have undergone a variety of transformations or reductions. This is a very interesting alternative because it requires us to look at the visual system in a radically different way. Hence, it is particularly important to examine the evidence on which this model rests. A careful inspection of the data on incomplete lesions in the visual system indicates that the support they provide for a model like Pribram's is tantalizing but by no means compelling.

The functional significance of spatial mapping in the brain has been challenged before. Lashley (1937) argued that it has none beyond providing control over intensity of response and spatial orientation. Yet he analyzed the capacity for pattern vision that he found in rats with small parts of striate cortex spared in terms of a corresponding sparing of the visual field (Lashley, 1939). He carefully estimated the properties of that visual island on the basis of anatomical data and concluded that the size of the island required the animal to reconstruct the test figures by a series of fixations. It is difficult to show that such an analysis, derivable from a local-feature model, cannot account for the sparing or recovery of function that animals with subtotal lesions exhibited in other studies as well. The difficulty lies in the limitations of the experimental conditions that were summarized above. It is simply not known in most cases to what aspects of the stimulus array the test animals were responding or how sensitive they were. Hence, it is not accurately known whether or to what extent the animals with subtotal lesions were better than the animals with total destruction of the target.

When quantitative data obtained under well-controlled stimulus conditions are available, they reveal significant features of what may be the underlying organization of the damaged system. The best example is Weiskrantz and Cowey's (1970) data, which show that acuity loss after lateral striate damage is less than predicted by the extent of the lesion in relation to the topographic organization of the visual pathways. They proposed that divergent projections from the retina provide the functional anatomical basis for this finding, though an alternative explanation in terms of the intact tectopulvinar system cannot be excluded.

Despite their technical limitations, there are data from incomplete lesions that can be considered in terms of competing models of visual function. A visual-island interpretation based on a local-feature model would predict the occurrence of abnormal orientation and head position to get the target stimulus into the functioning visual field. This behavior is rarely reported (e.g., Lashley, 1939; Hahn, cited by Snyder and Diamond, 1968), but it is also rarely carefully sought and specifically denied (e.g., Humphrey, 1974; Snyder and Diamond, 1968). But unless distributed processing models assume that each small portion of the retina is functionally connected to wide areas of the damaged structure, they would also require a similar process.

Patients with lesions in the visual projections exhibit subtle deficits in processing visual information in perimetrically normal parts of the visual field (Teuber, 1960, 1966). This fact appears to cause problems for local-feature model, but according to Pribram (1971), not for his holographic distributed model. However, the divergent projection of retina onto striage cortex inferable from Weiskrantz and Cowey's (1970) work and directly measurable in cortical physiology (Doty, 1961; Frommer et al., 1968; Teuber, 1966) provides a possible explanation in terms of a local-feature model. Destruction of a portion of the visual projection would reduce or remove a modulating input to neighboring undamaged tissue by eliminating the divergent output from the destroyed tissue. Parallel deficits can be found in the animal literature (e.g., Butter, 1969, 1972; Hamilton et al., 1973; Lashley, 1939). Butter interpreted features of his data as an attentional deficit.

Adding irrelevant background features to the stimulus display can disrupt pattern discrimination by animals with subtotal lesions in pulvinar (Chapula et al., 1976) and striate cortex (Atencio et al., 1975; Butter, 1969, 1972; Cornwell et al., unpublished), though the effect can be mild or nonexistent (Sprague et al., 1977; Towns and Stewart, 1972). It is not too difficult to explain this effect in terms of several models. It may reflect added difficulty in locating, detecting, and combining critical features with a spared visual island, in resolving critical features from degraded information available in a small portion of a distributed processor, or in attending to the critical features. The devastating effect that varying the hue of stripes in an orientation discrimination had on destriate tree shrews (Killackey et al., 1972) seems to fit best with an attentional loss.

There are two findings about subtotal lesions which appear to put significant constraints on what may be the underlying processes of pattern vision. One is the observation that varying the position of the critical stimulus disrupts performance on previously mastered discriminations (Atencio et al., 1975). This suggests that the stimulus must be picked up by a critical localized functioning portion of the visual representation. The second, which more directly leads to this interpretation, is work on combined retinal and striate lesions (Keating, 1977; Keating and Horel, 1976). Destruction of one part of the visual representation in the retina and the other part in the cortex resulted in a severe, lasting deficit in pattern vision. The monkeys that quickly relearned the discriminations were found to have overlapping sparing of a small portion of the visual representation. Chow's (1968, 1970) failure to find a lasting deficit after combined lesions of the optic tract and visual cortex in cat is probably due to the more diffuse arrangement of fibers in the tract than in the retina (Doty, 1961; Frommer *et al.*, 1968; McIlwain, 1964). Keating's results strongly indicate that the topographic representation of the visual field is preserved in the striate cortex and that it is necessary for pattern vision. It also puts a limit on the distance over which divergent conduction within the retinostriate projection may be effective in mediating pattern vision by itself.

In summary, the hypothesis of distributed processing of the sort Pribram (1971, 1974) has proposed is very interesting because of the novel conception of visual organization it presents. Data from incomplete lesions of the visual pathways represent an important support for this model. However, these data can be interpreted as satisfactorily in terms of a spared island of functional visual field because of limitations of the data. In order to obtain more useful and satisfactory data, it is necessary to test animals with stimuli that vary quantitatively over dimensions selected on the basis of information available on the anatomical and physiological organization of the target structures. The question seems important enough to warrant the time and effort required for this difficult program.

3.5.4. Electrical Recordings and Lesions in the Visual System

A few studies have reported evoked-potential recordings on behaviorally tested animals with lesions in visual structures (e.g., Cornwell *et al.*, 1976b; Frommer *et al.*, 1968; Hara *et al.*, 1974), but this measure cannot provide much information on the functional organization of the system. Unit data, which can, would provide data that can be compared much more directly to the behavioral discriminative capacities of the animals. For example, optic tract fibers receive input from wide areas of the retina (e.g., Krüger *et al.*, 1975). Yet combined partial lesions of the retina and striate cortex can destroy pattern vision in monkeys (Keating, 1977; Keating and Horel, 1976), setting functional limitations on what such fibers can do. Electrophysiological records from the intact portion of the striate cortex of such animals would provide evidence on unit properties that were abolished along with pattern vision and on properties that were spared and thus not sufficient for that function. Conversely, unit recordings from visual cortical cells in animals with subtotal optic tract lesions that spared pattern vision (Chow, 1968, 1970; Galambos *et al.*, 1967) would provide data on the features of functional organization that were preserved in association with preserved pattern vision. By systematically varying size and location of the lesions and making quantitative behavioral and electrophysiological observations in the same animals, it is possible to establish the features of the underlying anatomy and physiology that are associated with sparing different kinds or degrees of visual functioning. This is one kind of correlational analysis over a wide range of conditions that will ultimately establish relationships between psychophysical and neurophysiological processes (Jung, 1972; Mountcastle, 1975; Uttal, 1973).

There are promising signs of interest in using electrophysiological investigation of animals with lesions in the visual system as a tool for relating the underlying organization of the visual system to the behavioral effects of lesions. For example, Gross and co-workers (Gross, Bender, and Rocha-Miranda, 1974; Rocha-Miranda, Bender, Gross, and Mishkin, 1975), who have investigated extensively the effects of inferotemporal lesions on visual discrimination, have found that disconnecting the inferotemporal cortex from the striate by destroying the forebrain commissures and ipsilateral striate cortex abolished the response of inferotemporal units to photic stimuli. The visual input from the pulvinar appears to mediate only inhibitory effects, because its destruction generally expanded the receptive fields of the inferotemporal units. These data closely parallel neurobehavioral studies by Mishkin (1966, 1972) described above. Mohler and Wurtz (1977) recorded superior collicular units in the same monkeys that had served in their behavioral tests on the effects of lesions in striate cortex on detecting and looking toward brief light flashes. After functional recovery they found that the properties of collicular cells in the representation corresponding to the cortical lesions were grossly normal, but compared to cells in normal animals and in normal parts of the visual representation a greater percentage of them became more responsive when the monkey used the test stimulus as a saccade target.

Several studies have investigated the properties of superior collicular neurons after complete removal of the striate cortex. These data can be compared with the behavioral effects of these lesions. In cats, lesions destroying area 17 abolish directional selectivity of cells in the superficial superior colliculus, establish ocular dominance by the contralateral eye, and increase the proportion of cells responding to stationary spots of light (e.g., Mize and Murphy, 1976; Rosenquist and

Palmer, 1971). Extending the lesion to involve other cortical projections of the lateral geniculate had no additional effect. In contrast, removal of striate cortex in rabbits had no measurable effect on cells of the superior colliculus (Stewart, Birt, and Towns, 1973). Since destruction of area 17 has little effect on a simple visual discrimination in cats (e.g., Doty, 1971; Sprague *et al.*, 1977) but severely disrupts learning or transoperative retention in rabbits (Moore and Murphy, 1976; Murphy and Chow, 1974; Towns and Stewart, 1972), these unit properties are completely unrelated to the discriminative measures. In opossum Saraiva, Aragão, and Magalhães-Castro (1976) reported that unilateral striatectomies depressed responsiveness of tectal units to light stimuli, but subsequent destruction of input from the contralateral tectum largely reinstated it. This finding parallels the effects of these lesions on orienting and tracking responses in cat (Sherman, 1974; Sprague, 1966*b*) and rat (Kirvel *et al.*, 1974).

The effect of removing area 17 on unit activity of area 18 has been described (Dreher and Cottee, 1975). This lesion increased the proportion of cells responding to rapidly moving (as opposed to slowly moving) stimuli and reduced the proportion of cells that responded binocularly. These findings correspond to the anatomical organization of the inputs to area 18 from the Y cells in LGD, which are sensitive to rapidly moving stimuli, but do not parallel any of the neurobehavioral data. They suggest that discrimination of movement velocity should be affected by this lesion.

In summary, electrophysiological data should be obtained together with behavioral data from animals with lesions in the visual system to permit more direct comparison of the effect of the lesion on these two measures. By doing so the processes underlying coding and recovery can be more directly identified. Examples of successful and unsuccessful applications of this strategy are presented.

4. SENSORY SYSTEMS: SOMESTHESIS

In contrast to visual and auditory stimuli, somatosensory stimuli are difficult to specify and vary on rationally defined physical dimensions, except at the most elementary level. Despite the descriptive operationalism that must be used to define the stimuli, the functional organization of the somatosensory system is beginning to be understood. The afferent pathways are subdivided into anatomically segregated components, so there is ample opportunity to try to correlate selective destruction of individual components with specific discriminative deficits. Considerable overlap in functional organization between subdivisions has been found, but there is evidence for selectivity and specificity of function. However, in order to obtain lasting deficits, lesions must completely destroy (or nearly so) the target structure.

4.1. Peripheral Inputs

Kirk and Denny-Brown (1970) have demonstrated interactions between dorsal root inputs over a distance of several segments by using the classic method of remaining sensibility introduced by Sherrington to define the dermatome. They showed that the size of the dermatome decreased as the number of roots sectioned on either side of the spared root was increased. The size and affective quality of the spared sensibility also depended on whether the roots were sectioned distally or proximally to the dorsal root ganglion. If they were cut distally, the size of the dermatome was about twice as large and showed persistent hyperesthesia. These data indicated that the input from each dorsal root is influenced by tonic activity in neighboring roots. Selective lesions in the tract of Lissauer, which contains short axons of small cells traveling up and down the cord, showed that the medial portion of this pathway mediated facilitatory interactions while the lateral part carried inhibitory ones (Denny-Brown, Kirk, and Yanagisawa, 1973).

Wall and co-workers have electrophysiologically demonstrated similar interactions between neighboring roots and rootlets (Dostrovsky, Millar, and Wall, 1976; Merrill and Wall, 1972; Millar, Basbaum, and Wall, 1976). They sectioned or reversibly blocked dorsal roots or rootlets and measured the changes in the topographic representation of the body surface or in the receptive fields of cells in the spinal dorsal horn or in the dorsal column nuclei. These maneuvers produced an increase in the volume of the representation of the spared roots, widespread inhibitory fields, noncontinuous excitatory receptive fields, and/or changes in the position of the receptive field. These findings were interpreted as the unmasking of normally ineffective connections.

4.2. Afferent Pathways

Afferent pathways have been classified into two divisions, lemniscal and extralemniscal (Albe-Fessard, 1967; Bowsher, 1965). The former, which has physiological properties of the kind presumed to be required for mediating fine tactile discriminations (see Glassman and Glassman, 1977, and Semmes, 1969, for an alternate view), can be divided into three anatomically separable parts: dorsal columns; spinocervical tract in the dorsal lateral columns, which also contains fibers synapsing in the gracile nucleus; and neospinothalamic tract in the ventral quadrant of the cord. Although the populations of units traveling in each of these pathways respond to overlapping ranges of somatic stimulation, not all classes of primary afferents have access to each system (Brown, 1973; Vierck, 1974).

Some progress has been made in identifying the pathways that are necessary and/or sufficient to mediate various kinds of tactile discriminations. Lesions of the dorsal columns affect selectively only those discriminations that require spatiotemporal integration of either actively palpated or passively received stimuli (Azulay and Schwartz, 1975; Beck, 1976; Dubrovsky and Garcia-Rill, 1973; Melzak and Southmayd, 1974; Vierck, 1974; Wall and Dubner, 1972; see however Liu, Yu, Chambers, and Ha, 1975). Sparing part of the dorsal columns is associated with the retention of this kind of discrimination, even when other lemniscal pathways are extensively damaged (Azulay and Schwartz, 1975; Vierck, 1974).

Many other kinds of tasks guided by somatosensory input are little, if at all, affected by lesions restricted to the dorsal columns (see Vierck, 1974, and Wall and Dubner, 1972, for reviews). In primates these tasks include two-point limen (Levitt and Schwartzman, 1966); joint position (Schwartzman and Bogdonoff, 1969; Vierck, 1966); weight (DeVito, Ruch, and Patton, 1964); vibration (Schwartzman and Bogdonoff, 1968); moving versus stationary contact (Vierck, 1974); size (Vierck, 1973a); absolute and difference thresholds for light touch (Vierck, 1973b); roughness and three-dimensional shape (Azulay and Schwartz, 1975; Schwartz, Eidelberg, Marchok, and Azulay, 1972); and control of hand movements used to track a visual target (Eidelberg, Woolf, Kreinick, and Davis, 1976).

Some of these tasks have also been used on monkeys with lesions in other parts of the cord. Damage in the ventrolateral cord alone or in combination with dorsal column lesions has little lasting effect on several, including two-point limen (Levitt and Schwartzman, 1966), joint position (Vierck, 1966), and weight (DeVito et al., 1964). Combined destruction of the dorsal and dorsal lateral columns can have a substantial, lasting effect on some discriminations, including two-point limen (Levitt and Schwartzman, 1966); joint position (Vierck, 1966); detection, roughness, and shape (Azulay and Schwartz, 1975); size (Vierck, 1973a); absolute and difference thresholds (Vierck, 1973b); and moving versus stationary contact (Vierck, 1974). In the latter four tasks some animals showed no severe effect or a slow, progressive recovery. A human case (Noordenbos and Wall, 1976) presents a similar picture. The patient, who sustained a stab wound which at surgery was observed to transect the cord except for the ventral margin, could still appreciate tactile and thermal stimuli.

In other experiments the brainstem trajectory of the spinocervicothalamic and neospinothalamic systems was damaged together with the dorsal columns. These combined lesions had little or no effect on detection, shape, and roughness tasks (Azulay and Schwartz, 1975; Schwartz *et al.*, 1972). Finally, temperature discrimination was only transiently affected in monkeys sustaining lesions that destroyed the components of the afferent pathways in the cord, individually or in various combinations (Eidelberg and Rick, 1975).

Tactile discrimination in carnivores is often affected more severely by lesions in the dorsal lateral columns than in the dorsal columns. In cats, Kitai and Weinberg (1968) found only a minor reduction in sensitivity on roughness discriminations after lesions in the dorsal columns, but section of the decussation of the spinocervicothalamic tract in the cervical cord alone severely disrupted performance on this task. Tapper (1970) found that gentle pressure to single tactile pads, strong enough to initiate only a single impulse in the type I afferent which innervated it, could serve as a conditioned stimulus for cats, but only if the ipsilateral dorsal lateral column was intact. Other lesions had no effect. Midthoracic lesions of the dorsal columns in dogs did not reduce the effectiveness of airpuffs to the hindlegs as discriminative stimuli. Destruction of the spinocervical tract had only a transient effect. Combined lesions of these two pathways produced a marked, lasting deficit, though one of the three dogs eventually recovered fully (Norrsell, 1966, 1975).

Other workers have reported a somewhat different pattern of effects. Liu *et al.* (1975) found no deficit in their cats in tactile placing and tactile localization measured by orienting responses following damage in the dorsal lateral columns. Transient losses appeared on both measures after destruction of the dorsal columns. Combined lesions of the dorsal column–medial lemniscal and the spinocervicothalamic systems in the cord and/or the medulla produced a lasting deficit, though firm pressure could be localized. Incomplete destruction resulted in partial recovery, leaving localized areas to which orienting responses were not directed. None of the lesions abolished permanently the ability to walk on a horizontally oriented ladder. Dobry and Casey (1972*a*) found that lesions involving more than 90% of the cervical dorsal columns produced a reliable deficit on a roughness discrimination. The difference between the results of this study and Kitai and Weinberg's was attributed to the larger size of the effective lesions as well as to various procedural differences. Electrophysiological study of these lesioned cats revealed several significant correlates of the behaviorally effective lesions (Dobry and Casey, 1972*b*). Only the largest lesions reduced the proportion of driven cortical units, the proportion with short latencies, and the proportion with well-defined receptive fields. In addition, a characteristic "fatigue" appeared only after these lesions. In contrast, cortical evoked potentials did not exhibit any orderly variation with lesion size.

The converse lesion, sectioning the thoracic cord sparing only the dorsal columns, did not prevent cats from detecting low-intensity electrical stimuli to cutaneous afferent nerves from the hind legs (Myers, Hostetter, Bourrassa, and Swett, 1974). In a similar study, Frommer, Trefz, and Casey (1977) found that only a fraction of the dorsal columns was necessary to mediate the eventual recovery of the ability to detect innocuous cutaneous stimulation. The cat having the most sparing in the dorsal columns showed the least postoperative loss and learned a size discrimination as well. However, none of the lesioned animals ever oriented to any stimuli below the level of the lesion, confirming Wall's (1970) observation on rats prepared in the same manner. Such a dissociation between orienting and discriminative responses has not been found after lesions further centrally (see below). Unit recordings were also obtained. Ten or more days after the cord lesion was placed, there was a two-thirds reduction in the proportion of drivable units in the cortical hindpaw projection area, and of those that could be driven, several responded to foreleg stimulation above the level of the lesion (Frommer et al., 1977). Thus, a process analogous to that observed by Wall and coworkers (Dostrovsky et al., 1976; Merrill and Wall, 1972; Millar et al., 1976) in the dorsal horn and dorsal column nuclei is detectable in central units.

A number of purely physiological studies have been reported on animals with lesions of different components of the spinal cord. Dreyer, Schneider, Metz, and Whitsel (1974) found a massive loss of drivable units with lemniscal properties in specific zones of the monkey's hind leg projection after selective destruction of individual components of the lemniscal afferent system. The zones corresponded to specific portions of the single hind leg projection that this group had previously described, rather than to the cytoarchitectonic organization of the postcentral gyrus. In contrast, Eidelberg, Kreinick, and Langescheid (1975) obtained changes in the frequencies of different classes of units only after combined lesions in dorsal columns and in the spinocervicothalamic and spinothalamic pathways of the lateral lemniscus in the midbrain. These workers attributed the differences between their findings and those of Dreyer et al. to differences in sampling, lesion size, or interval between cord damage and recording. In cats, Levitt and Levitt (1968) found no changes in cortical SS I electrophysiology after *acute* destruction of the cord sparing only the dorsal columns, a finding since confirmed by Frommer et al. (1977). Destruction of the dorsal columns reduced the proportion of cells driven by hair movement and increased the proportion of undrivable cells. Adding hemisection of the ipsilateral cord to dorsal column lesions apparently released cells responding to light tap (Levitt and Levitt, 1968).

Extensive damage in the lateral midbrain destroying lemniscal pathways as well as other structures resulted in inattention to and poor localization of stimuli contralateral to the lesion in all modalities (Sprague, Chambers, and Stellar, 1961). If the lesions were localized to the somatosensory lemniscal pathways, the deficits were less severe and lasting, even to somatosensory stimuli (Sprague, Levitt, Robson, Liu, Stellar, and Chambers, 1963). Cats and rats with lesions placed under electrophysiological control in lemniscal pathways were able in most cases to learn or relearn a series of roughness discriminations (Frommer, unpublished). If training lasted long enough, performance returned to or exceeded preoperative levels despite major destruction of the lemniscal pathways. These lesions failed to destroy all the rapidly conducting afferents, as shown by the presence of normal or near-normal evoked potentials in SS I and SS II in response to peripheral electrical stimulation. Lesions extending well beyond the conventionally defined position of the lemniscal pathways were required to abolish these responses.

The research reviewed in this section attempted to determine the role that somatosensory afferent pathways in the cord and brain stem play in mediating different kinds of discriminative functions. Extensive data show the necessary role of the dorsal columns in mediating discriminations that require spatiotemporal integration of tactile information, even when other pathways are extensively damaged. Afferents in the dorsal lateral columns, presumably the spinocervical tract, appear to be important in several types of discriminations. However, no unifying stimulus dimensions have been identified, and in primates the effects of lesions restricted to this pathway are not established. In cats, damage in the spinocervical tract but not in the dorsal columns has been found to disrupt detection of stimuli restricted to Type I afferents and discrimination of roughness, but deficits on the latter task have also been reported after lesions restricted to the dorsal columns.

Taken as a whole, the evidence suggests that detection and localization of simple innocuous somesthetic stimuli activating a range of afferent fiber types can be mediated by more than one of the afferent pathways in the cord. In carnivores the ventral cord was ineffective in some tests, though recent evidence indicates that accurate orienting responses can be induced by firm pressure in cats with both dorsal pathways severed. The capacity of the severely compromised cord to function is dramatically illustrated by a recent case report (Ghatek,

Hirano, Lijtmaer, and Zimmerman, 1974) in which neurologic examination for a suspected metastatic tumor failed to reveal any sign of a
large, demyelinated plaque that included most of the dorsal columns
and substantial portions of the spinal gray and ventral columns at the
midcervical level. A similar "redundant" organization appears to exist
in the afferent systems mediating responsiveness to noxious stimulation. Pain perception returns in a substantial proportion of patients
after initially successful lesions placed in putative pain pathways to
relieve intractable pain (Noordenbos, 1959; White, 1966; White and
Sweet, 1969). A similar finding has been reported in cats (Orlowsky
and Glusman, 1969).

4.3. Forebrain Areas

Damage to the ventrobasal relay of the lemniscal pathways did
not abolish proprioceptive or vibratory discriminations in monkeys
(Schwartzman, 1970). In humans, such lesions placed under electrophysiological control produced significant but partly transient losses
in the appreciation of tactile stimuli (Tasker, 1969). Destruction in the
homologous structure of rats retarded but did not necessarily prevent
learning of a series of roughness discriminations (Finger, 1972, 1974;
Reyes, Finger, and Frye, 1973) and had little reliable effect on temperature discrimination (Finger and Frommer, 1970). Glassman, Forgus,
Goodman, and Glassman (1975) have reported that ventrobasal lesions
in cats produced deficits in discriminating between brushing and non-
moving contact with the fur and in orienting toward and localizing
light tactile stimuli. The extent to which the ventrobasal thalamus and
the lemniscal fibers immediately caudal to it were destroyed affected
the magnitude and duration of the effect. Damage limited to the posterior nuclear complex associated with extralemniscal afferents was ineffective, in agreement with Finger's data in rats.
The effect of somatosensory cortical lesions on measures of detection of innocuous somatic stimuli varies between studies that used different methods and species. Lesions in SS I and SS II of monkeys
produced at most a slight elevation in detection threshold as assessed
by a conditioning procedure (Schwartzman and Semmes, 1971). Cats
exhibited a deficit in orienting toward cutaneous stimuli after damage
to SS II but not SS I. (Glassman and Glassman, 1977). The response
usually recovered partially over the course of testing. Dogs showed a
modest, largely transient deficit on a similar task after selective bilateral
ablation of the hind-leg representation in SS I and SS II (Norrsell,
1967, 1975). Only when SS II lesions were added to preexisting ablations in somatic cortex was there evidence that this area was more important than SS I (Norrsell, 1971). Sensorimotor cortical lesions in rats

have been reported to produce a permanent loss of orienting toward stimuli to the affected areas of the body (Turner, 1975).

Finger (1974) has reviewed the research from his laboratory on the effects of forebrain lesions in rats on the discrimination between a smooth surface and a series of surfaces bearing grooves ranging from very coarse to very fine. The consequences of damage in the lemniscal projections ranged from the inability of many of the brain-damaged rats tested under particular conditions to master the discrimination in the allotted number (usually 200) of trials (see also Finger and Reyes, 1975; Walbran, 1976) to the absence of a reliable effect on retention (see also Finger and Simons, 1976). Lesions in SS I and SS II were equally effective in retarding acquisition, and combined lesions were no more effective. Temperature discrimination, on the other hand, was minimally affected. A number of variables were shown to influence the effectiveness of the lesion, but size and location within the somatosensory projections were rarely effective when the lesions were relatively large (Finger, Marshak, Cohen, Scheff, Trace, and Niemand, 1971).

However, recent studies (Finger, Simons, and Posner, 1977) on cortical lesions made in infnat rats demonstrated an association between structural and functional sparing. The lesions in some animals were incomplete, as indicated by unit recordings and anatomical analysis of the "barrel" organization of somatic cortex in rats (Welker, 1976). These rats performed better on the tactile discriminations and a neurologic battery than did animals with more complete lesions but less well than did control animals. These data suggested a hypothesis to explain why the consequences of brain damage can be ameliorated by factors such as placement of lesions early in life or in stages (see chapters by Johnson and Almli and by Finger in this volume). The effects may operate only if the lesions are incomplete and may do so by enabling animals to make more effective use of spared fragments than they ordinarily can when the lesions are placed at a single sitting in adulthood.

Several workers have reported that cats with lesions of the anterior ectosylvian gyrus (SS II) and of the postcruciate gyrus (SS I + part of motor-sensory cortex) are deficient in discriminating a variety of tactile stimuli (Benjamin and Thompson, 1959; Glassman, 1970, 1971; Sperry, 1959). Glassman found that his cats did perform above chance even with the most extensive lesions. He found that damage restricted to the postcruciate gyrus produced primarily postural deficits, while lesions in the anterior ectosylvian gyrus resulted primarily in tactile deficits (discrimination of a brushing contact from a brief, stationary one), albeit milder than those that followed combined lesions of these two somatic areas. Recently, Glassman and Glassman (1977) have reanalyzed these data and reported on additional subjects. They confirmed the ineffectiveness of lesions of SS I in disrupting tactile discrimination or orienting, but found that lesions of SS II in the anterior ectosylvian gyrus had to involve the neighboring orbital gyrus as well to be effective. The larger the lesion to this region the greater the deficit, but no critical focus could be identified. Orienting and discriminative measures were found to be highly correlated with each other. These results are consistent with the finding by Teitelbaum, Sharpless, and Byck (1968) that unilateral lesions restricted to SS I or to SS II did not affect acquisition or retention of tactile discriminations, though they did prevent interhemispheric transfer. Glassman and Glassman interpreted the effects of SS II lesions plus orbital lesions in terms of a loss in "higher sensorimotor integration" that requires a degree of flexibility of input–output coupling not present in the tightly coupled organization of SS I.

Early work on primates (e.g., Cole and Glees, 1954; Ruch, Fulton, and German, 1938) showed relatively mild, lasting effects of lesions in postcentral gyrus on tactile-discrimination tasks. Kruger and Porter (1958) found recovery on a tactile form discrimination with zero savings after destruction of SS I and SS II. A permanent deficit was obtained when the lesions encompassed precentral cortex as well. Orbach and Chow (1959) obtained positive savings on a series of roughness and form discriminations after removal of SS II. Removal of SS I alone or in combination with SS II resulted in more severe deficits, but in most cases the animals returned to preoperative level of performance after several hundred trials.

Recently, however, severe, lasting deficits have been found after lesions of either SS I or SS II. Semmes and coworkers presented evidence that the relatively mild and transient deficits on tactile discriminations previously reported following damage to SS I hand area may have reflected incomplete destruction of the projection of the finger tips in area 3 in the depths of the central sulcus. When this area was included in the lesion a profound, lasting deficit resulted in tactile shape and texture discriminations (Semmes and Porter, 1972; Semmes, Porter and Randolph, 1974). In contrast, temperature discrimination was unaffected by such lesions (Porter and Semmes, 1974). Performance on these tasks was unaffected by damage to the immediately adjacent area 4 on the anterior bank of the central sulcus (Semmes and Porter, 1972).

A more detailed neurobehavioral dissection of SS I has been provided by Randolph and Semmes (1974). Removal of area 3 on the posterior bank of the central sulcus resulted in severe, lasting deficits in discrimination between levers that were hard and soft, horizontally and vertically grooved, square and diamond shaped, and rough and smooth. The one animal in this group that showed electrophysiological evidence of some sparing of this part of the hand representation also showed less deficit than did the other two. Destruction of the hand representation in area 2 on the posterior half of the postcentral gyrus resulted in a different pattern of losses. Performance on the diamond–square and convex–concave discriminations was severely disrupted, while the other discriminations were learned normally. Damage to area 1 between areas 3 and 2 mildly retarded acquisition of the hard–soft, horizontal–vertical, and rough–smooth tasks but apparently accelerated acquisition of the square–diamond problem. Lesions of SS II have also been found to produce severe, lasting deficits on a battery of tactile discriminations (Ridley and Ettlinger, 1976). In the absence of anatomical verification of the brains, it is not possible to assess the relation of the size and location of the lesion to the magnitude of the deficit.

Lasting, severe deficits have also been found in humans contralateral to well-defined surgical excisions that involved the middle third of the postcentral gyrus (Corkin, Milner, and Rasmussen, 1970; Roland, 1976). Lesions sparing this area were largely ineffective. Roland found no effects on his task (forced choice between pairs of three-dimensional stimuli that varied quantitatively in size and shape) following any other lesion, and his most severe deficits occurred when the anterior portion of the critical area was involved. Lesions that encroached only on the posterior margin of the postcentral gyrus were largely ineffective. Corkin and coworkers reported no effects of precentral lesions on their tasks, and only transient effects of parietal lesions. There was one exception: Larger parietal lesions tended to produce a deficit in the ipsilateral hand. Corkin *et al.* also claimed that the deficit in recognition of common objects by touch was *not* disproportionate to simple sensory deficits they observed.

Anatomical (Graybiel, 1974) and neurobehavioral (Gross, 1973*a, b*) evidence indicates that the posterior parietal cortex adjacent to SS I plays a role in processing somatosensory information that is analogous to the role of prestriate and inferotemporal cortex in vision. This area receives input from SS I and from the somatosensory posteroventral portion of the pulvinar-posterior complex of the thalamus, and lesions in it disturb performance on somatosensory discriminations. A number of interpretations have been offered to explain the deficits, ranging from the suggestion that they are secondary to an ataxia to the claim that they represent a tactile agnosia. The evidence from the animal literature seems to indicate that whether or not there is an agnosia-like deficit, there is a deficit in reaching accurately with the hand contralateral to the damaged parietal cortex (Bates and Ettlinger, 1960; Mountcastle, 1975; Ratcliff, Ridley, and Ettlinger, 1977). Ettlinger and coworkers have investigated the possibility that more than one process might be disrupted by parietal lesions by comparing effects of selective damage to different parts of the posterior parietal cortex. Although Moffet, Ettlinger, Morton, and Piercy (1967) failed to obtain unambiguous evidence for localization within this area, their results suggested that the magnitude of deficits was related to both the location and the extent of the lesion. Damage to the anterior and lateral ventral margin was effective in disrupting acquisition of various shape discriminations, though total resections were more consistently effective. However, Ridley and Ettlinger (1975) obtained deficits on most tactile tasks after total removals, but failed to find impairment after partial lesions.

In summary, damage in the forebrain somatic areas produces substantial deficits on several tactually guided behaviors but at most minor losses on temperature discriminations. These findings hold for several species under a variety of test conditions, though some differences do exist that may reflect either species differences, differences in assessment techniques, or both. Simple detection appears to be markedly disrupted in cat and rat as measured by orienting responses, but much less so if at all in dog and monkey as determined by performance of conditioned responses. In addition, cats appear less affected on orienting and discrimination measures by destruction of SS I than of SS II and adjacent orbital cortex. Other species exhibit strong deficits in tactile discrimination after lesions in SS I, and destruction of SS II can result in comparable deficits. The effectiveness of the lesions depends on the completeness of destruction of the target areas. It has been suggested that sparing of target tissue may be necessary to mediate serial-lesion and early-lesion effects.

4.4. Summary and Conclusions

The neurobehavioral analysis of the somatosensory system has not progressed as far as in the visual system. Therefore, the conclusions that can be drawn from the data are even more limited. But even within these restrictions some parallels can be seen to the findings on the visual system, especially in the effects of subtotal lesions. Data can be marshaled to support the following statements:

1. Peripheral lesions markedly influence the functioning of undamaged neighboring afferent inputs.

2. Lesions restricted to subdivisions of the somatic afferent system in the cord can result in specific deficits. The clearest data are available for the extensively investigated dorsal columns which appear to mediate discriminations that require spatiotemporal integration. However,

simple detection and discriminations can be mediated by more than one subdivision, if the stimuli activate a wide enough range of afferent classes.

3. A remarkable redundancy can be observed after lesions in the cord and brain stem pathways, such that sparing of a fraction of the pathway(s) that appear to mediate a discrimination permits recovery of the discrimination performance to preoperative levels. The possible role of extralemniscal pathways in the recovery is obscure.

4. Despite the failure of early studies to find them, severe, lasting deficits on tactile discriminations can follow lesions in the cortical lemniscal projections if destruction of the target is complete. The relative importance of SS I and SS II is a matter of disagreement. Species and methodological differences contribute to the variation between experiments.

5. Spared tissue in the target areas of the forebrain appears to be able to mediate marked recovery.

6. Damage to somatosensory "association" cortex disrupts somatosensory discriminations, especially if areas 5 and 7 are completely removed. It is not clear whether the ablations produce a tactile "agnosia" or a deficit secondary to a deficit in reaching.

As in the visual system, the effects of lesions in the somatosensory system have been used to question the critical role commonly assigned to the lemniscal organization in mediating fine discriminative function (e.g., Eidelberg et al., 1975,; Glassman and Glassman, 1977; Semmes, 1969, 1973). The apparent redundancy of cord pathways, the relative ineffectiveness of cortical SS I ablations in permanently disrupting tactile discriminative performance, and the disruptive effects of cortical lesions outside the contralateral lemniscal projection on tactile functions have all been marshaled as evidence that the lemniscal organization is not the necessary coding scheme for tactile discriminative capacities. The data, while provocative, are not conclusive. Because of experimental limitations each of these three findings is subject to alternative interpretations.

The subtotal lesion effect in afferent lemniscal pathways may represent the action of an underlying organization not readily apparent in physiological recordings from intact animals on which the lemniscal concept is based. Electrophysiological data consistent with this idea are available (e.g., Dostrovsky et al., 1976; Eidelberg et al., 1975; Frommer et al., 1977; Millar et al., 1976). On the other hand, that effect may reflect the relatively normal functioning of the restricted input responding to stimuli that activate a sufficiently wide range of afferents. Stimulus control and response analysis are not adequate to decide between these (or other) alternatives.

Many early studies on the effects of lesions in the cortical somatic projections of monkeys found only mild or transient effects, especially if only one projection was the target. Similar findings have been reported for dog and cat, especially after ablation of SS I. These data suggested that the coding represented by the organization of the cortical projections, SS I in particular, may not be critical for tactile discriminations. Recent studies on monkeys and rats have found severe, lasting deficits after complete ablation of the target structures. Therefore, as in the visual system, recovery after somatic cortical lesions in some species at least may depend on the relatively normal function of spared cortex normally receiving projections from a relatively small but critical area of the sensory surface.

Electrophysiological data on lesioned animals are available. Some covariation between these measures and behavioral data can be found, but with rare exceptions there is enough difference between the test stimuli in the two experimental tasks that the relation is at best suggestive. As in the visual system, a future goal for research should be to test the same kinds of stimuli behaviorally and electrophysiologically in the same animals with lesions.

5. SENSORY FUNCTION: AUDITION

5.1. Frequency Discrimination

The apparent incongruity between aspects of the anatomical and physiological organization of the auditory system and the behavioral effects of lesions in it is marked. The difference is probably as clear as it is because the test stimuli used in the behavioral and physiological experiments are often very similar, permitting a much more direct comparison between the two kinds of experiments than is ordinarily achieved in visual and somesthetic experiments. Tonotopic organization exists at all levels of the auditory system, though authors disagree over its precision and significance especially at the cortical level (e.g., Evans, 1968; Merzenich, Knight, and Roth, 1975; Whitfield, 1971), perhaps because of differences in the methods used to demonstrate it (Goldstein and Abeles, 1975). Subtotal damage in the auditory system at any level does not prevent performance or recovery of simple discriminations based on changes in frequency. Although good correlations have been reported between deficits in behaviorally determined audiograms and cochlear damage produced by intense sounds or by ototoxic substances (Dolan, Ades, Bredberg, and Neff, 1975; Elliot, 1967; Stebbins, 1970; for a recent review see Bredberg and Hunter-

Duvar, 1975), no simple relationship between the part of the pathway or projection damaged within the nervous system and performance on frequency-dependent tasks is apparent. Even partial section of the auditory nerve that resulted in selective loss of spiral ganglion cells associated with specific parts of the basilar membrane failed to affect the audiogram or frequency difference thresholds in cats (Elliot, 1967).

Further centrally, only those sections of the brachium of the inferior colliculus that completely abolished auditory cortical evoked potentials in response to clicks were successful in preventing cats from relearning a simple frequency discrimination (Goldberg and Neff, 1961a; see also Randall, 1965). The story of the preservation or recovery of the capacity to make simple frequency discriminations following extensive ablations of the auditory portions of the cortex is well known (Diamond, 1967; Elliot and Trahiotis, 1972; Neff, Diamond, and Casseday, 1975). It should be added that recent data have demonstrated the importance of response variables (Cranford, Igarashi, and Stramler, 1976; Wingblade, 1977) as well as stimulus presentation variables (Goldberg and Neff, 1961b; Thompson, 1960) in determining the effects of these lesions on frequency discriminations.

When task variables are such that complete destruction of the auditory cortical target does produce lasting deficits on discriminations based on frequency differences, the size and completeness of the lesion does influence the magnitude of the effect. For example, Meyer and Woolsey (1952) found that cats with complete destruction of the auditory cortical projection in A I, A II, Ep, and SS II failed the task they used, but cats with sparing in any part could relearn, usually with positive savings. Diamond, Goldberg, and Neff (1962) found a similar effect using an interesting variant on the basic "filled background" (Elliot and Trahiotis, 1972) frequency-discrimination experiment. In this study the neutral intervals between the positive stimuli were filled with 0.8–1.0–0.8 kHz triads of tone bursts, and the positive signals were 0.8–0.8–0.8 kHz triads. This discrimination was much more difficult for normal cats than is the usual filled background task in which the positive triads vary in frequency and the interspaced neutral ones remain constant. It was also much more sensitive to auditory cortical ablation. Removal of A I, A II, and Ep abolished the discrimination and prevented its reacquisition. Sparing a functional fragment of A I that terminally showed evoked responses to tone pips between 8 and 32 kHz permitted eventual recovery of the discrimination.

Elliot and Trahiotis (1972) have summarized this aspect of the literature by concluding: ". . . if remnants of the auditory areas of either hemisphere remain, then discrimination may be affected little, if at all, provided that a single-response detection of a new frequency task is used and suprathreshold differences are presented" (p. 210). The suprathreshold qualification may be important. Although the threshold for detecting frequency differences was unaffected when sparing permitted the relearning of suprathreshold discriminations in Meyer and Woolsey's (1952) study, extensive lesions involving the middle third of the superior temporal gyrus and opercular and insular cortex as well produced a large increase in this threshold in monkeys (Massopust, Wolin, and Frost, 1971). An additional qualification should be added. Most studies have used frequencies below 2 kHz. At least one has found lasting deficits only at higher frequencies (Massopust, Barnes, and Verdura, 1965). Observations on normal cats suggest a significant difference between the processing of higher and lower frequencies (Neff, reported in Evans, 1968).

Attempts have been made to test the role of auditory cortex in processing frequency information by analyzing frequency generalization gradients. Thompson (1965) was able to predict the properties of the gradients his normal cats showed from features of the tonotopic organization of the auditory cortex and could account for the flattening of the gradient that followed ablation of that structure in his cats and those of Randall (1965). However, under other test conditions this lesion had no effect on the gradient's shape (Diamond, 1967).

Evidence for an effect of lesion size and location has been reported for discriminations between tones presented in triads that differed only in the pattern of the tones. In cats, Diamond and Neff (1957) found a negligible loss when the lesion was largely restricted to A I, a transient deficit following lesions confined to A I, A II, and Ep, and a permanent loss after destruction that encroached onto insular-temporal (I-T) cortex as well. However, the latter lesion did not prevent cats from reliably detecting the change from tone bursts that rose in frequency to bursts that fell (Kelly and Whitfield, 1971). If the lesions did not encroach onto I-T, this discrimination was acquired or reacquired more quickly and more reliably.

Other studies (see Neff et al., 1975) claim a critical role of I-T in mediating pattern discrimination. Kelly (1973) compared the effect of lesions in this area on the ability to detect the change from a low–high to a high–low pattern in tone pairs and from rising tone bursts to falling ones. Extensive damage to I-T prevented reacquisition of the former, but the latter discrimination was relearned with negative savings. Smaller lesions permitted recovery of both with positive savings. Colavita (1977) has summarized the evidence that damage to I-T disrupts discriminations of change in patterns of auditory, visual, and somesthetic intensity as well as of auditory frequency. Recent data from monkeys indicate that the discrimination of patterns of frequencies can be

relearned after lesions of primary auditory cortex on the caudal supratemporal plane or lesions of the anterior supratemporal plane, which
produce retrograde degeneration in the caudal medial geniculate as do
I-T lesions in cats (Wegener, 1976; unpublished data). The rate of recovery after primary auditory lesions was roughly proportional to the
extent of the lesion.

In summary, these data indicate little correspondence between the
functional tonotopic organization observable in auditory pathways and
projections and the effects of lesions in them. Complete removal of auditory areas often fails to abolish permanently discriminations based on
frequency differences. If complete removal is effective because a particular kind of task is used, then sparing of a portion of the target area
(cortical or subcortical) permits recovery even if the spared tissue responds physiologically to frequencies different from those tested behaviorally. Despite older and more recent demonstrations of precise
tonotopic organization under some experimental conditions, it has
been argued (Whitfield, 1971) that this organization represents only
the residue of anatomical organization without essential functional significance. Hence, insensitivity of frequency discriminations to damage
here can be expected.

5.2. Localization

Compared to simple frequency discriminations, auditory localization tasks appear relatively sensitive to damage throughout the auditory pathways (see Neff et al., 1975). For example, Casseday and Neff
(1975) found that extensive brainstem lesions that transected the trapezoid body or the lateral lemniscus or brachium of the inferior colliculus
bilaterally prevented cats from localizing sound sources even set 90°
apart. Sparing a portion of the lateral lemniscus or of the anterodorsal
trapezoid body left accuracy of localization virtually unchanged, even if
the noise bursts terminated before the response was permitted. Incomplete lesions of the brachium of the inferior colliculus had a substantially more severe effect.

Masterton, Jane, and Diamond (1967, 1968) have tested the effect
of brain stem lesions on the detection of change in two kinds of click
stimuli that humans perceive as shifting the source from the left ear to
the right. In the first, single clicks actually shifted from the left earphone to the right. In the second the phase relation of binaural click
pairs changed from the left earphone leading the right by 0.5 msec to
the right leading the left by that amount. Normal cats quickly trans-
ferred from the first discrimination to the second. Lesions that com-

pletely transected the trapezoid body had little effect on the first task but completely prevented transfer or acquisition of the second at interclick intervals of 0.5 msec or less, the range required for localizing a brief natural sound. Incomplete destruction of the trapezoid body preserved transfer from the first to the second task, but elevated the minimum detectable interclick interval in rough proportion to the degree of damage to the trapezoid body exceeding 50%. Incomplete section of the lateral lemniscus retarded transfer from the first to the second task and made performance on the latter less reliable, although it did not markedly elevate the minimum interclick interval.

Auditory cortical lesions also disrupt the ability to localize by approaching the source of a sound or to detect changes in the phase relation of binaural click pairs (Neff *et al.*, 1975). Cats with lesions including at least A I, A II, and Ep cannot reliably master the former task but can do the latter after special training with an added intensity cue (Masterton and Diamond, 1964). Wegener (1973) tested monkeys on a localizing task requiring them to reach toward a food box just below the sound source. Those with more than 80% of the primary auditory cortex destroyed were severely and permanently deficient at all angular separations tested (to 180°), but some did relearn at intermediate separations. Monkeys with more than 35% of the primary cortex spared exhibited milder and more transient deficits. Wegener (unpublished data) also trained monkeys to press a key on the side on which an auditory stimulus was presented. Auditory cortical lesions initially disrupted their ability to detect phase and intensity differences between binaural 1-kHz tones, but continued training, especially with more intense stimuli, reduced the deficit. Using a similar procedure Heffner and Masterton (1975) found that primary auditory cortical lesions produced no elevation in threshold for angular separation of sound sources but did mildly depress the reliability of detecting suprathreshold stimuli. Their monkeys could also approach the source of a continuing train of clicks, but again less reliably than before surgery. However, they were severely deficient in approaching a sound that terminated when the approach response was initiated. One animal with about one-third of A I spared on one side showed substantially less deficit than did the two with more than 90% of A I destroyed bilaterally.

Unilateral auditory cortical ablations affect localization of contralateral auditory stimuli. In otherwise intact cats, approach responses were disrupted only when the critical or leading element of a bilaterally originating stimulus pair was contralateral to the brain lesion (Cranford and Oberholtzer, 1976; Whitfield, Cranford, Ravizza, and Diamond, 1972). Cats with one cochlea destroyed, which can be trained to localize a sound source, though less accurately than can normal animals, were made more deficient in localizing sounds only if unilateral auditory cortical lesions were contralateral to the intact ear (Neff and Casseday, 1977).

5.3. Conclusions

Despite evidence for tonotopic organization which at many levels appears quite precise, damage to auditory targets must be complete and/or the discriminations must require relatively complex integration of frequency information in order for lesions to show an effect on tasks involving frequency differences. Perhaps this discrepancy reflects a preoccupation with the frequency analysis of pure tones as opposed to the sound features for which the auditory systems of different species may be specifically adapted (Gersuni and Vartanian, 1973). One such feature is localization in space. Although many neurons in auditory cortex, as well as in brain stem structures, respond to dimensions that can code spatial location (e.g., Evans, 1968; Starr, 1974; Whitfield, 1971), none of the auditory areas appears to be organized as a map of auditory space in relation to the animal. Maps of auditory space do exist elsewhere (Dräger and Hubel, 1975; Gordon, 1973; Morrell, 1972), but neither here nor within the auditory system are the units sharply enough tuned to account for the animals' abilities to localize sounds (Starr, 1974). Because of the absence of these properties, Starr (1974) has proposed that the difference between activity in populations of units sensitive to lateralized inputs controls the relative activity of the lateralized motor systems which produce the behavioral responses from which localization is inferred.

Another possibility also exists. The tonotopic organization of the auditory system may contribute significantly to the coding of other dimensions such as location. Masterton (1974) has demonstrated that the tonotopic organization of more peripheral structures in the auditory system can be viewed as adaptations for localizing brief sounds. Butler (1974) has presented evidence suggesting that frequency contributes to localization of the elevation of a sound source. Electrophysiological data from the auditory system of bats that emit orientation sounds containing a long, constant frequency component reveal an exceptionally intricate organization apparently specialized for analyzing the Doppler-shifted echos of that component (Suga, 1977). Thirty percent of the primary auditory cortex of these bats is devoted to the representation of the 2 kHz range of these echos. Within this area, columns of very sharply tuned cells with the same best frequency are organized in eccentric contours with best amplitude of stimulation superimposed radially on this tonotopic map. Such an arrangement is especially suited for detecting the relative velocity and the size of a moving target (Suga, 1973).

6. GENERAL CONCLUSIONS

Subtotal lesions lead to significant recovery or sparing of functions compared to complete destruction of targets in the nervous system. In some cases, as in recovery following bilateral destruction of the lateral hypothalamus, a plausible account of the mechanism of recovery can be made on the basis of the known properties of the spared tissue. But in sensory systems the mechanisms of the subtotal-lesion effect remain unclear. The problem lies in the often tenuous relation between behavioral tasks used to assess deficits and the models of sensory coding in the target structures. The data on behavioral effects of lesions, both complete and incomplete, do put significant constraints on physiologically based models of coding. Additional information about the mechanisms of coding that underlie recovery and sparing of function could be obtained by studying animals with lesions with combined behavioral and physiological techniques.

7. REFERENCES

Albe-Fessard, D. Organization of somatic central projections. In W. D. Neff (Ed.), *Contributions to sensory physiology*. Vol. 2. New York: Academic Press, 1967.

Anderson, K. V., and Symmes, D. The superior colliculus and higher visual functions in the monkey. *Brain Research*, 1969, *13*, 37–52.

Atencio, F. W., Diamond, I. T., and Ward, J. P. Behavioral study of the visual cortex of *Galago senegalensis*. *Journal of Comparative and Physiological Psychology*, 1975, *89*, 1109–1135.

Azulay, A., and Schwartz, A. S. The role of the dorsal funiculus of the primate in tactile discrimination. *Experimental Neurology*, 1975, *46*, 315–332.

Baden, J. P., Urbaitis, J. C., and Meikle, T. H., Jr. Effects of serial bilateral neocortical ablations on a visual discrimination by cats. *Experimental Neurology*, 1965, *13*, 233–251.

Barbas, H., and Spear, P. D. Effects of serial unilateral and serial bilateral visual cortex lesions on brightness discrimination relearning in rats. *Journal of Comparative and Physiological Psychology*, 1976, *90*, 279–292.

Barlow, H. B., Narasimhan, R., and Rosenfeld, A. Visual pattern analysis in machines and animals. *Science*, 1972, *177*, 567–575.

Barnes, P. J., Smith, L. M., and Latto, R. M. Orientation to visual stimuli and the superior colliculus in the rat. *Quarterly Journal of Experimental Psychology*, 1970, *22*, 239–247.

Bates, J. A. V., and Ettlinger, G. Posterior biparietal ablations in the monkey. *Archives of Neurology*, 1960, *3*, 177–192.

Beck, C. Forelimb performance by squirrel monkeys (*Saimiri sciureus*) before and after dorsal column lesions. *Journal of Comparative and Physiological Psychology*, 1976, *90*, 353–362.

Benjamin, R. M., and Thompson, R. F. Differential effects of cortical lesions in infant and adult cats on roughness discrimination. *Experimental Neurology*, 1959, *1*, 305–321.

Berkley, M. A. Cat visual psychophysics: Neural correlates and comparisons with man. In

J. M. Sprague and A. N. Epstein (Eds.), *Progress in psychobiology and physiological psychology.* Vol. 6. New York: Academic Press, 1976.

Berlucchi, G., Sprague, J. M., Levy, J., and DiBerardino, A. C. Pretectum and superior colliculus in visually guided behavior and in flux and form discrimination in the cat. *Journal of Comparative and Physiological Psychology Monograph,* 1972, *78,* 123–172.

Blake, L. The effects of lesions of the superior colliculus on brightness and pattern discrimination in the cat. *Journal of Comparative and Physiological Psychology,* 1959, *52,* 272–278.

Bowsher, D. The anatomophysiological basis of somatosensory discrimination. *International Review of Neurobiology,* 1965, *8,* 35–75.

Braun, J. J., Lundy, E. G., and McCarthy, F. V. Depth discrimination in rats following removal of visual neocortex. *Brain Research,* 1970, *20,* 283–291.

Braun, J. J., Meyer, P. M., and Meyer, D. R. Sparing of a brightness habit in rats following visual decortication. *Journal of Comparative and Physiological Psychology,* 1966, *61,* 79–82.

Bredberg, G., and Hunter-Duvar, I. Behavioral tests of hearing and inner ear damage. In W. D. Keidel and W. D. Neff (Eds.), *Handbook of sensory physiology.* Vol. V/2. *Auditory system.* Berlin: Springer Verlag, 1975.

Brown, A. G. Ascending and long spinal pathways: Dorsal columns, spino-cervical tract, and spinothalamic tract. In A. Iggo (Ed.), *Handbook of sensory physiology.* Vol. II. *Somatosensory system.* Berlin: Springer Verlag, 1973.

Butler, R. A. Does tonotopicity subserve the perceived elevation of a sound? *Federation Proceedings,* 1974, *33,* 1920–1923.

Butler, C. M. Impairment in selective attention to visual stimuli in monkeys with inferotemporal and lateral striate lesions. *Brain Research,* 1969, *12,* 374–383.

Butler, C. M. Detection of masked patterns in monkeys with inferotemporal, striate, or dorsolateral frontal lesions. *Neuropsychologia,* 1972, *10,* 241–243.

Butler, C. M. Effect of superior colliculus, striate, and prestriate lesions on visual sampling in rhesus monkeys. *Journal of Comparative and Physiological Psychology,* 1974a, *87,* 905–917.

Butler, C. M. Visual discrimination impairments in rhesus monkeys with combined lesions of superior colliculus and striate cortex. *Journal of Comparative and Physiological Psychology,* 1974b, *87,* 918–929.

Butter, C. M., Mishkin, M., and Rosvold, H. E. Stimulus generalization in monkeys with inferotemporal and lateral occipital lesions. In D. I. Mostofsky (Ed.), *Stimulus generalization.* Stanford, California: Stanford University Press, 1965.

Caldwell, R. B., and Ward, J. P. The effects of striate cortex lesions on visual function in bushbaby. Paper presented at the meeting of the Psychonomic Society, St. Louis, Nov. 1976.

Campbell, A. Deficits in visual learning produced by posterior temporal lesions in cats. *Journal of Comparative and Physiological Psychology,* 1977, in press.

Casagrande, V. A. and Diamond, I. T. Ablation study of the superior colliculus in the tree shrew *(Tupaia glis). Journal of Comparative Neurology,* 1974, *156,* 207–238.

Casseday, J. H., and Neff, W. D. Auditory localization: Role of auditory pathways in brain stem of the cat. *Journal of Neurophysiology,* 1975, *38,* 842–858.

Chapula, L. M., Coyle, R. S., and Lindsley, D. B. Effect of pulvinar lesions on visual pattern discriminations in monkeys. *Journal of Neurophysiology,* 1976, *39,* 354–369.

Chow, K. L. Visual discriminations after extensive ablation of optic tract and visual cortex in cats. *Brain Research,* 1968, *9,* 363–366.

Chow, K. L. Integrative functions of the thalamocortical visual system of cat. In K. Pribram and D. Broadbent (Eds.), *Biology of memory.* New York: Academic Press, 1970.

Christensen, C. A., and Pribram, K. H. The visual discrimination performance of monkeys with foveal prestriate and inferotemporal lesions. *Physiology and Behavior*, 1977, *18*, 403–407.

Colavita, F. B. Temporal pattern discrimination in the cat. *Physiology and Behavior*, 1977, *18*, 513–521.

Cole, J., and Glees, P. Effects of small lesions in sensory cortex in trained monkeys. *Journal of Neurophysiology*, 1954, *17*, 1–13.

Corkin, S., Milner, B., and Rasmussen, T. Somatosensory thresholds: Contrasting effects of post-central-gyrus and posterior parietal-lobe excisions. *Archives of Neurology*, 1970, *23*, 41–58.

Cornwell, P., Overman, W. H., and Campbell, A. Deficits in the discrimination of hidden figures following subtotal lesions of the visual cortex in cats. Unpublished manuscript, Animal Behavior Research Laboratory, Pennsylvania State University, University Park, Pennsylvania, Dec. 1975.

Cornwell, P., Overman, W., Levitsky, C., Shipley, J., and Lezynski, B. Performance on the visual cliff by cats with marginal gyrus lesions. *Journal of Comparative and Physiological Psychology*, 1976a, *90*, 996–1010.

Cornwell, P., Warren, J. M., and Nonneman, A. J. Marginal and extramarginal cortical lesions and visual discrimination by cats. *Journal of Comparative and Physiological Psychology*, 1976b, *90*, 986–995.

Cowey, A., and Gross, C. G. Effects of foveal prestriate and inferotemporal lesions on visual discrimination by rhesus monkeys. *Experimental Brain Research*, 1970, *11*, 128–144.

Cowey, A., and Weiskrantz, L. A comparison of the effects of inferotemporal and striate cortex lesions on visual behavior of rhesus monkeys. *Quarterly Journal of Experimental Psychology*, 1967, *19*, 246–253.

Cowey, A., and Weiskrantz, L. Contour discrimination in rats after frontal and striate cortical ablation. *Brain Research*, 1971, *30*, 241–252.

Cranford, J. L., Igarashi, M., and Stramler, J. H. Effect of auditory neocortex ablation on pitch perception in the cat. *Journal of Neurophysiology*, 1976, *39*, 143–152.

Cranford, J. L., and Oberholtzer, M. Role of auditory cortex in binaural hearing in the cat. II. The "precedence effect" in sound localization. *Brain Research*, 1976, *111*, 225–239.

Dalby, D. A., Meyer, D. R., and Meyer, P. H. Effects of occipital neocortical lesions upon visual discriminations in the cat. *Physiology and Behavior*, 1970, *5*, 727–734.

Dean, P. Choice reaction times for pattern discriminations in monkeys with inferotemporal lesions. *Neuropsychologia*, 1974, *12*, 465–476.

Dean, P. Effects of inferotemporal lesions on the behavior of monkeys. *Psychological Bulletin*, 1976, *83*, 41–71.

Dean, P., and Cowey, A. Inferotemporal lesions and memory for pattern discriminations after visual interference. *Neuropsychologia*, 1977, *15*, 93–98.

Denny-Brown, D., and Chambers, R. A. Physiological aspects of visual perception. I. Functional aspects of visual cortex. *Archives of Neurology*, 1976, *33*, 219–227.

Denny-Brown, D., and Fischer, E. G. Physiological aspects of visual perception. II. The subcortical visual direction of behavior. *Archives of Neurology*, 1976, *33*, 228–242.

Denny-Brown, D., Kirk, E. J., and Yanagisawa, N. The tract of Lissauer in relation to sensory transmission in the dorsal horn of spinal cord in the macaque monkey. *Journal of Comparative Neurology*, 1973, *151*, 175–199.

DeVito, J. L., Ruch, T. C., and Patton, H. D. Analysis of residual weight discriminatory capacity and evoked cortical potentials following section of dorsal columns in monkeys. *Indian Journal of Physiology and Pharmacology*, 1964, *8*, 117–126.

Diamond, I. T. The sensory neocortex. In W. D. Neff (Ed.), *Contributions to sensory physiology*. Vol. 2. New York: Academic Press, 1967.

Diamond, I. T. Organization of the visual cortex: Comparative anatomical and behavioral studies. *Federation Proceedings*, 1976, *35*, 60–67.

Diamond, I. T., and Hall, W. C. Evolution of neocortex. *Science*, 1969, *164*, 251–262.

Diamond, I. T., and Neff, W. D. Ablation of temporal cortex and discrimination of auditory patterns. *Journal of Neurophysiology*, 1957, *20*, 300–315.

Diamond, I. T., Goldberg, J. M., and Neff, W. D. Tonal discrimination after ablation of auditory cortex. *Journal of Neurophysiology*, 1962, *25*, 223–235.

Dobry, P. J. K., and Casey, K. L. Roughness discrimination in cats with dorsal column lesions. *Brain Research*, 1972a, *44*, 385–397.

Dobry, P. J. K., and Casey, K. L. Coronal somatosensory unit responses in cats with dorsal column lesions. *Brain Research*, 1972b, *44*, 399–416.

Dodwell, P. C., and Freedman, N. L. Visual form discrimination after removal of the visual cortex in cats. *Science*, 1968, *160*, 559–560.

Dolan, T. R., Ades, H. W., Bredberg, G., and Neff, W. D. Inner ear damage and hearing loss after exposure to tones of high intensity. *Acta Otolaryngologia*, 1975, *80*, 343–352.

Dostrovsky, J. O., Millar, J., and Wall, P. D. The immediate shift of afferent drive of dorsal column nucleus cells following deafferentation: A comparison of acute and chronic deafferentation in gracile nucleus and spinal cord. *Experimental Neurology*, 1976, *52*, 480–495.

Doty, R. W. Functional significance of the topographical aspects of the retino-cortical projection. In R. Jung and H. Kornhuber (Eds.), *The visual system: Neurophysiology and psychophysics*. Berlin: Springer Verlag, 1961.

Doty, R. W. Survival of pattern vision after removal of striate cortex in the adult cat. *Journal of Comparative neurology*, 1971, *143*, 341–369.

Doty, R. W. Ablation of visual areas in the central nervous system. In R. Jung (Ed.), *Handbook of sensory physiology*. Vol. VII/3B. *The visual centers in the brain*. Berlin: Springer Verlag, 1973.

Dräger, U. C., and Hubel, D. H. Responses to visual stimulation and relationship between visual, auditory, and somatosensory inputs in mouse superior colliculus. *Journal of Neurophysiology*, 1975, *38*, 690–713.

Dreher, B., and Cottee, L. J. Visual receptive-field properties of cells in area 18 of the cat's cerebral cortex before and after acute lesions in area 17. *Journal of Neurophysiology*, 1975, *38*, 735–750.

Dreyer, D. A., Schneider, R. J., Metz, C. B., and Whitsel, B. L. Differential contributions of spinal pathways to body representation in the post central gyrus of *Macaca mulatta*. *Journal of Neurophysiology*, 1974, *37*, 119–145.

Dubrovsky, B., and Garcia-Rill, E. Role of dorsal columns in sequential motor acts requiring precise forelimb projection. *Experimental Brain Research*, 1973, *18*, 165–177.

Dyer, R. S., Marino, M. F., Johnson, C., and Kruggel, T. Superior colliculus lesions do not impair orientation to pattern. *Brain Research*, 1976, *112*, 176–179.

Eidelberg, E., Kreinick, C. J., and Langescheid, C. On the possible functional role of afferent pathways in skin sensation. *Experimental Neurology*, 1975, *47*, 419–432.

Eidelberg, E., and Rick, C. Lack of effect of partial cord section upon thermal discrimination in the monkey. *Applied Neurophysiology*, 1975, *38*, 145–152.

Eidelberg, E., Woolf, B., Kreinick, C. J., and Davis, F. The role of the dorsal funiculi in movement control. *Brain Research*, 1976, *114*, 427–438.

Elliot, D. N. Effect of peripheral lesions on auditory acuity and discrimination in animals. In A. B. Graham (Ed.), *Sensorineural hearing processes and disorders*. Boston: Little, Brown, 1967.

Elliot, D. N., and Trahiotis, C. Cortical lesions and auditory discrimination. *Psychological Bulletin,* 1972, *77,* 198–222.

Ettlinger, G., Iwai, E., Mishkin, M., and Rosvold, H. E. Visual discrimination in the monkey following serial ablation of the inferotemporal and preoccipital cortex. *Journal of Comparative and Physiological Psychology,* 1968, *65,* 110–117.

Evans, E. F. Cortical representation. In A. V. S. DeReuck and J. Knight (Eds.), *Hearing mechanisms in vertebrates.* Boston: Little, Brown, 1968.

Ferrier, R. J., and Cooper, R. M. Striate cortex ablation and spatial vision. *Brain Research,* 1976, *106,* 71–85.

Finger, S. Lemniscal and extralemniscal thalamic lesions and tactile discrimination in the rat. *Experimental Brain Research,* 1972, *15,* 532–542.

Finger, S. Recovery after somatosensory forebrain damage. In D. G. Stein, J. J. Rosen, and N. Butters (Eds.), *Plasticity and recovery of function in the central nervous system.* New York: Academic Press, 1974.

Finger, S., and Frommer, G. P. Effects of cortical and thalamic lesions on temperature discrimination and responsiveness to foot shock in the rat. *Brain Research,* 1970, *24,* 69–89.

Finger, S., and Reyes, R. Long-term deficits after somatosensory cortical lesions in rats. *Physiology and Behavior,* 1975, *15,* 289–293.

Finger, S., and Simons, D. Effects of serial lesions of the somatosensory cortex and further neodecortication on retention of a rough-smooth discrimination in rats. *Experimental Brain Research,* 1976, *25,* 183–198.

Finger, S., Marshak, R. A., Cohen, M., Scheff, S., Trace, R., and Niemand D. Effects of successive and simultaneous lesions of somatosensory cortex on tactile discrimination in the rat. *Journal of Comparative and Physiological Psychology,* 1971, *77,* 221–227.

Finger, S., Simons, D., and Posner, R. The search for recovery of function after brain lesions in infancy: Somatosensory cortex of the rat. Paper presented at the meeting of the Midwestern Psychological Association, Chicago, May 1977.

Fischman, M., and Meikle, T. H., Jr. Visual intensity discrimination in cats after serial tectal and cortical lesions. *Journal of Comparative and Physiological Psychology,* 1965, *59,* 293–298.

Frommer, G. P., Galambos, R., and Norton, T. T. Visual evoked responses in cats with optic tract lesions. *Experimental Neurology,* 1968, *21,* 346–363.

Frommer, G. P., Trefz, B., and Casey, K. L. Somatosensory function and cortical unit activity in cats with only dorsal column fibers. *Experimental Brain Research,* 1977, *27,* 113–129.

Galambos, R., Norton, T. T., and Frommer, G. P. Optic tract lesions sparing pattern vision in cats. *Experimental Neurology,* 1967, *18,* 8–25.

Gerritts, H. J. M., and Vendrick, A. J. H. Simultaneous contrast, filling-in process and information processing in man's visual system. *Experimental Brain Research,* 1970, *11,* 411–430.

Gersuni, G. V., and Vartanian, I. A. Time dependent features of adequate sound stimuli and the functional organization of central auditory neurons. In A. Moller and P. Boston (Eds.), *Basic mechanisms in hearing.* New York: Academic Press, 1973.

Ghatek, N. R., Hirano, A., Lijtmaer, and Zimmerman, H. M. Asymptomatic demyelineated placque in the spinal cord. *Archives of Neurology,* 1974, *30,* 484–486.

Glassman, R. B. Cutaneous discrimination and motor control following somatosensory cortical ablations. *Physiology and Behavior,* 1970, *5,* 1009–1019.

Glassman, R. B. Discrimination of passively received kinesthetic stimuli following sensorimotor cortical ablations in cats. *Physiology and Behavior,* 1971, *7,* 239–243.

Glassman, R. B., and Glassman, H. N. Distribution of somatosensory and motor behavioral function in cat's frontal cortex. *Physiology and Behavior,* 1977, *18,* 1127–1152.

Moffet, A., Ettlinger, G., Morton, H. B., and Piercy, M. F. Tactile discrimination performance in the monkey: The effect of ablation of various subdivisions of posterior parietal cortex. *Cortex,* 1967, *3,* 59–96.

Mohler, C. W., and Wurtz, R. H. Role of striate cortex and superior colliculus in visual guidance of saccadic eye movements in monkeys. *Journal of Neurophysiology,* 1977, *40,* 74–94.

Moore, D. T., and Murphy, E. H. Differential effects of two visual cortical lesions in the rabbit. *Experimental Neurology,* 1976, *53,* 21–30.

Morrell, F. Visual system's view of acoustic space. *Nature,* 1972, *238,* 44–46.

Mountcastle, V. B. The view from within: Pathways to the study of perception. *The Johns Hopkins Medical Journal,* 1975, *136,* 109–131.

Murphy, E. H., and Chow, K. L. Effects of striate and occipital cortical lesions on visual discrimination in the rabbit. *Experimental Neurology,* 1974, *42,* 78–88.

Murphy, E. H., Mize, R. R., and Schechter, P. B. Visual discrimination following infant and adult ablation of cortical areas 17, 18, and 19 in the cat. *Experimental Neurology,* 1975, *49,* 386–405.

Myers, D. A., Hostetter, G., Bourassa, C. M., and Swett, J. E. Dorsal columns in sensory detection. *Brain Research,* 1974, *70,* 350–355.

Myers, R. E. Visual deficits after lesions of brain stem tegmentum in cats. *Archives of Neurology,* 1964, *11,* 73–90.

Neff, W. D., and Casseday, J. H. Effects of unilateral ablation of auditory cortex on monaural cat's ability to localize sound. *Journal of Neurophysiology,* 1977, *40,* 44–52.

Neff, W. D., Diamond, I. T., and Casseday, J. H. Behavioral studies of auditory discrimination: Central nervous system. In W. D. Keidel and W. D. Neff (Eds), *Handbook of sensory physiology.* Vol. V/2. *Auditory system.* Berlin: Springer Verlag, 1975.

Noordenboos, W. *Pain.* Amsterdam: Elsevier, 1959.

Noordenbos, W., and Wall, P. D. Diverse sensory functions with an almost totally divided spinal cord. *Pain,* 1976, *2,* 185–195.

Norrsell, U. The spinal afferent pathways of conditioned reflexes to cutaneous stimuli in the dog. *Experimental Brain Research,* 1966, *2,* 269–282.

Norrsell, U. A conditioned reflex study of sensory deficits caused by cortical somatosensory ablations. *Physiology and Behavior,* 1967, *2,* 73–81.

Norrsell, U. A comparison of function of the first and second somatosensory areas of the dog. *Experientia,* 1971, *27,* 1284.

Norrsell, U. Central nervous structures participating in the simple recognition of touch. *Acta Neurobiologiae Experimentalis,* 1975, *35,* 707–714.

Norton, T. T., Galambos, R., and Frommer, G. P. Optic tract lesions destroying pattern vision in cats. *Experimental Neurology,* 1967, *18,* 26–37.

Orbach, J., and Chow, K. L. Differential effects of resections of somatic areas I and II in monkeys. *Journal of Neurophysiology,* 1959, *22,* 195–203.

Orlowsky, W. J., and Glusman, M. Recovery of aversive thresholds following midbrain lesions in the cat. *Journal of Comparative and Physiological Psychology,* 1969, *67,* 245–251.

Pasik, T., and Pasik, P. The visual world of monkeys deprived of striate cortex: Effective stimulus parameters and the importance of the accessory optic system. *Vision Research Supplement #3,* 1971, 419–435.

Perenin, M. T., and Jeannerod, M. Residual vision in cortically blind hemifields. *Neuropsychologia,* 1975, *13,* 1–8.

Porter, L., and Semmes, J. Preservation of cutaneous temperature sensitivity after ablation of sensory cortex in monkeys. *Experimental Neurology,* 1974, *42,* 209–216.

Powley, T. L., and Keesey, R. E. Relationship of body weight to lateral hypothalamic feeding syndrome. *Journal of Comparative and Physiological Psychology,* 1970, *70,* 25–36.

Pribram, K. H. *Languages of the brain.* Englewood Cliffs, N. J.: Prentice-Hall, 1971.

Pribram, K. H. How is it that sensing so much we can do so little? In F. O. Schmitt and F. G. Wordon (Eds.), *The neurosciences, third study program*. Cambridge, Mass.: MIT Press, 1974.

Pribram, K. H., Spinelli, D. N., and Reitz, S. L. The effect of radical disconnection of occipital and temporal cortex on visual behavior of monkeys. *Brain*, 1969, *92*, 301–312.

Pritz, M. B., Mead, W. R., and Northcutt, R. G. The effects of Wulst ablations on color, brightness and pattern discrimination in pigeons (*Columba livia*). *Journal of Comparative Neurology*, 1970, *140*, 81–100.

Randall, W. L. Generalization after frequency discrimination in cats with central nervous system lesions. In D. I. Mostofsky (Ed.), *Stimulus generalization*. Stanford, Calif.: Stanford University Press, 1965.

Randolph, M., and Semmes, J. Behavioral consequences of selective subtotal ablations in the postcentral gyrus of *Macaca mulatta*. *Brain Research*, 1974, *70*, 55–70.

Ratcliff, G., Ridley, R. M., and Ettlinger, G. Spatial disorientation in the monkey. *Cortex*, 1977, *13*, 62–65.

Reyes, R., Finger, S., and Frye, J. Serial thalamic lesions and tactile discrimination in the rat. *Behavioral Biology*, 1973, *8*, 807–813.

Ridley, R. M., and Ettlinger, G. Tactile and visuospatial performance in the monkey: The effects of total and partial posterior parietal removals. *Neuropsychologia*, 1975, *13*, 191–206.

Ridley, R. M., and Ettlinger, G. Impaired learning and retention after removals of the second somatic sensory projection (SII) in the monkey. *Brain Research*, 1976, *109*, 656–660.

Ritchie, G. D., Meyer, P. M., and Meyer, D. R. Residual spatial vision of cats with lesions of the visual cortex. *Experimental Neurology*, 1976, *53*, 227–253.

Rocha-Miranda, C. E., Bender, D. B., Gross, C. G., and Mishkin, M. Visual activity of neurons in inferotemporal cortex depends on striate cortex and forebrain commissures. *Journal of Neurophysiology*, 1975, *38*, 475–491.

Roland, P. E. Astereognosis. Tactile discrimination after localized hemispheric lesions in man. *Archives of Neurology*, 1976, *33*, 543–550.

Rosenquist, A. C., and Palmer, L. A. Visual receptive field properties of cells of the superior colliculus after cortical lesions in the cat. *Experimental Neurology*, 1971, *33*, 629–652.

Rosner, B. S. Brain functions. *Annual Review of Psychology*, 1970, *21*, 555–594.

Ruch, T. C., Fulton, J. F., and German, W. J. Sensory discrimination in monkey, chimpanzee, and man after lesions of the parietal lobe. *Archives of Neurology and Psychiatry*, 1938, *39*, 919–938.

Saraiva, P. E. S., Aragão, A. S., and Magalhães-Castro, B. Recovery of depressed superior colliculus activity in neodecorticate opossum through the destruction of the contralateral superior colliculus. *Brain Research*, 1976, *112*, 168–175.

Schallert, T., Whishaw, I. Q., and Flannigan, K. P. Gastric pathology and feeding deficits induced by hypothalamic damage in rats: Effects of lesion type, size, and placement. *Journal of Comparative and Physiological Psychology*, 1977, *91*, 598–610.

Schiller, P. H. Some functional characteristics of the superior colliculus of monkey. In J. Dichgans and E. Bizzi (Eds.), *Cerebral control of eye movements and motion perceptions*. Basel: Karger, 1972.

Schiller, P. H., and Koerner, F. Discharge characteristics of single units in superior colliculus of the alert rhesus monkey. *Journal of Neurophysiology*, 1971, *34*, 920–936.

Schiller, P. H., Pasik, P., and Pasik, T. Extrageniculostriate vision in the monkey. III. Circle vs. triangle and "red vs. green" discrimination. *Experimental Brain Research*, 1972, *14*, 436–448.

Schneider, G. E. Two visual systems. *Science*, 1969, *163*, 895–905.

Schwartz, A. S., Eidelberg, E., Marchok, P., and Azulay, A. Tactile discrimination in the monkey after section of the dorsal funiculus and lateral lemniscus. *Experimental Neurology*, 1972, *37*, 582–596.

Schwartzman, R. J. Thalamic sensory nuclear ablations in trained monkeys. *Archives of Neurology*, 1970, *23*, 419–429.

Schwartzman, R. J., and Bogdonoff, M. D. Behavioral and anatomical analysis of vibration sensibility. *Experimental Neurology*, 1968, *20*, 43–51.

Schwartzman, R. J., and Bogdonoff, M. D. Proprioception and vibration sensibility discrimination in the absence of the posterior columns. *Archives of Neurology*, 1969, *20*, 349–353.

Schwartzman, R. J., and Semmes, J. The sensory cortex and tactile sensitivity. *Experimental Neurology*, 1971, *33*, 147–158.

Semmes, J. Protopathic and epicritic sensation. In A. L. Benton (Ed.), *Contributions to clinical neuropsychology*. Chicago: Aldine Press, 1969.

Semmes, J. Somesthetic effects of damage to the central nervous system. In A. Iggo (Ed.) *Handbook of sensory physiology*. Vol. II. *Somatosensory system*. Berlin: Springer Verlag, 1973.

Semmes, J., and Porter, L. A comparison of precentral and postcentral cortical lesions on somatosensory discrimination in monkey. *Cortex*, 1972, *8*, 249–264.

Semmes, J., Porter, L., and Randolph, M. Further studies of anterior postcentral lesions in monkeys. *Cortex*, 1974, 10, 55–68.

Sherman, S. M. Visual fields of cats with cortical and tectal lesions. *Science*, 1974, *185*, 355–357.

Smith, K. U. Visual discrimination in the cat: V. The post-operative effects of removal of the striate cortex upon intensity discrimination. *Journal of Genetic Psychology*, 1937, *51*, 329–369.

Smith, K. U. Visual discrimination in the cat. VI. The relation between pattern vision and visual acuity and the optic projection centers of the nervous system. *Journal of Genetic Psychology*, 1938, 53, 251–272.

Snyder, M., and Diamond, I. T. The organization and function of the visual cortex in the tree shrew. *Brain, Behavior, and Evolution*, 1968, *1*, 244–288.

Spear, P. D., and Barbas, H. Recovery of pattern discrimination ability in rats receiving serial or one-stage visual cortex lesions. *Brain Research*, 1975, *94*, 337–346.

Spear, P. D., and Braun, J. J. Pattern discrimination following removal of visual neocortex in the cat. *Experimental Neurology*, 1969, *25*, 331–348.

Sperry, R. W. Preservation of high-order function in isolated somatic cortex in callosum-sectioned cat. *Journal of Neurophysiology*, 1959, *22*, 78–87.

Sprague, J. M. Visual, acoustic, and somesthetic deficits in the cat after cortical and midbrain lesions. In D. P. Purpura and M. D. Yahr (Eds.), *The thalamus*. New York: Columbia University Press, 1966a.

Sprague, J. M. Interaction of cortex and superior colliculus in mediating visually guided behavior in the cat. *Science*, 1966b, *153*, 1544–1547.

Sprague, J. M., and Meikle, T. H., Jr. The role of superior colliculus in visually guided behavior. *Experimental Neurology*, 1965, *11*, 115–146.

Sprague, J. M., Chambers, W. W., and Stellar, E. Attentive, affective, and adaptive behavior in the cat. *Science*, 1961, *133*, 165–173.

Sprague, J. M., Levitt, M., Robson, K., Liu, C. N., Stellar, E., and Chambers, W. W. A neuroanatomical and behavioral analysis of the syndromes resulting from midbrain lemniscal and reticular lesions in the cat. *Archives Italiennes de Biologie*, 1963, *101*, 225–295.

Sprague, J. M., Berlucchi, G., and Rizzolatti, G. The role of the superior colliculus and pretectum in vision and visually guided behavior. In R. Jung (Ed.), *Handbook of sensory physiology*. Vol. VII/3B. *The visual centers in the brain*. Berlin: Springer Verlag, 1973.

Sprague, J. M., Levy, J., DiBerardino, A., and Berlucchi, G. Visual cortical areas mediating form discrimination in the cat. *Journal of Comparative Neurology,* 1977, *172,* 441–488.

Starr, A. Neurophysiological mechanisms of sound localization. *Federation Proceedings,* 1974, *33,* 1911–1914.

Stebbins, W. C. Studies of hearing and hearing loss in the monkey. In W. C. Stebbins (Ed.), *Animal psychophysics: The design and conduct of sensory experiments.* New York: Appleton-Century-Crofts, 1970.

Stewart, D. L., Birt, D., and Towns, L. C. Visual receptive-field characteristics of superior colliculus neurons after cortical lesions in the rabbit. *Vision Research,* 1973, *13,* 1965–1977.

Suga, N. Feature extraction in the auditory system of bats. In A. R. Møller and P. Boston (Eds.), *Basic mechanisms in hearing.* New York: Academic Press, 1973.

Suga, N. Amplitude spectrum representation in the Doppler-shifted-CF-processing area of the auditory cortex of the mustache bat. *Science,* 1977, *196,* 64–67.

Stricker, E. M., and Zigmond, M. J. Recovery of function after damage to central catecholamine containing neurons: A neurochemical model for the lateral hypothalamic syndrome. In J. M. Sprague and A. Epstein (Eds.), *Progress in psychobiology and physiological psychology.* Vol. 6. New York: Academic Press, 1976.

Tapper, D. N. Behavioral evaluation of the tactile pad receptor system in hairy skin of the cat. *Experimental Neurology,* 1970, *26,* 447–459.

Tasker, R. R. Thalamotomy for pain: Lesion localization by detailed thalamic mapping. *Canadian Journal of Surgery,* 1969, *12,* 62–74.

Teitelbaum, H., Sharpless, S. K., and Byck, R. Role of somatosensory cortex in interhemispheric transfer of tactile habits. *Journal of Comparative and Physiological Psychology,* 1968, *66,* 623–632.

Teitelbaum, P., and Epstein, A. N. The lateral hypothalamic syndrome. *Psychological Review,* 1962, *69,* 74–90.

Teuber, H.-L. Perception. In J. Field (Ed.), *Handbook of physiology, section 1: Neurophysiology.* Vol. 3. Washington, D.C.: American Physiological Society, 1960.

Teuber, H.-L. Alterations of perception after brain injury. In J. C. Eccles (Ed.), *Brain and conscious experience.* New York: Springer Verlag, 1966.

Thompson, R. Localization of the "visual memory system" in the white rat. *Journal of Comparative and Physiological Psychology Monograph,* 1969, *69.* (4, pt. 2)

Thompson, R., and Myers, R. E. Brainstem mechanisms underlying visually guided responses in the rhesus monkey. *Journal of Comparative and Physiological Psychology Monograph,* 1971, *74,* 479–512.

Thompson, R. F. Function of auditory cortex of cats in frequency discrimination. *Journal of Neurophysiology,* 1960, *23,* 321–334.

Thompson, R. F. The neural basis of stimulus generalization. In D. I. Mostofsky (Ed.), *Stimulus generalization.* Stanford, Calif.: Stanford University Press, 1965.

Towns, L. C., and Stewart, D. L. Role of striate and extrastriate cortex in visual discriminations in rabbits. Paper presented at the meeting of the Western Psychological Association, Portland, Ore., Apr. 1972.

Trachtenberg, M. C., and Gower, E. C. Exacerbation of cortical visual discrimination deficits by pulvinar lesion in the macaque. *Neuroscience Abstracts,* 1975, *1,* 70.

Turner, B. H. Functional capacities of rat sensorimotor cortex. *Neuroscience Abstracts,* 1975, *1,* 510.

Tunkl, J. E., and Berkley, M. A. Form discrimination and localization performance in cats with superior colliculus ablations. *Proceedings of the Society for Neuroscience,* 1974, *4,* 454.

Tusa, R. J., Palmer, L. A., and Rosenquist, A. C. The retinotopic organization of the visual cortex in the cat. *Neuroscience Abstracts, 1975, 1,* 52.

Ungeleider, L. G., Ganz, L., and Pribram, K. H. Size constancy in rhesus monkeys: Effects of pulvinar, prestriate, and inferotemporal lesions. *Experimental Brain Research, 1977, 27,* 251–269.

Urbaitis, J. C., and Meikle, T. H., Jr. Relearning a dark-light discrimination by cats after cortical and collicular lesions. *Experimental Neurology, 1968, 20,* 295–311.

Uttal, W. R. *The psychobiology of sensory coding.* New York: Harper and Row, 1973.

Vierck, C. J., Jr. Spinal pathways mediating limb position sense. *Anatomical Record, 1966, 154,* 437.

Vierck, C. J., Jr. Alteration of spatio-tactile discrimination after lesions of primate spinal cord. *Brain Research, 1973a, 58,* 69–79.

Vierck, C. J., Jr. Absolute and differential sensitivities to touch stimuli after spinal cord lesions in monkeys. *Proceedings of the Society for Neuroscience, 1973b, 3,* 208.

Vierck, C. J., Jr. Tactile movement detection and discrimination following dorsal column lesions in monkeys. *Experimental Brain Research, 1974, 20,* 331–346.

Villablanca, J. R., Marcus, R. J., and Olmstead, C. E. Effects of caudate nuclei or frontal cortical ablations in cats. I. Neurology and gross behavior. *Experimental Neurology, 1976, 52,* 389–420.

Walbran, B. B. Age and serial ablations of somatosensory cortex in the rat. *Physiology and Behavior, 1976, 17,* 13–18.

Wall, P. D. The sensory and motor role of impulses traveling in the dorsal columns towards cerebral cortex. *Brain, 1970, 93,* 505–524.

Wall, P. D., and Dubner, R. Somatosensory pathways. *Annual Review of Physiology, 1972, 44,* 315–336.

Ward, J. P., and Masterton, B. Encephalization and the visual cortex in the tree shrew (*Tupaia glis*). *Brain, Behavior, and Evolution, 1970, 3,* 421–469.

Ward, J. P., Frank, J., and Moss, M. Visual acuity deficits in destriate tree shrews as a function of stimulus area and stripe separation. *Neuroscience Abstracts, 1975, 1,* 71.

Ware, C. B., Diamond, I. T., and Casagrande, V. A. Effects of ablating the striate cortex of a successive pattern discrimination: Further study of the visual system in the tree shrew (*Tupaia glis*). *Brain, Behavior, and Evolution, 1974, 9,* 264–279.

Wegener, J. G. The sound localizing behavior of normal and brain damaged monkeys. *Journal of Auditory Research, 1973, 13,* 191–219.

Wegener, J. G. Auditory and visual discrimination following lesions of the anterior supratemporal plane in monkeys. *Neuropsychologia, 1976, 14,* 161–173.

Weiskrantz, L. Encephalization and the scotoma. In W. H. Thorpe and O. L. Zangwill (Eds.), *Current problems in animal behavior.* London: Cambridge University Press, 1961.

Weiskrantz, L. Behavioral analysis of the monkey's visual nervous system. *Proceedings of the Royal Society* (London), Series B, 1972, 182, 427–455.

Weiskrantz, L. The interaction between occipital and temporal cortex in vision: An overview. In F. O. Schmitt and F. G. Worden (Eds.), *The neurosciences, third study program.* Cambridge, Mass.: MIT Press, 1974.

Weiskrantz, L., and Cowey, A. Filling in the scotoma: A study of residual vision after striate cortex lesions in monkeys. In E. Stellar and J. M. Sprague (Eds.), *Progress in physiological psychology.* Vol. 3. New York: Academic Press, 1970.

Weiskrantz, L., and Passingham, C. Equivalent stimuli for stripes in rats with striate cortex ablations. *Brain Research, 1975, 86,* 389–397.

Weiskrantz, L., Warrington, E. K., Sanders, M. D., and Marshall, J. Visual capacity in the hemianopic field following a restricted occipital ablation. *Brain, 1974, 97,* 709–728.

Welker, C. Receptive fields of barrels in the somatosensory neocortex of the rat. *Journal of Comparative Neurology,* 1976, *166,* 173–190.

Werner, G. Neural information processing with stimulus feature extractors. In F. O. Schmitt and F. G. Worden (Eds.), *The neurosciences, third study program.* Cambridge, Mass.: MIT Press, 1974.

Wetzel, A. B. Visual cortical lesions in the cat: A study of depth and pattern discrimination. *Journal of Comparative and Physiological Psychology,* 1969, *68,* 580–588.

White, J. C. Cordotomy: Assessment of its effectiveness and suggestions for its improvement. *Clinical Neurosurgery,* 1966, *13,* 1–19.

White, J. C., and Sweet, W. H. *Pain and the neurosurgeon.* Springfield, Ill.: Thomas, 1969.

Whitfield, I. C. Auditory cortex: Tonal, temporal or topical? In M. B. Sachs (Ed.), *Physiology of the auditory system.* Baltimore, Md.: National Educational Consultants, 1971.

Whitfield, I. C., Cranford, J. L., Ravizza, R., and Diamond, I. T. Effects of unilateral ablation of auditory cortex in cat on complex sound localization. *Journal of Neurophysiology,* 1972, *35,* 718–731.

Wilson, W. A., Jr., and Mishkin, M. Comparison of the effects of inferotemporal and lateral occipital lesions on visually guided behavior in monkeys. *Journal of Comparative and Physiological Psychology,* 1959, *52,* 10–17.

Winans, S. S. Visual form discrimination after removal of the visual cortex in cats. *Science,* 1967, *158,* 944–946.

Winans, S. S. Visual cues used by normal and visual-decorticate cats to discriminate figures of equal luminous flux. *Journal of Comparative and Physiological Psychology,* 1971, *74,* 167–178.

Wingblade, L. C. Auditory temporal cortex lesions and frequency discriminations in the rabbit and cat. Unpublished doctoral dissertation, Indiana University, Bloomington, 1977.

Winterkorn, J. M. S. Visual discrimination between spatially separated stimuli by cats with lesions of the superior colliculus-pretectum. *Brain Research,* 1975, *100,* 523–541.

Wood, C. C., Spear, P. D., and Braun, J. J. Effects of sequential lesions of suprasylvian gyri and visual cortex on pattern discrimination in the cat. *Brain Research,* 1974, *66,* 443–466.

Zangwill, O. Lashley's concept of cerebral mass action. In W. H. Thorpe and O. L. Zangwill (Eds.), *Current problems in animal behavior.* London: Cambridge University Press, 1961.

Zeigler, H. P. Effects of endbrain lesions upon visual discrimination learning in pigeons. *Journal of Comparative Neurology,* 1963, *120,* 161–182.

11

Pharmacological Modification of Brain Lesion Syndromes

STANLEY D. GLICK AND BETTY ZIMMERBERG

The study of the interaction of drugs with lesions has usually been approached from two points of view, depending upon whether the investigator is primarily interested in where drugs act or in how the effects of lesions can be ameliorated. Site of action studies have been reviewed previously (Glick, 1976, 1977). This chapter will focus on how drugs can be used to understand behavioral syndromes following brain damage and, how, in some cases, recovery of function can be facilitated by drugs. However, before discussing the data, a very brief review of some methodological considerations is in order.

1. METHODOLOGICAL CONSIDERATIONS

Lesion Size and Behavioral Baselines. Lesion size is a potentially critical variable in determining the nature of a postoperative drug response. Quite different conclusions can be reached depending upon whether the lesions under consideration are very large or very small. "Very large" or "very small" refers to the relative size of the lesion, that is, the size of the lesion in relationship to the size of the structure in which the lesion is made. A lesion 1 mm in diameter might be very

STANLEY D. GLICK AND BETTY ZIMMERBERG • Department of Pharmacology, Mount Sinai School of Medicine, City University of New York, Fifth Avenue and 100th Street, New York, N.Y. 10029

large if placed in the substantia nigra of the rat but very small if placed in the striatum of the rat. Different degrees of behavioral effects produced by large and small lesions may *a priori* determine the range of possible drug responses. For example, suppose we are testing the behavioral effects of a drug known to inhibit synthesis of dopamine in the striatum. If we test the drug in an animal with a small striatal lesion, we might find that the drug produces a larger behavioral effect than in the normal animal. We might interpret this result to indicate that, since we had destroyed some dopaminergic striatal neurons with the lesion, there were fewer neurons to inhibit with the drug, and hence the result of increased postoperative drug sensitivity. In the case of an animal with a large striatal lesion, our behavioral baseline might differ considerably; in fact, such an animal might exhibit behaviors similar to those induced by the inhibitor of dopamine synthesis in normal animals. When the inhibitor is administered to the animal with the large lesion, there might be no measurable effect of the drug. A conclusion of decreased drug sensitivity might then be reached. This conclusion would seem to be erroneous or at least prejudiced because the lesion had already produced a maximal or "ceiling" effect in the same system affected by the drug. Thus, the kind of drug response is in part determined by behavioral baselines, and behavioral baselines may be different in animals with lesions of different extent (e.g., Glick, 1975).

Postoperative Intervals. The time between surgery and postoperative testing with drugs should be either critically controlled or systematically varied since, as will become evident later, different changes in drug sensitivity may occur at different postoperative intervals. Such information may be particularly useful in providing inferences about recovery mechanisms (e.g., Glick, 1974).

Dose–Response Curves. It is usually essential to conduct complete dose–response curves if any interpretation of a lesion–drug interaction is to be made. This is especially true if the normal dose–response curve is nonmonotonic (e.g., Glick and Marsanico, 1974).

Schedule of Drug Administration. It is frequently desirable to test an animal several times, either to confirm a particular result or to gather as much information about a phenomenon as possible with a minimum amount of expense and effort. This is often the case when testing drug responses in animals with brain lesions; if a different animal had to be used each time one dose of a drug was tested, an experiment might require an enormous number of subjects requiring an enormous number of brain lesions. Sometimes, this is exactly what is required to prove a particular point. However, when the experimental design does involve repeated testing of the same animal with different doses of the same or different drugs, some consideration must be given to the schedule of drug administration. Unless one specifically intends to study effects of chronic drug administration, successive doses must be spaced far apart so that the animal is in approximately the same state during each testing session. Two points are of special significance for drug testing in the brain-damaged animal: (1) Drugs may have more persistent effects than in normal animals; this may occur because more drug is getting into the brain as a result of a lesion-induced impairment in the blood–brain barrier. (2) Drug administration may affect the time course of processes under study. For example, as a function of some hypothetical mechanism, changes in drug sensitivity might progressively occur with increasing time after surgery. If drug administration itself affected the responsible mechanism, then different results might occur if the same animals were tested at several different time points than if different animals were each tested once at different time points (e.g., Glick and Greenstein, 1973).

2. LATERAL HYPOTHALAMIC SYNDROME

It is well established that bilateral lesions of the lateral hypothalamus (LH) in the rat produce a syndrome of aphagia and adipsia. If kept alive by intragastric tube feedings for several days or weeks, recovery of spontaneous feeding may eventually occur, although residual deficits, particularly in the regulation of water intake, remain indefinitely (Teitelbaum and Epstein, 1962). An important role of catecholamines has been implicated in both normal feeding behavior (e.g., Grossman, 1962; Leibowitz, 1971; Margules, 1970) and in the aphagic-adipsic syndrome following LH lesions (e.g., Berger, Wise and Stein, 1971; Zigmond and Stricker, 1972). However, there is some controversy as to which catecholamine—norepinephrine or dopamine— is primarily involved in feeding and to what extent the LH syndrome is attributable to damage of noradrenergic pathways within the hypothalamus or of dopaminergic nigrostriatal fibers adjacent to the hypothalamus (e.g., Marshall, Richardson, and Teitelbaum, 1974). The administration of drugs has been useful in examining both the localization problem and possible mechanisms responsible for the partial recovery of function that usually occurs in LH animals.

One approach has been to mimic the LH syndrome with drug treatments that differentially deplete the brain of norepinephrine and dopamine. Most commonly used is 6-hydroxydopamine, an agent which destroys catecholamine-containing neurons when injected intraventricularly or intracisternally. If combined with other drugs, for example, desipramine or pargyline (Breese and Traylor, 1971), the relative depletion of brain norepinephrine and dopamine can be altered. Desipramine inhibits presynaptic uptake of amines at noradrenergic, but not at dopaminergic, terminals. Since 6-hydroxydopamine enters neurons via the membrane amine transport mechanism, the concurrent administration of desipramine results in the normal degree of dopamine depletion but less norepinephrine depletion. In contrast, when combined with pargyline, 6-hydroxydopamine produces the same degree of norepinephrine depletion as it would alone but a greater degree of dopamine depletion. Although the mechanism of pargyline's interaction is not clear, the combination of pargyline and 6-hydroxydopamine induces much more severe symptoms of the LH syndrome than does 6-hydroxydopamine alone (e.g., Zigmond and Stricker, 1972). Since pargyline only increases the depletion of dopamine, the behavioral result indicates that impairment of dopaminergic, rather than noradrenergic, function is more critical in producing the LH syndrome. In several studies of this kind, a better correlation of the LH syndrome with dopamine levels than with norepinephrine levels has been consistently observed.

The process of recovery after LH lesions appears to depend on time after surgery *per se* rather than on any postoperative experience (DiCara, 1970). Recovery can be facilitated by administering drugs before making the lesion. α-Methyl-p-tyrosine (aMT), a reversible inhibitor of tyrosine hydroxylase, depletes the brain of both dopamine and norepinephrine. When aMT was administered to rats for 3 days before LH surgery, postoperative recovery was facilitated. In fact, rats with LH lesions recovered spontaneously, without having been kept alive with intragastric tube feedings (Glick, Greenstein, and Zimmerberg, 1972). Other investigators observed a similar facilitatory effect with haloperidol, a dopamine-receptor blocking agent (Hynes, Anderson, Gianutsos, and Lal, 1975). The sequential nature of these drug–lesion interactions may be analogous to a two-stage lesioning procedure (see Finger, this volume). The first stage is a pharmacological lesion, which initiates the recovery process. This action was revealed by the more rapid recovery from the surgical lesion, which is the second stage.

Although the mechanism responsible for the recovery process is not known (see Laurence and Stein, this volume), one mechanism consistent with these pharmacological data would be the development of denervation supersensitivity (Trendelenburg, 1963). *Denervation supersensitivity* generally refers to the observation that when a postsynaptic membrane is deprived of input, either by destruction of presynaptic neurons (i.e., denervation) or by pharmacological intervention (Emmelin, 1961), then postsynaptic sensitivity to chemical stimulation, either by the neurochemical that normally mediates synaptic transmission or by others, increases (i.e., supersensitivity) as a function of time after denervation. This phenomenon has been directly demonstrated in the peripheral nervous system, and much evidence suggests that it also occurs in the central nervous system (e.g., Ungerstedt, 1971b). In the present context, by administering drugs prior to surgery, the neurons subserving recovery should have been functionally denervated before surgery and sufficiently supersensitive sooner after surgery for recovery to be apparent. Termination of drug treatment before surgery should have allowed intact inputs remaining after surgery to become functional again. If aMT or haloperidol were first administered after the lesion, it might be expected that the deficits would be worse than if the drug were not administered. However, upon termination of drug treatment, recovery should proceed faster than if the drug were not administered because, as a result of the initially greater denervation induced by the drug, the compensatory mechanism (i.e., denervation supersensitivity) mediating recovery would develop faster. At least in the case of aMT, these predictions have been verified: LH-lesioned animals lost more weight initially but recovered faster when given aMT after surgery (Glick, 1974; Glick and Greenstein, 1974).

3. UNILATERAL NIGROSTRIATAL LESIONS AND ROTATION

It is now well documented (e.g., Crow, 1971; Ungerstedt and Arbuthnott, 1970) that a unilateral lesion in any part of the nigrostriatal system (i.e., the substantia nigra, the nigrostriatal bundle, and the corpus striatum) will induce rats and mice to turn in circles toward the side of the lesion (ipsilateral rotation). An imbalance in dopaminergic nigrostriatal function on the two sides of the brain appears to be the primary cause of such rotation, although there is evidence for modulation by other pathways (Glick, Jerussi, and Fleisher, 1976). If the lesions are incomplete, animals will gradually recover from the tendency to rotate spontaneously. Amphetamine, an agent which releases dopamine from presynaptic terminals, will reelicit ipsilateral rotation in recovered animals as well as potentiate the spontaneous rotation occurring earlier after surgery (e.g., Ungerstedt, 1971a). By acting predominantly on the intact side, amphetamine enhances the imbalance between the two nigrostriatal systems. Apomorphine, a drug that directly stimulates dopamine receptors, also induces rotation, but its effects differ, depending upon the location of the lesion within the nigrostriatal system. Following a unilateral lesion of the corpus striatum, apomorphine, like amphetamine, will always potentiate or induce ipsilateral rotation (e.g., Jerussi and Glick, 1975). However, the action of apomorphine varies with time after a unilateral lesion of the substantia nigra or nigrostriatal bundle (Ungerstedt, 1971*b*). Although producing very little effect immediately after such a lesion, apomorphine increasingly induces contralateral rotation (i.e., toward the side opposite the lesion) thereafter. This result has been attributed to the development of denervation supersensitivity. The nigral lesion denervates dopamine receptors in the striatum, which become progressively supersensitive as a function of time following the denervation. As supersensitivity occurs, therefore, apomorphine has a progressively greater effect on the denervated striatum than on the intact striatum. Since amphetamine's action depends upon intact presynaptic terminals containing dopamine, its effect varies little with time after surgery. The effects of both amphetamine and apomorphine are antagonized by haloperidol, a drug that blocks dopamine receptors. Comparable results have been reported with other dopamine agonists and antagonists (Glick *et al.*, 1976). Hence, a pharmacological approach has elucidated the physiological mechanism underlying at least one aspect of a brain-lesion syndrome.

4. LESIONS OF THE MEDIAL FOREBRAIN BUNDLE AND HYPERALGESIA

Lesions of the medial forebrain bundle (MFB) in rats result in a persistent increase in sensitivity to painful stimuli (Harvey and Lints, 1965, 1971). This hyperalgesia first appears 3 days after surgery and reaches maximum at 10 days. Damage to the MFB (which contains ascending serotonergic fibers) lowers telencephalic serotonin, and the time course of the neurochemical effect parallels that of the development of hyperalgesia (Lints and Harvey, 1969*a*). Administration of *p*-chlorophenylalanine (an agent that blocks serotonin synthesis by inhibition of tryptophan hydroxylase) also causes an increase in pain sensitivity (Tenen, 1967). If the absence of serotonin is responsible for the altered response to pain, then "replacement" of the transmitter should ameliorate the syndrome. 5-Hydroxytryptophan is converted in the brain to serotonin; administration of this drug several weeks after surgery was found to normalize both the serotonin content and the pain sensitivity in MFB rats (Lints and Harvey, 1969*b*; Yunger and Harvey, 1973). Recently, Yunger and Harvey (1976) reported that the restoration of normal pain sensitivity by 5-hydroxytryptophan was prevented if catecholamine–containing neurons were also destroyed by pretreatment with intraventricular 6-hydroxydopamine. The authors suggest that the catecholaminergic terminals decarboxylate 5-hydroxy-tryptophan to serotonin and release it as a false transmitter. Evidence for such a possibility has been reported in the reverse situation: *l*-DOPA was found to be taken up by serotonergic terminals and released where dopamine would not be physiologically present (Ng, Chase, Colburn and Kopin, 1970; Ng, Colburn and Kopin, 1971).

At this point it should be mentioned that another time-dependent mechanism, known as "sprouting" (see Laurence and Stein, this volume), has recently been implicated in the recovery process. Evidence for at least two types of sprouting in the CNS has been reported. When some neuronal inputs to a structure are damaged, it appears that collaterals from intact neighboring inputs will sprout and reinnervate the same structure (e.g., Moore, Björklund, and Stenevi, 1971). Or, when distal axons are damaged, it appears that other collateral axons of the same neuron may sprout; these sprouts may not necessarily innervate the same structure that was denervated (e.g., Lynch, Stanfield, and Cotman, 1973). Both kinds of sprouting, particularly the first, could underlie recovery of normal function. In the case of MFB lesions, Yunger and Harvey suggest that after serotonergic input to common structures is lost, the catecholaminergic fibers may sprout and form new functional connections. These sprouts may take up the administered 5-hydroxytryptophan and release newly synthesized serotonin, thereby mediating the therapeutic effect of the drug. Subsequent loss of these sprouts after destruction of the catecholamine system by 6-hydroxy-dopamine thus eliminates the mechanism responsible for the recovery. It is possible that such a mechanism may have more general significance in terms of "vicarious function" (see Laurence and Stein, this volume).

5. SEPTAL-RAGE SYNDROME

Lesions in the septal area in the rat have been found to cause a hyperreactivity syndrome (Brady and Nauta, 1953). The hyperreactivity is characterized by an exaggerated escape or attack response to normally neutral stimuli such as an air puff or an approaching object; it appears almost immediately after surgery and gradually diminishes over 2 weeks (Gage and Olton, 1975; King, 1958). Septal lesions cause significant reductions in hypothalamic catecholamines and in limbic dopamine (Bernard, Berchek, and Yutzey, 1975). Catecholamine depletion produced by intraventricular 6-hydroxydopamine or 6-hydroxydopa also results in hyperreactivity (Nakamura and Thoenen, 1972; Richardson and Jacobowitz, 1973), but the behavioral effects last far longer than those induced by septal ablation (at least 4 months, or 42 days, in the respective studies). Gage and Olton (1976) found that post-operative administration of L-DOPA caused a dose-dependent decrease in septal hyperreactivity and an increased rate of recovery from the hyperreactivity. This finding was interpreted as evidence that the rage syndrome is caused by a lesion-induced deficit in catecholamines, and that "replacement" of the missing transmitter will lead to both an ameliorated behavioral syndrome and more rapid recovery. Unfortunately, there is as yet no evidence that the reported decreases in catecholamine levels seen two days after septal lesions (Bernard, et al., 1975) also recover to preoperative levels as the behavior returns to normal. Administration of α-methyl-p-tyrosine preoperatively (which would be expected to decrease brain catecholamines and thus enhance supersensitivity development) had no effect on either the intensity or time course of recovery from septal hyperreactivity (Dominguez and Longo, 1970).

There is also some evidence that serotonin plays a role in mediating septal hyperreactivity. Septal lesions cause a 12–14% decrease in brain serotonin (Heller, Harvey, and Moore, 1962), which, however, persists after behavioral recovery is apparent (Heller and Moore, 1965). p-Chloro-phenylalanine (PCPA), an agent that inhibits serotonin synthesis, decreases septal rage within 30 min after administration on the second postoperative day (Dominguez and Longo, 1969). Since the maximum effect of this drug in reducing serotonin synthesis is not reached for 2–3 days, it appears that this taming effect is not due to a direct action of PCPA on serotonergic pathways. Pretreatment with PCPA for 5 days prior to septal ablation (but not 2 days) will cause an amelioration of the hyperreactivity and a faster recovery rate (Harrell and Balagura, 1975); this course of treatment would insure almost total serotonin depletion at the time of surgery and is consistent with a supersensitivity model of recovery. However, PCPA also depletes brain catecholamines, though to a lesser extent, and an effect on catecholaminergic systems cannot be ruled out.

Acetylcholine may also play a role in recovery from the septal-rage syndrome. There is a decrease in brain acetylcholine after septal lesions (Sorensen and Harvey, 1971). Stark and Henderson (1972) reported that physostigmine (an anticholinesterase agent that acts to increase acetylcholine levels in the brain) will diminish hyperreactivity after septal lesions, while a noncentrally acting anticholinesterase agent, neostigmine, will not. These findings indicate that a hypofunctional cholinergic system mediates the septal-rage syndrome, and that a "replacement" of the deficient transmitter by inactivation of its metabolism will result in recovered function; this study is thus analogous to the "replacement" of decreased catecholamines after septal lesions by administration of L-DOPA in the previously cited study by Gage and Olton (1976). Although these two studies appear to suggest two different neurochemical mechanisms, they are not directly comparable. Gage and Olton administered the drug 1 day after surgery and tested the subjects daily until recovery appeared (within 12 days), while Stark and Henderson did not test their subjects nor inject a drug until 2 weeks after surgery (when other investigators have found recovery to have occurred without pharmacological intervention).

6. CHANGES IN DRUG SENSITIVITY AFTER FRONTAL CORTICAL LESIONS

Several years ago it was first reported that rats with bilateral ablations of frontal cortex became increasingly sensitive to the activity-stimulant effect of amphetamine with increasing time following surgery (Adler, 1971). This result was attributed to denervation supersensitivity. Frontal cortical lesions were envisioned as partially denervating subcortical structures; amphetamine presumably released catecholamines from remaining input to such structures and activated supersensitive postsynaptic receptors. In subsequent studies by others, the increasing sensitivity of frontal rats to amphetamine-induced hyperactivity was sometimes replicated (Glick, 1970; Iversen, Wilkinson and Simpson, 1971; Iversen, 1971) and sometimes not (Lynch, Ballantine, and Campbell, 1969, 1971). Eventually, it was shown that negative results occurred only when a long period of habituation to the testing apparatus preceded drug administration (Glick, 1972). Thus, testing variables which influence the baseline rate of activity may alter or obscure a drug–lesion interaction.

Postoperative changes in sensitivity to amphetamine have been sought in several other experimental situations involving lesions of frontal cortex. Frontal monkeys that had recovered from an initial deficit in delayed-response performance were found to be less sensitive than control monkeys to an amphetamine-induced impairment (Glick and Jarvik, 1970a). But, like frontal rats, frontal monkeys were hypersensitive to the effect of amphetamine on locomotor activity (Glick and Jarvik, unpublished results; Miller, 1976). Moreover, frontal rats were less sensitive than sham-operated rats to an impairment of spatial-discrimination performance when tested long after a postoperative deficit had subsided (Glick, 1971). Similarly, mice with frontal lesions were hypersensitive to enhancement of activity by amphetamine and hyposensitive to impairment of passive-avoidance learning by amphetamine when tested after recovery from an early decrement (Glick, Nakamura and Jarvik, 1971; Glick and Zimmerberg, 1972). In all three species there were no changes in sensitivity to scopolamine, an anticholinergic agent (Glick, 1974). Results with other agents tested in monkeys suggested that frontal cortical lesions selectively interfered with catecholaminergic functions (Glick and Jarvik, 1970*b*), and recent studies with rats have indicated that dopaminergic, rather than noradrenergic, pathways are primarily affected (Glick and Greenstein, 1973; Glick and Cox, 1976). Despite the specificity of the drug–lesion interactions, with respect to neurochemical mediation, the problem remained as to why frontal animals were hypersensitive to amphetamine in some experiments and hyposensitive to amphetamine in others.

Dose–response considerations have suggested that the discrepancy may be more apparent than real. In all instances of amphetamine hypersensitivity in frontal animals, amphetamine has enhanced performance of normal animals while frontal animals have been more sensitive to this facilitation. In all instances of amphetamine hyposensitivity in frontal animals, amphetamine has impaired or depressed performance of normal animals while frontal animals have been less sensitive to this depression. However, in normal animals amphetamine usually both increases and decreases performance at low and high doses, respectively, in most tasks (Glick and Muller, 1971). The exact doses that produce each of these effects may vary tremendously depending upon the task and particular testing parameters. If, after a lesion, supersensitivity occurred uniformly throughout the dosage range, the curve would simply shift to the left. But if amphetamine has two actions, one predominating in the ascending and the other in the descending phases of the dose–response curve, then supersensitivity to both actions need not occur uniformly. A greater increase in sensitivity to low doses would produce an *apparent* decrease in sensitivity to high doses. This seems to be the case in frontal animals. When a whole dose–response curve was examined in a bar-pressing experiment with frontal rats, the results indicated that frontal cortical lesions differentially enhanced sensitivity to different actions of amphetamine (Glick and Marsanico, 1974).

7. DEGREE OF FUNCTIONAL RECOVERY AND AMPHETAMINE SENSITIVITY

If responsiveness to drugs after brain damage changes in relation to recovery phenomena, it would be expected that animals with persistent deficits and little functional recovery would respond differently to drugs than animals which have showed nearly complete recovery. In an experiment designed to test this idea, rats trained to bar-press were administered amphetamine several weeks after receiving either small or large lesions of the caudate nuclei (Glick, 1975). Although both lesions produced initial impairment of bar-pressing rates, only the larger lesions resulted in a persistent impairment. The entire amphetamine dose–response curve was shifted to the right by large lesions and to the left by small lesions. Hence, lesion-induced hypo- and hypersensitivity to amphetamine were associated with lesser and greater degrees of functional recovery, respectively. The data suggested that, following small lesions which damage some nigrostriatal fibers, supersensitivity of the remaining caudate to remaining nigral input may develop, whereas, following large lesions, amphetamine is less potent because its site of action has been excessively damaged (Glick, 1977).

In another study (Glick, Marsanico, and Greenstein, 1974) bilateral lesions of either the caudate nucleus, septum, or hippocampus initially (1–2 days postoperatively) impaired one-trial passive-avoidance learning in mice. Recovery occurred within a month after caudate lesions but not at all after septal or hippocampal lesions. When determined at 1–2 days after surgery, mice with either of the three lesions were less sensitive than sham-operated controls to amphetamine-induced impairment of passive-avoidance learning. By 1 month after surgery, mice with caudate lesions became hypersensitive to amphetamine, whereas mice with either septal or hippocampal lesions remained hyposensitive to amphetamine. Thus, an acute change in drug sensitivity reversed only when behavioral recovery occurred; when a deficit persisted, the acute change in amphetamine sensitivity also persisted.

8. FACILITATION OF SERIAL-STAGE SAVINGS

As reviewed by Finger (this volume), bilateral brain lesions performed sequentially may, under particular experimental conditions, result in less severe postoperative deficits than bilateral lesions performed in one operation. In addition to other factors, the amount of sensory stimulation available to the animal in the interoperative interval may influence the magnitude of the serial lesion effect (Meyer, Isaac, and Maher, 1958; Isaac, 1964; Petrinovich and Bliss, 1966; Petrinovich and Carew, 1969). Amphetamine has been shown to enhance the savings produced by serial lesions of occipital cortex if injected during the interoperative interval (Cole, Sullins, and Isaac, 1967). The interpretation of this finding is usually that amphetamine produces an effect equivalent to "stimulation" (e.g., auditory or visual). Little attention has been directed toward understanding the mechanism of this drug action; indeed, it is interesting that the rather simple equation of "stimulation" and "stimulant" (i.e., drug) has resulted in a somewhat remarkable result.

9. CLINICAL IMPLICATIONS

Consideration of the ways in which drugs may interact with brain damage suggests a basis for some current as well as potential therapeutic practices. For example, although L-DOPA is thought to restore dopaminergic function in Parkinsonism, the question arises as to how such restoration is possible if, as a result of the disease process, there are many fewer presynaptic terminals left in the corpus striatum to synthesize dopamine. Several explanations have been proposed to account for this (e.g., Hornykiewicz, 1974). One very plausible reason for the efficacy of L-DOPA is denervation supersensitivity. Supersensitivity of dopamine receptors, resulting from the loss of many nigrostriatal neurons, would partially compensate for the greatly reduced input; further compensation would occur if, by the administration of L-DOPA, remaining nigrostriatal neurons could synthesize and release moderately increased amounts of dopamine to activate the supersensitive receptors.

Using special regimens of administration, drugs may eventually be of benefit in some specific cases of stroke or tumor surgery. As a precondition for such drug administration, extensive knowledge of the damaged brain area would be required, to the extent that the functional roles of particular neurotransmitters could be evaluated. If damage to such a brain area is anticipated (e.g., in tumor surgery), then a drug or drugs interfering with the actions of the most relevant neurotransmitters might be administered before the damage was to occur in order to promote the development of supersensitivity in the system to be affected by the damage. Faster recovery following the damage might then be expected. If the damage occurs unexpectedly (e.g., stroke), the drug might be administered for a short period of time after the damage. Clinical symptomatology might temporarily be worse than if the drug were not administered, inasmuch as the drug would produce a functional, but reversible, lesion summating with the actual lesion. However, upon termination of drug treatment, recovery should occur faster than if the drug were not administered because, as a result of the initially greater denervation induced by the drug, the compensatory mechanism (i.e., denervation supersensitivity) mediating recovery would develop faster. This kind of prediction is, of course, still at a very hypothetical stage. Other mechanisms, e.g., collateral sprouting and axonal proliferation (see Laurence and Stein, this volume), may also modify or mediate altered sensitivity to drugs after brain injury. In addition, drugs may affect some aspects of a lesion syndrome but not others (e.g., de Castro and Balagura, 1976; Lanier, Petit, and Isaacson, 1974).

ACKNOWLEDGMENT

Stanley D. Glick was supported by NIDA Research Scientist Award DA70082. Betty Zimmerberg was supported by NINCDS Research Fellowship NS05125.

10. REFERENCES

Adler, M. W. Changes in sensitivity to amphetamine in rats with chronic brain damage. *Journal of Pharmacology and Experimental Therapeutics,* 1961, *134,* 214–221.

Berger, B. D., Wise, D. C., and Stein, L. Norepinephrine: reversal of anorexia in rats with lateral hypothalamic damage. *Science,* 1971, *172,* 281–284.

Bernard, B. K., Berchek, J. R., and Yutzey, D. A. Alterations in brain monoaminergic functioning associated with septal lesion induced hyperactivity. *Pharmacology, Biochemistry and Behavior,* 1975, *3,* 121–126.

Brady, J. V., and Nauta, W. J. H. Subcortical mechanisms in emotional behavior: Affective changes following septal lesions in the albino rat. *Journal of Comparative and Physiological Psychology,* 1953, *46,* 339–346.

Breese, G. R., and Taylor, T. D. Depletion of brain noradrenaline and dopamine by 6-hydroxydopamine. *British Journal of Pharmacology,* 1971, *42,* 88–89.

Cole, D., Sullins, W. R., and Isaac, W. Pharmacological modification of the effects of spaced occipital ablations. *Psychopharmacologia,* 1967, *11,* 311–316.

Crow, T. J. The relationship between lesion site, dopamine neurones and turning behavior in the rat. *Experimental Neurology,* 1971, *32,* 247–255.

de Castro, J. M., and Balagura, S. Insulin pretreatment facilitates recovery after dorsal hippocampal lesions. *Physiology and Behavior,* 1976, *16,* 517–520.

DiCara, L. Role of postoperative feeding experience in recovery from lateral hypothalamic damage. *Journal of Comparative and Physiological Psychology.* 1970, *72,* 60–65.

Dominguez, M., and Longo, V. G. Taming effects of para-chlorophenylalanine on septal rats. *Physiology and Behavior,* 1969, *4,* 1031–1033.

Dominguez, M., and Longo, V. G. Effects of *p*-chlorophenylalanine, α-methylparatyrosine and of other indol- and catechol-amine depletors on the hyperirritability syndrome of septal rats. *Physiology and Behavior,* 1970, *5,* 607–610.

Emmelin, N. Supersensitivity following "pharmacological denervation." *Pharmacological Review,* 1961, *13,* 17–37.

Gage, F. H., and Olton, D. S. Hippocampal influence on septal hyperreactivity. *Brain Research,* 1975, *98,* 311–325.

Gage, F. H., and Olton, D. S. L-DOPA reduces hyperreactivity induced by septal lesions in rats. *Behavioral Biology,* 1976, *17,* 213–218.

Glick, S. D. Change in sensitivity to d-amphetamine in frontal rats as a function of time: shifting of the dose-response curve. *Psychonomic Science,* 1970, *19,* 57–58.

Glick, S. D. Differential sensitivity of frontal rats to d-amphetamine and scopolamine. *Communications in Behavioral Biology,* 1971, *4,* 341–346.

Glick, S. D. Changes in amphetamine sensitivity following frontal cortical damage in rats and mice. *European Journal of Pharmacology,* 1972, *20,* 351–356.

Glick, S. D. Change in drug sensitivity and mechanisms of functional recovery after brain damage. In D. G. Stein, J. J. Rosen, and N. Butters (Eds.), *Plasticity and recovery of function in the central nervous system.* New York: Academic Press, 1974, pp. 339–372.

Glick, S. D. Recovery of function and changes in sensitivity to amphetamine following caudate lesions in rats. *Behavioral Biology,* 1975, *13,* 239–244.

Glick, S. D. Brain damage and changes in drug sensitivity. In S. D. Glick, and J. Goldfarb (Eds.), *Behavioral Pharmacology.* St. Louis: C. V. Mosby Company, 1976, pp. 317–338.

Glick, S. D. Behavioral effects of amphetamine in brain damaged animals: Problems in the search for sites of action. In E. Ellinwood (Ed.), *Cocaine and other stimulants.* New York: Plenum Press, 1977, pp. 77–96.

Glick, S. D., and Cox, R. D. Differential sensitivity to apomorphine and clonidine following frontal cortical damage in rats. *European Journal of Pharmacology,* 1976, *36,* 241–245.

Glick, S. D., and Greenstein, S. Possible modulating influence of frontal cortex on nigro-striatal function. *British Journal of Pharmacology,* 1973, *49,* 316–321.

Glick, S. D., and Greenstein, S. Facilitation of lateral hypothalamic recovery by post-operative administration of α-methyl-p-tyrosine. *Brain Research,* 1974, *73,* 180–183.

Glick, S. D., and Jarvik, M. E. Differential effects of amphetamine and scopolamine on matching performance of monkeys with lateral frontal lesions. *Journal of Comparative and Physiological Psychology,* 1970a, *53,* 56–61.

Glick, S. D., and Jarvik, M. E. Differential impairment by drugs of delayed matching performance in frontal and normal monkeys. *Federation Proceedings,* 1970b, *29,* 279.

Glick, S. D., and Marsanico, R. G. Shifting of the d-amphetamine dose-response curve in rats with frontal cortical ablations. *Psychopharmacologia,* 1974, *36,* 109–115.

Glick, S. D., and Muller, R. U. Paradoxical effects of low doses of d-amphetamine in rats. *Psychopharmacologia,* 1971, *22,* 396–402.

Glick, S. D., and Zimmerberg, B. Comparative recovery following simultaneous- and successive-stage frontal brain damage in mice. *Journal of Comparative and Physiological Psychology,* 1972, *79,* 481–487.

Glick, S. D., Nakamura, R. K., and Jarvik, M. E. Recovery of function following frontal brain damage in mice: Changes in sensitivity to amphetamine. *Journal of Comparative and Physiological Psychology,* 1971, *76,* 454–459.

Glick, S. D., Greenstein, S., and Zimmerberg, B. Facilitation of recovery by α-methyl-p-tyrosine after lateral hypothalamic damage. *Science,* 1072, *177,* 534–535.

Glick, S. D., Marsanico, R. G., and Greenstein, S. Differential recovery of function following caudate, hippocampal and septal lesions in mice. *Journal of Comparative and Physiological Psychology,* 1974, *86,* 787–792.

Glick, S. D., Jerussi, T. P., and Fleisher, L. N. Turning in circles: The neuropharmacology of rotation. *Life Sciences,* 1976, *18,* 889–896.

Grossman, S. P. Direct adrenergic and cholinergic stimulation of hypothalamic mechanisms. *American Journal of Physiology,* 1962, *202,* 872–882.

Harrell, L. E., and Balagura, S. Septal rage: Mitigation by pre-surgical treatment with p-chlorophenylalanine. *Pharmacology, Biochemistry and Behavior,* 1975, *3,* 157–159.

Harvey, J. A., and Lints, C. E. Lesions in the medial forebrain bundle: Delayed effects on sensitivity to electric shock. *Science,* 1965, *148,* 250–252.

Harvey, J. A., and Lints, C. E. Lesions in the medial forebrain bundle: Relationship between pain sensitivity and telencephalic content of serotonin. *Journal of Comparative and Physiological Psychology*, 1971, *74*, 28–36.

Heller, A., Harvey, J. A., and Moore, R. Y. A demonstration of a fall in brain serotonin following central nervous system lesions in the rat. *Biochemical pharmacology*, 1962, *11*, 859–866.

Heller, A., and Moore, R. Y. Effect of central nervous system lesions on brain monoamines in the rat. *Journal of Pharmacology and Experimental Therapeutics*, 1965, *150*, 1–9.

Horneykiewicz, O. The mechanisms of action of L-dopa in Parkinson's disease. *Life Sciences*, 1974, *15*, 1249–1259.

Hynes, M. D., Anderson, C. D. Gianutsos, G., and Lal, H. Effects of haloperidol, methyltyrosine and morphine on recovery from lesions of lateral hypothalamus. *Pharmacology, Biochemistry and Behavior*, 1975, *3*, 755–759.

Isaac, W. Role of stimulation and time in the effects of spaced occipital ablations. *Psychological Reports*, 1964, *14*, 151–154.

Iversen, S. D. The effect of surgical lesions to frontal cortex and substantia nigra on amphetamine responses in rats. *Brain Research*, 1971, *31*, 295–311.

Iversen, S. D., Wilkinson, S., and Simpson, B. Enhanced amphetamine responses after frontal cortex lesions in the rat. *European Journal of Pharmacology*, 1971, *13*, 387–390.

Jerussi, T. P., and Glick, S. D. Apomorphine-induced rotation in normal rats and interaction with unilateral caudate lesions. *Psychopharmacologia*, 1975, *40*, 329–334.

King, F. A. Effects of septal and amygdaloid lesions on emotional behaviior and conditioned avoidance responses in the rat. *Journal of Nervous and Mental Diseases*, 1958, *126*, 57–63.

Lanier, L. P., Petit, T. L., and Isaacson, R. L. Protection against effects of brain damage by catecholamine depletion is test dependent. *Brain Research*, 1974, *82*, 374–377.

Leibowitz, S. F. Hyypothalamic alpha- and beta-adrenergic systems regulate both thirst and hunger in the rat. *Proceedings of the National Academy of Sciences*, 1971, *68*, 332–334.

Lints, C. E., and Harvey, J. A. Altered sensitivity to foot shock and decreased brain content of serotonin following brain lesions in the rat. *Journal of Comparative and Physiological Psychology*, 1969a, *67*, 23–31.

Lints, C. E., and Harvey, J. A. Drug induced reversal of brain damage in the rat. *Physiology and Behavior*, 1969b, *4*, 29–31.

Lynch, G., Ballantine, P., and Campbell, B. A. Potentiation of behavioral arousal after cortical damage and subsequent recovery. *Experimental Neurology*, 1969, *23*, 195–206.

Lynch, G., Ballantine, P., and Campbell, B. A. Differential rates of recovery following frontal cortical lesions in rats. *Physiology and Behavior*, 1971, *7*, 731–741.

Lynch, G., Stanfield, B., and Cotman, C. W. Developmental differences in post-lesion axonal growth in the hippocampus. *Brain Research*, 1973, *59*, 155–168.

Margules, D. L. Alpha-adrenergic receptors in hypothalamus for suppression of feeding behavior by satiety. *Journal of Comparative and Physiological Psychology*, 1970, *73*, 1–12.

Marshall, J. F., Richardson, J. S., and Teitelbaum, P. Nigrostriatal bundle damage and the lateral hypothalamic syndrome. *Journal of Comparative and Physiological Psychology*, 1974, *87*, 808–830.

Meyer, D. R., Isaac, W., and Maher, R. The role of stimulation in spontaneous reorganization of visual habits. *Journal of Comparative and Physiological Psychology*, 1958, *51*, 546–548.

Miller, M. H. Behavioral effects of amphetamine in a group of rhesus monkeys with lesions of dorsolateral frontal cortex. *Psychopharmacology*, 1976, *47*, 71–74.

Moore, R. Y., Björklund, A., and Stenevi, U. Plastic changes in the adrenergic innervation of the rat septal area in response to denervation. *Brain Research,* 1971, *33,* 13–35.

Nakamura, K., and Thoenen, H. Increased irritability: A permanent behavior change induced in the rat by intraventricular administration of 6-hydroxydopamine. *Psychopharmacologia,* 1972, *24,* 359–372.

Ng, K. Y., Chase, T. N., Colburn, R. W., and Kopin, I. J. L-dopa-induced release of cerebral monoamines. *Science,* 1970, *170,* 76–77.

Ng, K. Y., Colburn, R. W., and Kopin, I. J. Effect of *L*-dopa on efflux of cerebral monoamines from synaptosomes. Nature, 1971, *230,* 331–332.

Petrinovich, L., and Bliss, D. Retention of a learned brightness discrimination following ablations of the occipital cortex in the rat. *Journal of Comparative and Physiological Psychology,* 1966, *61,* 136–138.

Petrinovich, L., and Carew, T. J. Interaction of neocortical lesion size and interoperative experience in retention of a learned brightness discrimination. *Journal of Comparative and Physiological Psychology,* 1969, *68,* 451–454.

Richardson, J. S., and Jacobowitz, D. M. Depletion of brain norepinephrine by intraventricular injection of 6-hydroxydopa: A biochemical, histochemical and behavioral study in rats. *Brain Research,* 1973, *58,* 117–133.

Sorensen, J. P., and Harvey, J. A. Decreased brain acetylcholine after septal lesions in rats: Correlation with thirst. *Physiology and Behavior,* 1971, *6,* 723–725.

Stark, P., and Henderson, J. K. Central cholinergic suppression of hyperreactivity and aggression in septal-lesioned rats. *Neuropharmacology,* 1972, *11,* 839–847.

Teitelbaum, P., and Epstein, A. N. The lateral hypothalamic syndrome: Recovery of feeding and drinking after lateral hypothalamic lesions. *Psychological Review,* 1962, *69,* 74–90.

Tenen, S. S. The effects of *p*-chlorophenylalanine, a serotonin depletor, on avoidance acquisition, pain sensitivity and related behavior in the rat. *Psychopharmacologia,* 1967, *10,* 204–219.

Trendelenburg, U. Supersensitivity and subsensitivity to sympathomimetic amines. *Pharmacological Review,* 1963, *14,* 225–277.

Ungerstedt, U. Striatal dopamine release after amphetamine or nerve degeneration revealed by rotational behaviour. *Acta Physiologica Scandinavia,* 1971a, Suppl. *367,* 49–68.

Ungerstedt, U. Postsynaptic supersensitivity after 6-hydroxydopamine induced degeneration of the nigro-striatal dopamine system in the rat brain. *Acta Physiologica Scandinavia,* 1971b, Suppl. *367,* 69–93.

Ungerstedt, U., and Arbuthnott, G. W. Quantitative recording of rotational behavior in rats after 6-hydroxydopamine lesions of the nigrostriatal dopamine system. *Brain Research,* 1970, *24,* 485–493.

Yunger, L. W., and Harvey, J. A. Effect of lesions in the medial forebrain bundle on three measures of pain sensitivity and noise-elicited startle. *Journal of Comparative and Physiological Psychology,* 1973, *83,* 173–183.

Yunger, L. M., and Harvey, J. A. Behavioral effects of *L*-5-hydroxytryptophan after destruction of ascending serotonergic pathways in the rat: The role of catecholaminergic neurons. *Journal of Pharmacology and Experimental Therapeutics,* 1976, *196,* 307–315.

Zigmond, M. J., and Stricker, E. M. Deficits in feeding behavior after intraventricular injection of 6-hydroxydopamine in rats. *Science,* 1972, *177,* 1211–1214.

12

Environmental Attenuation of Brain-Lesion Symptoms

STANLEY FINGER

1. INTRODUCTION

The present chapter deals with the possibility that some behavioral manifestations of brain damage can be modified by general environmental conditions. Specifically, it examines the hypothesis that brain-lesion effects might be increased or decreased in severity as a function of the level of environmental stimulation before or after damage, or between successive injuries. It might be expected that marked changes in brain lesion symptomatology would follow severe deprivation or exposure to aberrant or very restrictive stimulus conditions. However, deprivation effects, while interesting in their own right, shed only indirect light on how maximum recovery might be achieved. In contrast, exposure to stimulating environments could reveal more information about the recovery potential of an organism after a specific brain lesion. Hence, the effects of enhanced stimulation will be emphasized in this review.

With regard to nomenclature, terms such as *enrichment, impoverishment, restriction,* and *complexity* are commonly used to describe environmental conditions in this area of research. For the rat, these terms can be operationally defined in relation to a "standard" colony condition in which animals are maintained in relatively small group cages with no special stimulation. In the enriched, or complex, experimental

STANLEY FINGER • Department of Psychology, Washington University, St. Louis, Missouri 63130

condition, stimulation is enhanced above the standard level by housing more animals together in larger cages or arenas and/or by providing them with a variety of stimulus objects ("toys") that can be seen, manipulated, and explored. Conversely, in the restricted or impoverished condition, stimulation is lowered by housing the animals individually in smaller cages, and sometimes by manipulations such as inserting opaque dividers between the cages. Figure 12-1 shows rats living in isolated and complex home cage environments; this figure also shows the free-play area which was experienced by the enriched rats in one set of experiments (Greenough, Volkmar, and Fleishmann, 1976c; for additional photographs see Bennett, Diamond, Krech, and Rosenzweig, 1964; Greenough, 1975; and Rosenzweig, Bennett, and Diamond, 1972a).

As Rosenzweig and Bennett (1976) have emphasized, the specifics of the experimental environments may vary somewhat from one study to another. For example, illumination and noise levels may be controlled by some investigators and not by others; some may change the objects in the enriched environment regularly, while others may keep them constant. This being the case, it is not contended that these environments are directly comparable across studies, although they may have much in common. Furthermore, it should be stressed that "en-

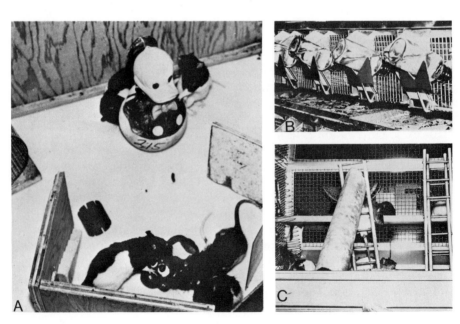

Figure 12-1. (A) Complex environment: free-play area; (B) isolated environment; (C) complex environment; home cage. (From Greenough et al., 1976a. Photograph courtesy of Wm. Greenough, and reprinted by permission of Prentice-Hall, Inc.).

richment" and "complexity" are not states which can be equated with natural conditions for the species under study. Rather, these are artificial environments which *at best* might only begin to approximate feral conditions, at least to a greater degree than would more barren laboratory cages.

Since brain-lesion research with complex environments is relatively new and limited in scope, the current case for lesion–environment interactions will not be treated as an established set of facts, but rather will be presented as a series of preliminary findings. Nevertheless, two sources of *indirect* evidence would suggest that environmental attenuation of brain-lesion symptoms can be expected under some conditions. First, the fact that changes in both neurochemical and neuroanatomical measures have been correlated with the degree of environmental complexity is indicative of the possibility that the environment can play a role in brain-lesion syndromes. Second, a large behavioral literature on normal laboratory animals reared in complex environments prior to testing would signify that some of the same experiential effects (e.g., faster problem solving after enrichment) might be noted with brain-damaged subjects as well. In view of the relevance of these data, some introductory statements will be made about the anatomical, biochemical, and behavioral correlates of environmental enrichment and restriction prior to examining the brain-lesion findings, their interpretation, and their significance.

2. ANATOMICAL AND BIOCHEMICAL CORRELATES OF DIFFERENT REARING CONDITIONS

Recent papers by Bennett (1976), Globus (1975), Greenough (1975, 1976), and Rosenzweig and Bennett (1976) have summarized some of the anatomical and biochemical changes associated with different rearing conditions. Although the majority of relevant experiments involve rats, a growing number of studies now indicate that at least some of the same environmental effects can be seen with mice (Henderson, 1970; LaTorre, 1968) and Mongolian gerbils (Rosenzweig and Bennett, 1970). Species other than rodents, however, remain to be evaluated under conditions comparable to those described for rats and mice.

When animals reared in enriched environments are compared to those from standard or mildly impoverished conditions, the brains of the enriched subjects generally display greater cortical depth (Diamond, Law, Rhodes, Lindner, Rosenzweig, Krech, and Bennett, 1966), increased cortical weight (Bennett, Rosenzweig, and Diamond, 1969), and more glial proliferation (Diamond *et al.*, 1966). In addition, several investigators have shown that dendritic branching increases with environmental complexity (Greenough and Volkmar, 1973; Greenough, Volkmar, and Juraska, 1973; see also the earlier report by Holloway, 1966), and that other pre- and postsynpatic effects such as larger synaptic contacts can be observed in some regions of the brain (e.g., occipital cortex) when rats are raised under enriched rearing conditions (West and Greenough, 1972; Møllgaard, Diamond, Bennett, Rosenzweig, and Lindner, 1971).

RNA/DNA ratios also have been found to increase with environmental stimulation (Bennett, 1976; Ferchmin, Eterovic, and Caputto, 1970; Rosenzweig, Bennett, and Diamond, 1972*b*). Moreover, there are changes in total acetylcholinesterase activity levels in the cortex after exposure to complex environments (Bennett *et al.*, 1964; Rosenzweig, 1971; Rosenzweig *et al.*, 1972*b*). The exact pattern of these and other biochemical changes (e.g., choline acetyltransferase and hexokinase levels) depends upon the brain region sampled, the age of the subject, and the duration of the enriched-housing period (cf. Greenough, 1976). However, recent comparisons with animals raised under "standard" colony conditions now indicate that at least some of the enzymatic differences between enriched and mildly impoverished rats could be more a consequence of isolation than of enrichment (see Rosenzweig *et al.*, 1972*b*), whereas the opposite may be the case with at least some anatomical measures when sexually mature animals serve as subjects (Diamond, Ingham, Johnson, Bennett, and Rosenzweig, 1976).

Many of these anatomical and biochemical changes do not require long periods of exposure to these environments (Rosenzweig, 1971), group housing (Rosenzweig and Bennett, 1972), or complexity throughout the daily cycle (Rosenzweig, Love, and Bennett, 1968) to be seen. However, Ferchmin, Bennett, and Rosenzweig (1975), working with "observer" rats, have shown that active contact with an enriched environment is essential for these differences to be obtained.

Some anatomical changes are demonstrable subcortically as well as at the cortical level. In particular, a number of researchers have studied the effects of complexity on the hippocampus because of the apparent association between this structure and long-term learning and memory (Isaacson, 1974). For example, Walsh, Budtz-Olsen, Penny, and Cummins (1969) noted that the medial region of the hippocampus was 5.7% thicker in rats reared in complex environments than in isolated animals, and that there were also significant differences in neuroglia cell counts between these groups. In related research, Fleishmann (1972) found larger synaptic contacts in the hippocampi of rats housed in complex environments, and Greenough, Snow, and Fiala (1976*b*) noted a 25% difference in dendritic branching in dentate granule cells between rats raised for 30 days in complex cages and those in individual cages (see, however, Diamond *et al.*, 1976, for negative data concerning hippocampal depth differences).

The degree to which the cortical and subcortical environmental effects may vary over time (e.g., Ferchmin *et al.*, 1970) or change with a later modification in environmental conditions (cf. Bennett, 1976), is only beginning to be fully explored. Also, it should be emphasized that even within the same laboratory some environmental effects have been difficult to replicate (e.g., AChe total activity levels; see Rosenzweig *et al.*, 1972*b*). Nevertheless, there now appears to be strong overall support for the hypothesis that the brains of animals housed under diverse conditions may not be equivalent across a variety of anatomical and biochemical dimensions, and for the contention that such changes can take place in sexually mature subjects.

3. REARING CONDITIONS AND PROBLEM-SOLVING PERFORMANCE

A sizable literature now exists in which the *behavioral* effects of environmental complexity and impoverishment have been evaluated. Many of these experiments have examined emotionality, reproduction, gregarious behaviors, consummatory acts, and perceptual responses in both specific and general situations (cf. Beach and Jaynes, 1954; Thompson and Grusec, 1970). Among the most interesting behavioral studies are those which have assessed the learning and memory capabilities of animals raised under different housing conditions.

In his classic monograph, *The Organization of Behavior,* Hebb (1949) presented some preliminary data which he felt showed that exposing rats to complex environments improved performance on an "intelligence test" for rodents (Hebb and Williams, 1946; see Figure 12-2):

> Two litters were taken home to be reared as pets. . . . While this was being done, 25 cage-reared rats from the same colony were tested. When the pet group was tested, all 7 scored in the top third of the total distribution for cage-reared and pets. More important still, the pets improved their relative standing in the last 10 days of testing. . . . One explanation of the better scores of the pets is just that they were tamer, more used to handling, and less disturbed by testing. But if this were so, the longer the cage-reared animals were worked with the closer they would come to the pet group, as the cage-reared became tamer with prolonged handling. On the contrary, the pets improved more than the cage-reared. This means that *the richer experience of the pet group during development made them better able to profit by new experiences at maturity*—one of the characteristics of the "intelligent" human being (Hebb, 1949, pp. 298–299; Hebb's italics).

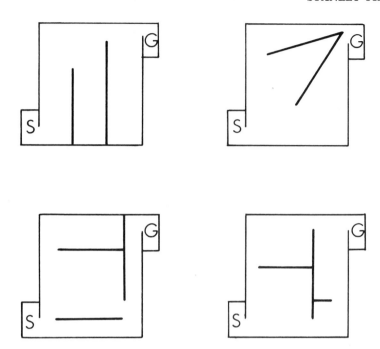

Figure 12-2.   Four mazes from the series described by Hebb and Williams (1946). These mazes have been used to study the effects of environmental complexity on problem-solving abilities. Rabinovich and Rosvold (1951) modified the patterns and standardized the procedures for testing rats in these mazes. (S, start area; G, goal box)

Forgays and Forgays (1952) and Denenberg, Woodcock, and Rosenberg (1968) are among the many investigators who have explored in greater detail the role of the environment on problem-solving abilities. Their experiments on rats will be briefly summarized since they are in many ways representative of a larger population of studies using learning measures. Together, these efforts have been viewed as a significant challenge to Tryon's (1940) contention that "intelligence" is primarily determined by heredity.

In the investigation conducted by Forgays and Forgays (1952), rats were assigned at the time of weaning to small laboratory cages or to large communal ones ("free-environment") with (or without) a variety of playthings for added stimulation. The rats were tested on the Hebb–Williams series of mazes when they were 90 days old. Forgays and Forgays found that animals raised in free environments performed significantly better than littermates housed under more traditional laboratory conditions. As predicted, the rats from the communal environments with access to playthings were superior to all other groups.

Denenberg *et al.* (1968) also raised rats in standard laboratory cages or under complex conditions which, in this case, consisted of a 34 sq. in. (approximately 0.7 m²) arena with a wood block, a tin can, a ramp, and a running disk. Some animals experienced the free environment before weaning (day 21), some were exposed to it after weaning, and some were kept in this environment both before and after weaning. When the animals were 50 days old, all were put into standard laboratory cages for approximately 1 year, after which they were tested on the series of 12 Hebb–Williams maze problems. These investigators reported that enriched experience either before or after weaning enhanced later problem-solving behavior, with postweaning enrichment being more effective. The rats exposed to the large arena both before and after weaning had the best performance scores. These results were interpreted in the context of the hypothesis that problem-solving performance can be permanently affected by early experience (Hebb, 1949, p. 299).

Other studies (cf. Greenough, 1976) have revealed that a large number of variables can affect the outcomes of experiments such as these. Age at the time of exposure to the experimental environment, for example, can play a role, with the most consistent results occurring when enrichment is initiated at about the time of weaning (Denenberg, 1962; Hymovitch, 1952; Nyman, 1967). The particular type of task used to evaluate the effects of environmental conditions also appears to be an important factor, as was noted in a relatively early study using a visual problem (Bingham and Griffiths, 1952) and in a more recent experiment using tactile stimuli (Finger and Fox, 1971). Among other factors that may influence the results of such studies are the duration of exposure to the complex environment (Forgays and Read, 1962; Nyman, 1967), the degree of environmental complexity and restriction, and the duration and amount of testing. With regard to this last variable, Rosenzweig and his colleagues (cf. Rosenzweig, 1971) and Lewis (1975) have now reported that these behavioral effects may diminish with repeated exposures to some behavioral tests including Lashley mazes, visual reversal problems, Hebb–Williams mazes, extinction tasks, and spatial-reversal tasks.

Strain differences also have been reported in this behavioral literature. In one frequently cited study (Cooper and Zubek, 1958), McGill bright and dull strains (F_{13}) of rats were reared under enriched or restricted conditions. Enrichment was found to be beneficial to the dull group, but not to the bright animals, while restriction affected the bright group, but not the dull animals.

Although nonrodent species are rarely chosen for enrichment research with behavioral measures, when such reports do appear they typically have confirmed the rat data (see Thompson and Grusec, 1970). One example of this is a study by Wilson, Warren, and Abbott (1965) in which it was found that cats exposed to a complex environment were superior in learning a series of Hebb–Williams mazes to a group of animals who did not have this experience. In addition to this type of investigation, there is a related group of less rigorously controlled studies which suggests that pets, especially household dogs, are superior in learning to animals raised in laboratory cages. Some of these reports are mentioned by Beach and Jaynes (1954) and by Thompson and Grusec (1970) in their reviews.

As might be expected, there are some studies which show that enriching the environments of laboratory animals will not always improve their learning scores relative to those of animals housed in small laboratory cages (LeBoeuf and Peeke, 1969; Peeke, LeBoeuf, and Herz, 1971; Wilson *et al.*, 1965). In addition, as in the anatomical and biochemical literatures (e.g., Rosenzweig *et al.*, 1972b), there also are findings which have been difficult to replicate, as well as conditions under which the effects of complexity remain to be explored (cf. Greenough, 1976). Nevertheless, the overwhelming majority of experiments utilizing learning paradigms clearly support the hypothesis that animals from complex environments can outperform conspecifics raised under less stimulating and more sterile laboratory conditions.*

4. ENVIRONMENTAL MODIFICATION OF BRAIN-LESION SYNDROMES: EMPIRICAL FINDINGS

The fact that antomical, biochemical, and behavioral measures can be affected by the environment would suggest that animals reared under complex, standard, or restricted conditions might also respond differently to some types of brain damage. The data described in the preceding sections (especially those which show that these effects can be observed in mature animals) also generate the related hypothesis

---

* Recently, attempts have been made to correlate learning measures with some of the anatomical and enzymatic indices described in Section 2. Although significant relationships have appeared in a number of experiments, some investigators have cautioned that these correlations take on major significance only when one variable (e.g., maze performance) changes concomitantly with another (e.g., cortical depth) across *a wide variety* of experimental conditions known to affect one of the factors. Indeed, with reference to the many enrichment studies that have come out of the Berkeley laboratories, Rosenzweig (1971, pp. 326–327) was careful to state that there does not appear to be a *simple* relationship between the brain and behavioral measures that have been investigated.

Table 12-1.   Three Basic Designs for Assessing the Effects of Environmental Variables on Brain-Lesion Syndromes

Prelesion Manipulation	Postlesion Manipulation	Serial-Lesion Manipulation
Different Environments	Identical Environments	Identical Environments
↓	↓	↓
Surgery	Surgery	Surgery 1
↓	↓	↓
Testing	Different Environments	Different Environments
	↓	↓
	Testing	Surgery 2
		↓
		Testing

that brain-damaged subjects exposed *postoperatively* to stimulating environments might be expected to show fewer deficits on some tasks than matched subjects that had been housed under standard or more impoverished conditions. Surprisingly, neither the first ("protection") nor the second ("therapy") hypothesis has received much attention in laboratory situations.

Greenough, Fass, and DeVoogd (1975a), in their recent theoretical review, made reference to three basic paradigms that characterize experiments designed to assess the interaction between "experience" (broadly defined to include handling, training, drug treatments, etc.) and acute brain lesions. The experimental designs involve: (1) an experiential manipulation prior to brain damage and later testing; (2) brain damage followed by the experiential factor and subsequent training; and (3) different experiences interposed between repeated surgeries on the same animals (i.e., "serial lesions"; Finger, Walbran, and Stein, 1973). Although some lesion experiments are not easily classified, these same three divisions will be used to categorize and present material dealing specifically with the effects of environmental complexity on brain-lesion syndromes. These basic paradigms are outlined in Table 12-1.

4.1. Prelesion Enrichment and Performance

Some investigators have enriched the preoperative environment in order to determine whether such manipulations would spare animals from some of the debilitating effects of brain damage. In one of the earliest of these experiments, Smith (1959) examined Hebb–Williams maze performance in a large population of rats, some of which were raised from day 18 to day 90 under "free-environment" conditions (large arena with tunnels, barriers, etc.) while others were housed in standard laboratory cages. Some of these rats experienced small (7% total cortex) posterior cortical lesions, larger (14% total cortex) anterior cortical lesions, or sham operations when they were 100 days old. When the *cage-reared* animals were tested, those with the large anterior cortical lesions were the worst performers, while the rats with the posterior ablations were statistically comparable to the control animals. The *enriched* rats, in contrast, displayed a different pattern of scores. In this case, the animals sustaining posterior cortical lesions were the most debilitated and the least affected by preoperative stimulation. These puzzling results led Smith to conclude that Lashley's (1929) mass-action principle held only for rats raised in standard laboratory cages (see also Lansdell, 1953). Importantly, as can be seen in Figure 12-3, the anterior cortical and sham-operated free-environment groups out-performed their matched cage-reared groups by significant margins, although this difference was much less impressive for rats with posterior cortical injury.

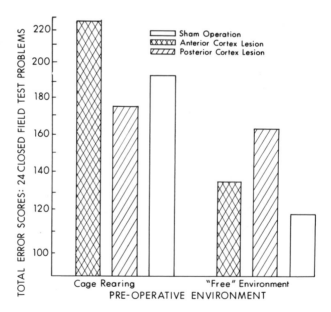

Figure 12-3. Performance of 6 groups of rats on the Hebb–Williams test of "animal intelligence." Data taken from Smith (1959). (Although most animals in each group were operated upon on days 95–100, some had surgery on days 20–25. Smith pooled this factor when presenting the data shown here, since age differences failed to approach statistical significance.)

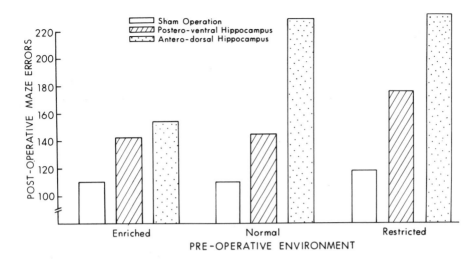

Figure 12-4.   Performance of 9 groups of rats on a series of Hebb–Williams mazes. Data taken from Hughes (1965).

In a closely related experiment, Hughes (1965) raised rats from day 33 to day 66 in standard, restricted, or enriched laboratory environments and then subjected them to one of two types of hippocampal lesions or to control operations. Using the Hebb–Williams series of problems, he found that enrichment was most beneficial prior to anterodorsal hippocampal lesions, and that restricting the level of sensory stimulation below baseline was most debilitating when it preceded posteroventral hippocampal lesions (Figure 12-4). In contrast to the findings of Smith (1959), however, the enriched lesion groups never achieved a level of performance equal to that of any control group, and the sham-operated groups were relatively unaffected by environmental conditions.*

Preoperative enrichment has also been studied with rats subjected to septal lesions (Donovick, Burright, and Swidler, 1973). Although environment and lesion effects were found on consummatory (drinking) and exploratory measures, the use of a spatial-alternation task as a measure of learning failed to reveal a difference between the brain-

---

*Wittrig's (1966) finding that there is a main effect of preoperative enrichment on Lashley III maze learning may be relevant here. Unfortunately, this author only presents a figure for pooled groups of rats (posterior cortical lesion + sham operation; enucleated early or late in life) and an incomplete statistical summary table, making it impossible to separate the data of each treatment group from the mass. Nevertheless, it is stated that no first-order or second-order interaction effects were noted on this problem.

damaged groups: both enriched and restricted rats with septal lesions performed poorly relative to the control groups on this task.

Data comparable to those of Donovick *et al.* (1973) were recently compiled by Lewis (1975) with rats raised from the time of weaning until 4 months of age in enriched or isolated cages and then given large lesions of the hippocampi. The rats with enrichment and one-stage bilateral lesions were hyperreactive (biting, vocalizing, resistance to handling, etc.) longer than the impoverished rats with comparable lesions, and they also gained more weight during the 45-day postoperative period than did the restricted rats. Neither trend was significant among the control groups. On learning tasks, however, Lewis, like Donovick *et al.*, found that the effects of enrichment were limited to the sham-operated animals. In general, both one-stage lesion groups either performed poorly (spatial reversals, extinction) or did not differ significantly from the control rats (brightness discrimination, brightness reversal) on the measures.

It should also be noted that enucleated rats reared in group cages with a variety of objects to explore and to manipulate tactually were no better off than littermates from relatively barren cages when it came to mastering a series of tactile discriminations after large, somatosensory cortical lesions inflicted at maturity (Finger, 1978). Although there was little learning among the animals with lesions, the enriched and traditionally housed control animals quickly acquired the tactile problems that were presented to them. In this study the experiential variable, introduced at the time of weaning, was maintained throughout surgical recovery and testing.

These results, together with those of Donovick *et al.*, (1973) on the spatial learning task and the learning data provided by Lewis (1975), show that under some conditions where environmental effects might be expected, enhanced preoperative environmental stimulation may not affect performance after brain damage.

4.2. Postlesion Enrichment and Performance

A number of investigators have chosen to assess the postoperative environmental contribution to recovery after brain damage. One impetus for this type of experiment is that enriching the experiences of laboratory animals that have already sustained brain injuries can be considered a "therapeutic" procedure. Thus, this paradigm may have greater relevance than preoperative environmental designs for clinical problems, especially in the field of rehabilitation. Furthermore, these investigations can be related to a great number of anecdotal and case-study accounts which have suggested that experiential factors after trauma can affect recovery in man (e.g., Luria, Naydin, Tsvetkova, and Vinarskaya, 1969).

Some postlesion enrichment experiments have examined general learning abilities of subjects operated upon in infancy. Schwartz (1964) and Will, Rosenzweig, and Bennett (1976), for example, subjected 1-day-old rats to posterior (occipital) cortical surgery and tested them on a series of Hebb–Williams problems after prolonged enrichment or more restricted conditions. Many of the results in these experiments were similar. Most importantly, both reported that rats exposed to conditions permitting greater peceptual and motor exploration performed significantly better than animals reared after weaning in individual (Will *et al.*, 1976) or standard community cages (Schwartz, 1964). This outcome appears to be extremely robust in that these two reports cover (1) different strains of laboratory rats, (2) both sexes, (3) various exposure durations, (4) different ages at the time of introduction to the complex environment, (5) large and small lesions, and (6) differing subcortical involvement. In the Schwartz experiment, however, the enriched lesion group actually did better than the standard-colony control group, whereas in the Will *et al.* study the scores of the enriched lesion group did not match the level attained by either the enriched or the impoverished control group. Figure 12-5 shows the findings that were obtained by Schwartz.

Although the results presented above involve brain damage in infancy, there is evidence to suggest that a stimulating environment can

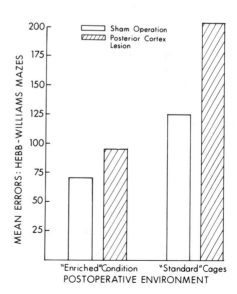

Figure 12-5. Data collected by Schwartz (1964) on housing rats postoperatively in one of two environments prior to testing them on a series of maze problems.

also overcome some of the effects of brain lesions inflicted after sexual maturity. In one such experiment (Will and Rosenzweig, 1976), groups of 4-month-old rats underwent occipital cortex lesions or sham operations and then were housed in large group cages with a variety of stimulus objects or in small individual cages with no special stimulation. Two months later they were tested on the Hebb–Williams battery. Statistical analyses showed that exposure to the enriched environment enhanced performance for both brain-damaged and control animals. Furthermore, the enriched lesion group performed as well as the deprived control group on one of the measures in this study.

Will *et al.* have now extended these findings to rats operated upon at 30 days of age, and have shown that 2 hours per day of postoperative enrichment can produce an effect as great as that seen with continuous daily exposure to the complex environment. The animals with posterior cortical lesions benefited more than the sham-operated animals from the stimulating environments in this study.

Negative findings, indicative of no environmental effects, also appear in the postoperative-enrichment literature. Specifically, the experiments of Bland and Cooper (1969, 1970) provide data which stand in contrast to the results just described. These investigators studied the effects of visual cortex lesions in infant and adult rats on their ability to make visual-pattern and brightness discriminations. In spite of the fact that some of the animals were permitted as much as 11 months of postsurgical enrichment, the only environmental effect that emerged in the individual experiments was on an intensity discrimination with rats operated upon in adulthood. Significantly, this proved to be attributable to restriction rather than to a difference between the enriched and standard-colony groups. Restriction in this case was very severe, involving only 15 min of 1 footcandle illumination every second day (see also Tees, 1976).

4.3. Interlesion Enrichment and Performance

Because a brain structure can be damaged in two or more successive operations, experimenters can also vary the nature and amount of environmental stimulation that is experienced in the "interoperative interval" when "serial lesions" are made (see Finger, this volume). Successive unilateral lesions of a bilateral structure are attempted most frequently in these studies, although other paradigms (e.g., enlarging incomplete bilateral lesions) are now becoming more common. Typically, when the experiment calls for two successive lesions, a period of 10 days to 1 month separates the surgeries.

Unfortunately, there are no experiments utilizing nonspecific enrichment conditions *between* multiple surgeries in the serial-lesion literature (see, however, Lewis, 1975). Nevertheless, there are some studies which have demonstrated that *more specific* interoperative experiences can be important determinants of behavior in the staged-lesion paradigm. Most relevant is an experiment by Dru, Walker, and Walker (1975) on pattern discrimination performance after two-stage cortical lesions in rats. These investigators claimed that self-produced locomotion during interoperative exposure to visual patterned stimuli allowed the rats to relearn a visual-pattern discrimination after the second surgery. Animals that had 4 hours of interoperative exposure per day to the same visual stimuli while being passively transported in a special "gondola" did not relearn the problem; nor did two-stage animals that did not see the stimuli at all. The descriptions and quality of the lesions in this study, however, have been subject to criticism, and some investigators appear to be withholding acceptance of these findings pending replication of this experiment (see Lewis and Stein, 1975).

Experimenters studying staged lesion effects have concerned themselves to a greater degree with the consequences of *specific sensory restriction* during the interoperative period (see review by Finger *et al.*, 1973). Typically, these studies have evaluated brightness discrimination performance after staged visual cortex lesions in rats. Following the lead of Meyer, Isaac, and Maher (1958), a number of investigators have now shown that the serial-lesion effect (i.e., minimal loss of function) may be prevented by keeping the animals in darkness during the interoperative period. Some of the deleterious effects of interoperative darkness, however, can be overcome with intensive stimulation in the auditory modality (Isaac, 1964), or by administering stimulant drugs to the animals (Cole, Sullins, and Isaac, 1967). The hypothesis that these stimuli are acting upon the reticular formation is central to one explanation for these findings (Isaac, 1964).

5. ANALYSIS OF BRAIN-LESION STUDIES

The results of the experiments summarized in the preceding section show that housing animals preoperatively under conditions more stimulating than the relatively barren group or individual cages that characterize most laboratory environments has the *potential* for improving some postoperative performance scores appreciably. The data also reveal that an enriched environment can be "therapeutic" to some subjects that have already sustained brain damage. However, since these results were not obtained by all investigators, it is important to examine the contingencies upon which symptom-attenuation effects appear to be dependent.

The point can be made that a meaningful analysis of a phenomenon such as this one will ultimately depend upon at least one of two conditions being satisfied. First, there should be a reasonable number and variety of experiments in the field. If this is not the case, the relevant factors that may differentiate the successful from the unsuccessful demonstrations may not readily stand apart from many less significant variables. Second, the use of complex factorial designs in which some variables are increased or decreased systematically while others are held constant can do much to clarify the conditions upon which the effects are based, even when the literature itself is of limited size.

At the present time the lesion experiments with environmental manipulations fall short of meeting the criteria for more than a preliminary analysis. Looking first at the number of experiments that have been conducted, this literature, as has been shown, is composed of only a limited number of studies. In fact, two of the experiments (Bland and Cooper, 1969; Finger, 1978) report negative enrichment data, and in only two other investigations (Hughes, 1965; Schwartz, 1964) were *enrichment versus standard colony effects* observed with learning measures. The absence of a standard colony group in the investigations of Will and his coworkers makes it difficult to say whether their maze-learning differences are due to enrichment *per se,* or whether they can be attributed to the fact that comparisons were made between enriched and isolated animals (i.e., due at least in part to restriction).* The same is the case with the nonlearning differences described by Lewis (1975) and Donovick *et al.* (1973). Furthermore, only minimal information and pooled data are given in one investigation (Wittrig, 1966), and no mention is made of whether the enriched animals were compared to communal or isolated cage-reared rats in another study (Smith, 1959). With small samples, these limitations clearly minimize the conclusions that can be drawn about environmental enrichment and postoperative performance.

With reference to the designs of the individual experiments, one finds that when brain ablation is excluded, the typical experiment in this field stands as a single-factor in which only one level of the critical variable (i.e., enriched or restricted rearing) is assessed. In brief, there have been no attempts to manipulate such factors as the time of obser-

---

* Research currently being prepared for publication by Rosenzweig and his colleagues now indicates that standard colony groups with cortical lesions are essentially comparable to isolated groups on the maze tasks (Rosenzweig, personal communication).

vation after environmental treatment or the effects of repeated testing, although brief daily exposures to enriched environments have recently been studied by Will, Rosenzweig, and Bennett (1977). Of paramount importance, there have been no studies in which the investigators systematically removed objects or contracted the enriched environments in order to determine which stimuli or conditions are essential for enhancing recovery among the brain-damaged animals. In contrast, some initial attempts to restrict "proprioception" (Forgus, 1954) or stimulus objects (Bernstein, 1973; Forgays and Forgays, 1952) have provided mixed but interesting results with unoperated rats, and related work with normal mice also has been published (Manosevitz and Pryor, 1975).

In spite of the fact that both the paucity and simplicity of these experiments limit a thorough analysis of these effects at the present time, there still are some methodological conditions which recommend themselves for special consideration on the basis of the limited results that have been published, and, to some extent, because they are known to be important in brain-lesion experiments in general. For example, the type of behavior that is being evaluated after a particular lesion and how difficult the learning task is for the brain-damaged animals are factors which may account for much of the variance in this field, regardless of whether the enriched subjects are compared to standard colony or socially isolated animals. These and other "task" variables that have the potential to underlie some of the differences in the outcomes of these experiments will now be described, as will a number of other factors that might also prove to be important in these studies. The non-task variables arbitrarily will be pooled into environmental, surgical, and species categories.

5.1. Task Variables

Examination of the various experiments in which significant differences between enriched and standard colony or mildly impoverished animals have been reported shows that these studies involve consummatory responses (Donovick et al., 1973), emotional reactivity (Lewis, 1975), exploratory behaviors (Donovick et al., 1973), and the ability to negotiate simple mazes with a limited number of blind passages (Hughes, 1965; Schwartz, 1964; Will and Rosenzweig, 1976; Will et al., 1976, 1977; Wittrig, 1966). In comparison, the two cortical lesion studies that failed to demonstrate any beneficial effects of preoperative or postoperative enrichment appear on closer examination to be more concerned with specific sensory capabilities known to be dependent upon small regions of the brain. Specifically, the experimental investigations of Bland and Cooper (1969) are based on a large number of studies which have shown that severe deficits in pattern vision follow visual cortex damage, while the research of Finger (1978) followed many experiments demonstrating markedly impaired tactile learning after large, one-stage lesions of the somatosensory cortex.

In short, the maze-learning data and some of the positive findings with the other measures raise the possibility that nonspecific enrichment may be affecting a general factor and/or a host of specific factors which may relate to the "general adaptive capacity" of the organism, i.e., to its ability to respond appropriately to, and to cope with, a variety of situations and problems of a general nature. With specific sensory tasks having focal cortical involvement, however, this may have limited functional significance because an appropriately placed lesion can prevent the subject from processing or utilizing the only sensory information which may be relevant for the particular problem. That is, even if highly stimulating conditions lead to something like a superior "intellect," its utility after a lesion would be expected to be restricted to cases where a critical level of afferent input or central processing (possibly due to redundant circuitry or multiple representation; Rosner, 1970) remains functional. With the Hebb–Williams series of mazes, for example, it would be difficult to damage all of the alternative information channels with anything less than an enormous lesion (see Section 6; also Orbach, 1959), and this could be why enrichment is effective here.

Task difficulty *for the brain-damaged animals* represents a covarying factor of immense importance (e.g., Lashley, 1929) which could also be significant in many of these experiments. In this case, task difficulty might best be defined, not with regard to control-group performance, but in terms of whether the animals with lesions exhibited any learning after being on a problem for a reasonable period of time. Using these guidelines, inspection of the data shows that hippocampal and cortical lesions merely delayed learning on the battery of Hebb–Williams mazes (Hughes, 1965; Schwartz, 1964; Smith, 1959; Will and Rosenzweig, 1976; Will et al., 1976, 1977; Wittrig, 1966). In these studies the differences between the animals with and without lesions were quantitative, and enrichment effects were observed.

In contrast, there may have been a qualitative difference between the lesion and control animals on the visual-pattern discrimination after destruction of the striate cortex (Bland and Cooper, 1969), and perhaps on some items of the tactile battery after large, somatosensory cortical ablations (Finger, 1977). These tasks proved too difficult for the animals with these lesions, and the possibility of differentiating between the enriched and restricted ablation groups was effectively precluded when maximum learning scores were assigned after a sustained period of testing. In this context it is important to remember that it is not unusual to find animals reverting to stereotyped behaviors (e.g., position habits, freezing) when confronted with very difficult problems, although fading-out procedures and gradually working them onto such discriminations may sometimes show that they are in fact capable of some learning (Norrsell, this volume).

Task difficulty, as defined by the lesion group scores, could also explain the results of the lesion experiment conducted by Donovick *et al.* (1973). Only 2 of 19 animals with septal lesions mastered their spatial-alternation problem, and this was the only one of three measures on which there was no environmental modification of the lesion effect. The converse situation, where the task may have been too easy for the animals with brain lesions, can account for at least some of the negative data that were obtained by Lewis (1975) with rats that were tested on a variety of learning problems after sustaining hippocampal lesions. Together, these findings strongly suggest that environmental effects are dependent upon task difficulty, with best results appearing with problems that are neither too taxing nor too easy for the animals with brain insult.

It is also necessary to ask whether the testing situation has features which closely resemble the enriched environment. If this is the case, as it is believed to be for some of the tasks described here, many of the effects of nonspecific enrichment can be explained in terms of learning and stimulus-generalization concepts (cf. Kimble, 1961). In fact, with reference to the relationship between the environment and the task, Greenough *et al.* (1976*a*) probably understated the issue when they concluded that "it seems clear that a better understanding of the generality of preoperative experience effects on recovery could be gained through multiple assessment procedures, including tasks which differ from the experimental manipulation" (p. 20). This important issue is considered more fully in Section 6.

Other task variables that could be important in enrichment studies, but about which little can be concluded at the present time, include whether the animals are handled prior to, and/or during testing (Denenberg, 1964; Fuller, 1967; Gotsick and Marshall, 1972; Wilson *et al.*, 1965) and whether they are allowed to "stabilize" to the testing situation prior to the start of formal testing.

5.2. Environmental Variables

An equally important set of parameters relates to the characteristics of the environments to which the animals are exposed. As already stated, investigators have not varied the length of the environmental stimulation within a single study while keeping *all* other factors constant (see, however, Will *et al.*, 1976). Nevertheless, differences in exposure duration can be seen across studies. Hughes (1965), for example, used a 33-day enrichment period, whereas Lewis (1975) exposed his rats to the environmental treatment for 95 days before operating upon them. On the surface at least, differences of this magnitude do not by themselves appear to be the distinguishing features of the successful and unsuccessful experiments in this field. Furthermore, Will *et al.* (1977) have shown that complexity effects are not eliminated when enrichment is restricted to 2 hours per day over a 60-day period.

The degree and variety of enrichment could, however, be extremely important in these studies (see Bennett, 1976; Brown and King, 1971; Kuenzle and Knüsel, 1974), and it is possible that a trade-off could exist between the quality and the duration of stimulation. Related to this is the fact that some investigators (e.g., Schwartz, 1964; Finger, 1978) have chosen to keep the objects in the enriched environment constant, while others (e.g., Will *et al.*, 1976) have exposed their rats to different objects from a common pool every day. Although Rosenzweig and Bennett (1976) did not find that the latter procedure affected normal animals, it should be remembered that in at least two studies (Hughes, 1965; Lewis, 1975) the environmental effects were essentially limited to the animals with lesions.

The treatment group used for comparison with the enriched group could also account for some of the variability witnessed among these studies, and a considerable literature has built up around the "isolation syndrome" as opposed to the effects of group housing (cf. Fuller, 1967; Greenough, 1976; Thompson and Grusec, 1970). Hughes (1965), for example, would not have found an environmental interaction effect after posteroventral hippocampal lesions if his enriched animals had been compared to a standard colony group, whereas a significant difference did appear when they were matched against a restricted group. (In contrast, his enriched animals with anterodorsal lesions showed a difference when compared to the standard group.) Nevertheless, with cortical lesions and maze learning, statistically significant differences with enriched animals have been found in comparisons with mildly impoverished and communal colony groups (e.g., Schwartz, 1964; Will and Rosenzweig, 1976; Rosenzweig, personal communication), indicating that this factor might be of only minor importance in some experimental situations.

Whether enrichment and restriction come before or after surgery may also prove to be critical in specific cases, although the present literature clearly shows that enrichment effects can be observed in both preoperative and postoperative situations, especially with general learning measures. Less can be said about the significance of the interval between the termination of stimulation and the start of testing or about whether the animals are receiving other stimulation or special care in addition to being housed in a particular environment (see Will *et al.*, 1977). Regarding the latter factor, however, it should be noted that some experimenters have attempted to keep handling and related variables constant across the various groups, whereas Donovick *et al.* (1973) may represent the opposite extreme in terms of caring for and feeding the enriched animals differently from the other animals in a study (see pp. 544–545).

5.3. Surgical Variables

With regard to lesion locus, environmental effects of one type or another have been found with hippocampal (Hughes, 1965; Lewis, 1975) and septal placements (Donovick *et al.*, 1973), as well as with lesions in different areas of the cortex (e.g., Smith, 1959). Thus, with at least some behavioral measures, the symptom attenuation phenomena do not appear to be limited to just one or two brain areas. Nevertheless, differences due to anatomical placement have been observed both cortically (Smith, 1959) and subcortically (Hughes, 1965), indicating that the locus factor cannot be taken too lightly. As for lesion size, Will *et al.* (1976) found larger environmental effects with smaller cortical lesions in their two experiments.* The data of Smith (1959), however, show convincingly that it can be a mistake to consider lesion size as a variable independent of lesion locus.

Whether the animals receive damage in addition to the brain lesions can also affect results, and this might account for at least one failure to find an enrichment effect after a brain lesion. Specifically, in the experiment conducted by Finger (1978) the animals were enucleated prior to undergoing somatosensory cortical ablations. Blinding is known to cause hypertrophic changes in the somatosensory cortex (Krech, Rosenzweig, and Bennett, 1963), and the severe deficits that

---

* In this context it is interesting to consider the possiblity that enriched animals can make better use of spared fragments of target tissue than restricted animals; this is possibly reflected in part in the ease with which the animals in the various environmental treatment groups can shift to different but related systems (e.g., paws versus vibrissae) to solve problems after brain insult (see Section 6). On the basis of this hypothesis one would predict that differences between enriched and impoverished animals would decrease with larger, more complete lesions.

were observed in this ablation study may have reflected greater than
normal dependence upon the integrity of the ablated areas in the enucleated animals (see Wittrig, 1966).

Age at the time of surgery is a frequently discussed factor in this
field, and while it may eventually prove to be important under some
conditions, it is clear that it will not be critical under others since environmental effects have been found with neonatal (Schwartz, 1964; Will
et al., 1976), young (Will *et al.*, 1977), and adult operates (Will and
Rosenzweig, 1976) in postoperative enrichment paradigms with comparable tasks. Notably, very old animals have not been tested in these enrichment studies, although data on aged subjects could clarify a
number of important issues (see Gilbert, 1935; Harlow, 1949).

A final surgical variable that deserves at least some mention is the
length of the postoperative recovery period. This may not assume
major importance when long periods of environmental stimulation follow the surgery, but in the preoperative-enrichment paradigm there is
the possibility that environmental effects could be negated by testing
the animals before they have had time to recover from the general effects of surgery. This factor, however, cannot account for differences
among the studies thus far conducted.

5.4. Species Variables

The nonspecific enrichment lesion literature, as has been shown,
contains only rat studies, and within these experiments strain differences cannot account for the positive and negative findings that
have thus far appeared. Some experimenters, however, appear willing
to assume that data such as these are applicable to nonrodent species as
well. For example, with reference to man, Harlow (1949, p. 63) surmised that "the educated man can face arteriosclerosis with confidence,
if the results of brain-injured animals are applicable to man." He also
argued from animal data that experiential factors could explain "why
educated people show less apparent deterioration with advancing age
than uneducated people" (Harlow, 1949, p. 63; see also Gilbert, 1935).

In a preliminary test of Harlow's first contention, Weinstein and
Teuber (1957) examined men with cerebral loss due to penetrating
trauma and found that higher levels of preinjury education were not
associated with smaller losses on the Army General Classification Test:

> Our results give no support to the assumption that education before brain injury
> can influence the extent to which performance on an intelligence test is affected
> after injury. Correlations between preinjury educational level and deficit in
> AGCT performance after injury were of zero order. Correspondingly, groups
> with divergent degrees of education showed nondifferential change in score

when their pre- and postinjury scores were compared. These results not only fail to indicate a trend in the expected direction, but rather show the opposite tendency, since the grammar-school group gained 4.9 points and the college group lost 5.8 points on retesting. (p. 538)

Thus, whether the effects of nonspecific sensory stimulation with rats or even more specific experiential manipulations, such as the training procedures used with monkeys (Harlow, 1949), can generalize to brain-injured man is far from settled.

5.5. Comment

Although it may seem perfectly reasonable to conclude that the nature of the task relative to the lesion, problem difficulty, and the degree and amount of environmental stimulation are among the most critical variables underlying environmental attenuation of brain lesion symptomatology, it should be emphasized that it is not yet possible to state that these are the only factors that may account for the presence or absence of environmental effects, or even that these always represent unmodifiable conditions, since many other variables may prove to be operative in each of these experiments. Clearly, additional experiments, especially some using complex multifactor designs, are needed before the role of these and other manipulations such as handling and the consequences of repeated testing can be evaluated in more than a preliminary or superficial way. Furthermore, if this lesion-effect literature follows in the footsteps of some of the other lesion literatures, complex interaction effects among the various factors will undoubtedly emerge. The interaction of different variables is just beginning to be understood in the infant-lesion field (Johnson and Almli, this volume) and in staged-lesion paradigms (Finger, this volume) in spite of a much larger number of studies in these areas.

6. THEORETICAL FORMULATIONS

There is a lack of understanding of the mechanisms by which greater environmental stimulation is able to modify the symptoms that follow brain injury, and this subject is likely to remain speculative until the methodological conditions upon which these events are contingent can be better delineated. In part because the limiting conditions are not clear, the issue of underlying factors is not even discussed in the large majority of these lesion experiments. A related reason for the sparsity of theory with the lesion preparation is that the types of behavior that seem most affected by enrichment (i.e., exploration, emotionality, simple maze learning) are typically those which are least amenable to the kinds of analyses which would allow one to distinguish among the various possible explanations (for comparison, see discussion of visual-pattern experiments by Bland and Cooper, 1969, 1970). One thing which seems reasonably clear, however, is that *the environment may not necessarily affect the brain damaged and the sham-operated animals equivalently* (e.g., Hughes, 1965; Lewis, 1975). This means that some of the hypotheses that have been presented and evaluated in the case of normal animals (e.g., Greenough, 1976; Rosenzweig, 1971; Rosenzweig and Bennett, 1976) must be reevaluated, amended, or sometimes even discarded, when reference is made to brain-injured subjects. The significance of interaction effects in this field is discussed by Greenough *et al.* (1976*a*).

6.1. Behavioral Models

Explanations for recovery phenomena with brain-damaged organisms can be classified as falling into either of two categories. One group of models stresses behavioral or psychological factors such as emotionality and exposure to stimuli similar to those previously encountered. The other is more concerned with anatomical and physiological changes that are believed to be taking place in the nervous system as a result of experience. Little *direct* support can be found for either type of model in the enrichment literature, although considerable *indirect* evidence can be brought forth to warrant serious consideration for both of these positions.

Representative of the theories stressing behavioral factors are those which hold that exposure to enriched settings allows the animals to learn many different strategies and hypotheses for dealing with complex situations (Forgus, 1954; see also general formulations by Krechevsky, 1932, and Witkin, 1941). From this premise it could be argued that a focal brain lesion in an enriched subject would have a lower probability of affecting all known solutions or approaches to a general type of problem. Maze learning, of course, is precisely the type of task that could be approached in many ways (e.g., visually, tactually, proprioceptively; selective sampling versus go–no-go solutions, etc.), and animals raised in complex environments may come into the maze situation with learning sets and strategy hierarchies that the restricted animals do not have. However, a successful shift from a preferred strategy to a less preferred and possibly less efficient one after a brain lesion may require time, and this could explain why these animals sometimes take longer to reach criterion on some problems than unoperated subjects who can rely on their original strategies. In contrast, only a limited number of solutions may be possible when tactile and visual problems are presented in a controlled manner (Bland and Cooper, 1969; Finger, 1977). In this case, no lesion group may be able to utilize relevant alternative cues after an appropriately placed ablation. It can be added that if there are alternate strategies or solutions that rely on the same brain area, the effect might not be different from that observed with a problem that could be approached in only one way. In short, enrichment should not be effective in either case.

A different model emphasizing learned factors is based on hypothesized differences in the probability of an animal's displaying maladaptive responses during testing:

> The apparent importance of emotional trauma to behavioral studies involving gross changes in environmental stimulation . . . strongly suggests that emotional factors not directly related to the effects of the lesion on brain function should be considered in interpretation of results, particularly when testing closely follows the operation. Moreover, this factor could be critical to the evaluation of the role of experience in behavioral recovery from brain damage (Greenough et al., 1976a, p. 36).

The emotionality factor might be expected to be most important when brain-damaged animals are exposed to novel stimuli. In brief, because the testing environment may contain many stimuli like those previously encountered, the enriched rats could be showing fewer maladaptive responses on some of the measures than the restricted animals (see Forgus, 1954). The similarity of the enriched condition relative to the Hebb–Williams maze environment is significant in this regard, as is the fact that the enriched animals may not view a large arena, such as the one used for exploratory testing, as being especially novel. This might not be the case for subjects reared in small cages with little room for movement and exploration.

This interpretation of the data stems from Fuller's (1967) "emergence-as-stress" formulation: "In the emergence–stress model, excessive arousal in an organism exposed to a myriad of unfamiliar stimuli is assumed to produce an overload in the neural systems underlying many forms of behavior" (p. 1650). Fuller (1967) presents evidence to show that emergence shock in animals (e.g., dogs) without brain lesions can be cushioned in a number of ways, including (1) handling and stroking the animals prior to exposure; (2) first tranquilizing them with drugs such as chlorpromazine; and (3) modifying the new environment to make the changes seem less abrupt.

Additional support for emotionality differences among the lesion groups, although not necessarily for the emergence-as-stress model, comes from Lewis (1975). He noted that enriched rats with hippocampal lesions (or control operations) were hyperreactive relative to restricted animals on an index of emotional responsivity. His scale included (1) resistance to capture, (2) resistance to handling, (3) biting, (4) reflexive head jerk to nose tap, (5) vocalization, (6) urination and defecation, and (7) startle to air-puff stimuli. Although he did not find differences among the animals with lesions when they were later tested on learning tasks, this could be due to the fact that some emotional responses are transient and are readily overcome with extensive handling (see Bernstein, 1957; Bernstein, Borda-Bossana, Atkinson, and Elrick, 1961). Also, as mentioned, some of his problems may have been too easy for the animals with these lesions. In brief, one might expect this factor to vary in importance with the specifics of each experiment.

The major argument that has been raised against some stress hypotheses comes primarily from studies of endocrine function. It has been found, for example, that adrenal weight/body ratios do not differ between enriched and impoverished animals, and that hypophysectomy does not eliminate the anatomical and enzymatic differences that appear between these two environmental groups (cf. Rosenzweig, 1971; Rosenzweig et al., 1972b). These and related experiments (e.g., Riege and Morimoto, 1970), however, may not bear on the emergence-trauma notion or reliably reflect the situation with the subjects described in this chapter. First, the endocrine samples were not taken from the animals soon after they started the maze series. Equally important, these measurements did not involve animals with brain injuries.

6.2. Anatomical Models

In contrast to explanations based on strategy selection, familiarity, or emotionality, some investigators refer to the structural changes that are known to take place in the brain as a result of enrichment (Section 2) and contend that these changes are directly or indirectly involved in superior performance after brain damage (see Will et al., 1977). Stated somewhat differently, the enriched animals may be thought of as having neural circuitry that the standard colony or isolated animals do not have, and theoretically it is this anatomy which enables them to outperform their counterparts under certain test conditions.

With reference to this idea, at least two basic models may be suggested. One is that functional reorganization follows some types of brain damage but not others, and that the capacity for posttraumatic reorganization is in part dependent upon the organization of the brain (this differing between enriched and restricted subjects) at the time of injury. Reorganization of function is frequently discussed in the serial-lesion literature on visual performance after striate cortex lesions (e.g., Dru *et al.*, 1975; Meyer *et al.*, 1958; Scheff and Wright, 1977) and in the infant-lesion field. The basic concept, however, need not be restricted to young animals or those with serial lesions.

The related model, which would appear to have more adherents among the workers in this field, is based upon the supposition that more synapses are formed (or become capable of effective transmission) under enriched conditions (Hebb, 1949) and contends that these new connections can be involved in the critical behavioral functions even before injury. Indirect evidence for this comes from the superior scores of normal animals that have been exposed to nonspecific enrichment procedures. From this premise it is argued that the new circuitry assumes even greater significance after brain damage since its presence may allow a brain-injured animal to continue to perform satisfactorily on the task being examined.

The environmental interactions that are witnessed when brain-damaged animals are tested on alley mazes or on exploratory measures but not on specific sensory problems could be explained if one is willing to accept the possibility that the new synapses that result from exposure to complex environments (cf. Greenough, 1975, 1976) will have the greatest probability of supporting or protecting multiply represented or lower-order behaviors and the lowest probability of mediating higher-order discriminative acts that have more limited representation. Stated somewhat differently, visual- and tactile-pattern problems may require qualitatively or quantitatively different changes in the brain than those needed for maze learning before the scores of these animals can rise above chance levels after injury to striate or somatosensory cortices, respectively. Needless to say, many other assumptions could be made to account for the observation that specific sensory discriminative acts seem to be relatively unaffected by enrichment in these lesion investigations. Hence, the idea that under certain anatomical conditions one solution could be substituted for another on some types of problems but not on others could also account for these data.

It should be stressed that the hypotheses presented in the preceding paragraphs may not be mutually exclusive and that they do not represent all of the behavioral and biological theories that could be advanced to explain how environmental conditions can affect the performance scores of brain-damaged subjects. Thus, these interpretations should be looked upon as illustrative and not as exhaustive. In particular, the reader is referred to Greenough *et al.* (1976a) for a further analysis of some of these ideas and presentation of other models that may also be applicable to the subjects in these experiments.

7. CONCLUSIONS

While there is strong support for the hypothesis that generalized environmental experience has the potential to attenuate some brain-lesion effects, a number of unknowns limit the significance of this finding:

1. The extent to which the results from maze-learning studies are generalizable to other learning situations is not certain.
2. Whether the degree of recovery demonstrated by the enriched rats is even approximating that which may be possible under feral conditions has yet to be ascertained.
3. The extent to which these findings are rat- or rodent-specific is not known.
4. The conditions limiting these phenomena have yet to be defined.
5. The mechanisms underlying the effects remain to be elucidated.

Further experimentation with different organisms, more varied environments, and a greater range of behavioral measures should clarify some of these issues, and multifactor designs may be especially useful in this regard.

Although more questions may be raised than are answered by the studies that have already been conducted, the presence of "positive instances" with brain-damaged animals strongly suggests that more attention should be paid to environmental and experiential variables in behavioral research, especially when neurological manipulations are employed. These factors may affect the capacities of laboratory animals and man to recover from damage to the central nervous system, and they could account for at least some of the variability that is characteristically witnessed both among subjects and between studies in the behavioral sciences.

Acknowledgment

The preparation of this chapter was supported in part by NINCDS Grant NS-11002.

8. REFERENCES

Beach, F. A., and Jaynes, J. Effects of early experience upon the behavior of animals. *Psychological Bulletin*, 1954, *51*, 239–263.

Bennett, E. L. Cerebral effects of differential experience and training. In M. R. Rosenzweig and E. L. Bennett (Eds.), *Neural mechanisms of learning and memory*. Cambridge, Mass.: M.I.T. Press, 1976, pp. 279–287.

Bennett, E. L., Diamond, M. C., Krech, D., and Rosenzweig, M. R. Chemical and anatomical plasticity of the brain. *Science*, 1964, *146*, 610–619.

Bennett, E. L., Rosenzweig, M. R., and Diamond, M. C. Rat brain: Effects of environmental enrichment on wet and dry weights. *Science*, 1969, *163*, 825–826.

Bernstein, L. The effects of variations in handling upon learning and retention. *Journal of Comparative and Physiological Psychology*, 1957, *50*, 162–167.

Bernstein, L. A study of some enriching variables in a free-environment for rats. *Journal of Psychosomatic Research*, 1973, *17*, 85–88.

Bernstein, L., Borda-Bossana, D., Atkinson, H. An experimental test of the permanence of learning deficits in the environmentally restricted rat. *Journal of Psychosomatic Research*, 1961, *5*, 127–131.

Bingham, W. E., and Griffiths, W. J., Jr. The effect of different environments during infancy on adult behavior in the rat. *Journal of Comparative and Physiological Psychology*, 1952, *45*, 307–312.

Bland, B. H., and Cooper, R. M. Posterior neodecortication in the rat: Age at operation and experience. *Journal of Comparative and Physiological Psychology*, 1969, *69*, 345–354.

Bland, B. H., and Cooper, R. M. Experience and vision of the posterior neodecorticate rat. *Physiology and Behavior*, 1970, *5*, 211–214.

Brown, C. P., and King, M. G. Developmental environment: Variables important for later learning and changes in cholinergic activity. *Developmental Psychobiology*, 1971, *4*, 275–286.

Cole, D. D., Sullins, W. R., and Isaac, W. Pharmacological modifications of the effects of spaced occipital ablations. *Psychopharmacologia* (Berlin), 1967, *11*, 311–316.

Cooper, R. M., and Zubek, J. P. Effects of enriched and restricted early environments on the learning ability of bright and dull rats. *Canadian Journal of Psychology*, 1958, *12*, 159–164.

Denenberg, V. H. An attempt to isolate critical periods for development in the rat. *Journal of Comparative and Physiological Psychology*, 1962, *55*, 813–815.

Denenberg, V. H. Critical periods, stimulus input, and emotional reactivity: A theory of infantile stimulation. *Psychological Review*, 1964, *71*, 335–351.

Denenberg, V. H., Woodcock, J. M., and Rosenberg, K. M. Long-term effects of preweaning and postweaning free-environment experience on rats' problem-solving behavior. *Journal of Comparative and Physiological Psychology*, 1968, *66*, 533–535.

Diamond, M. C., Law, F., Rhodes, H., Lindner, B., Rosenzweig, M. R., Krech, D., and Bennett, E. L. Increases in cortical depth and glia numbers in rats subjected to enriched environment. *Journal of Comparative Neurology*, 1966, *128*, 117–125.

Diamond, M. C., Ingham, C. A., Johnson, R. E., Bennett, E. L., and Rosenzweig, M. R. Effects of environment on morphology of rat cerebral cortex and hippocampus. *Journal of Neurobiology*, 1976, *7*, 75–85.

Donovick, P. J., Burright, R. G., and Swidler, M. A. Presurgical rearing environment alters exploration, fluid consumption, and learning of septal lesioned and control rats. *Physiology and Behavior*, 1973, *11*, 543–553.

Dru, D., Walker, J. P., and Walker, J. B. Self-produced locomotion restores visual capacity after striate lesion. *Science,* 1975, *187,* 265–266.

Ferchmin, P. A., Bennett, E. L., and Rosenzweig, M. R. Direct contact with enriched environment is required to alter cerebral weights in rats. *Journal of Comparative and Physiological Psychology,* 1975, *88,* 360–367.

Ferchmin, P. A., Eterovic, V. A., and Caputto, R. Studies of brain weight and RNA content after short periods of exposure to environmental complexity. *Brain Research,* 1970, *20,* 49–57.

Finger, S. Postweaning environmental stimulation and somesthetic performance in rats sustaining cortical lesions at maturity. *Developmental Psychobiology,* 1978, in press.

Finger, S., and Fox, M. W. Effects of early tactile enrichment on open field activity and tactile discriminative ability in the rat. *Developmental Psychobiology,* 1971, *4,* 269–274.

Finger, S., Walbran, B., and Stein, D. G. Brain damage and behavioral recovery: Serial lesion phenomena. *Brain Research,* 1973, *63,* 1–18.

Fleishmann, T. B. Effects of differential rearing complexity on synapses of the rat hippocampus. Unpublished Masters thesis, University of Illinois, 1972.

Forgays, D. G., and Forgays, J. W. The nature of the effect of free-environmental experience in the rat. *Journal of Comparative and Physiological Psychology,* 1952, *45,* 322–328.

Forgays, D. G., and Read, J. M. Crucial periods for free-environmental experience in the rat. *Journal of Comparative and Physiological Psychology,* 1962, *55,* 816–818.

Forgus, R. H. The effect of early perceptual learning on the behavioral organization of adult rats. *Journal of Comparative and Physiological Psychology,* 1954, *47,* 331–336.

Fuller, J. L. Experiential deprivation and later behavior. *Science,* 1967, *158,* 1645–1652.

Gilbert, J. G. Mental efficiency in senescence. *Archives of Psychology* (New York), 1935, *27* No. 188.

Globus, A. Brain morphology as a function of presynaptic morphology and activity. In A. H. Riesen (Ed.), *The developmental psychology of sensory deprivation.* New York: Academic Press, 1975, pp. 9–91.

Gotsick, J. E., and Marshall, R. C. Time course of the septal rage syndrome. *Physiology and Behavior,* 1972, *9,* 685–687.

Greenough, W. T. Experiential modification of the developing brain. *American Scientist,* 1975, *63,* 37–46.

Greenough, W. T. Enduring brain effects of differential experience and training. In M. R. Rosenzweig and E. L. Bennett (Eds.), *Neural mechanisms of learning and memory.* Cambridge, Mass.: M.I.T. Press, 1976, pp. 255–278.

Greenough, W. T., and Volkmar, F. R. Pattern of dendritic branching in occipital cortex of rats reared in complex environments. *Experimental Neurology,* 1973, *40,* 491–504.

Greenough, W. T., Volkmar, F. R., and Juraska, J. M. Effects of rearing complexity on dendritic branching in frontolateral and temporal cortex of the rat. *Experimental Neurology,* 1973, *41,* 371–378.

Greenough, W. T., Fass, B., and DeVoogd, T. J. The influence of experience on recovery following brain damage in rodents: Hypotheses based on development research. In R. N. Walsh and W. T. Greenough (Eds.), *Environments as therapy for brain dysfunction. Advances in behavioral biology.* Vol. 17. New York: Plenum, 1976a, pp. 10–50.

Greenough, W. T., Snow, F. M., and Fiala, B. A. Environmental complexity versus isolation: A sensitive period for effects on cortical and subcortical dendritic branching in rats? *Society for Neuroscience Abstracts,* 1976b, Vol. II, part 2, p. 824.

Greenough, W. T., Volkmar, F. R., and Fleishmann, T. B. Environmental effects on brain connectivity and behavior. In D. I. Mostofsky (Ed.), *Behavior control and modification of physiological activity.* Englewood Cliffs, N.J.: Prentice-Hall, 1976c, pp. 220–245.

Harlow, H. F. The formation of learning sets. *Psychological Review,* 1949, *56,* 51–65.

Hebb, D. O. *The organization of behavior.* New York: John Wiley and Sons, Inc., 1949.

Hebb, D. O., and Williams, K. A method of rating animal intelligence. *The Journal of General Psychology,* 1946, *34,* 59–65.

Henderson, N. D. Brain weight increases resulting from environmental enrichment: A directional dominance in mice. *Science,* 1970, *169,* 776–778.

Hughes, K. R. Dorsal and ventral hippocampus lesions and maze learning: Influence of preoperative environment. *Canadian Journal of Psychology,* 1965, *19,* 325–332.

Hymovitch, B. The effects of experimental variations on problem solving in the rat. *Journal of Comparative and Physiological Psychology,* 1952, *45,* 313–321.

Isaac, W. Role of stimulation and time in the effects of spaced occipital ablations. *Psychological Reports,* 1964, *14,* 151–154.

Isaacson, R. L. *The limbic system.* New York: Plenum, 1974.

Kimble, G. A. *Hilgard and Marquis' conditioning and learning.* New York: Appleton-Century-Crofts, 1961.

Krech, D., Rosenzweig, M. R., and Bennett, E. L. Effects of complex environments and blindness on rat brain. *Archives of Neurology,* 1963, *8,* 403–412.

Kreschevsky, I. "Hypotheses" in rats. *Psychological Review,* 1932, *39,* 516–532.

Kuenzle, C. C., and Knüsel, A. Mass training of rats in a superenriched environment. *Physiology and Behavior,* 1974, *13,* 205–210.

Lansdell, H. C. Effect of brain damage on intelligence in rats. *Journal of Comparative and Physiological Psychology,* 1953, *46,* 461–464.

Lashley, K. S. *Brain mechanisms and intelligence.* Chicago: University of Chicago Press, 1929.

LaTorre, J. C. Effect of differential environmental enrichment on brain weight and on acetylcholinesterase and cholinesterase activities in mice. *Experimental Neurology,* 1968, *22,* 493–503.

LeBoeuf,B. J., and Peeke, H. V. S. The effect of strychnine administration during development on adult maze learning in the rat. *Psychopharmacologia* (Berlin), 1969, *16,* 49–53.

Lewis, M. E. The influence of early experience on the effects of one- and two- stage hippocampal lesions in male rats. Unpublished Masters thesis, Clark University, 1975.

Lewis, M. E,., and Stein, D. G. Pattern discrimination after lesions of the visual cortex. *Science,* 1975, *190,* 914–915.

Luria, A. R., Naydin, V. L., Tsvetkova, L. S., and Vinarskaya, E. N. Restoration of higher cortical function following local brain damage. In K. J. Vinken and G. W. Bruyn (Eds.), *Handbook of clinical neurology.* Vol. 3. Amsterdam: North Holland, 1969, pp. 368–433.

Manosevitz, M., and Pryor, J. B. Cage size as a factor in environmental enrichment. *Journal of Comparative and Physiological Psychology,* 1975, *89,* 648–654.

Meyer, D. R., Isaac, W., and Maher, B. The role of stimulation in spontaneous reorganization of visual habits. *Journal of Comparative and Physiological Psychology,* 1958, *51,* 546–548.

Møllgaard, K., Diamond, M. C., Bennett, E. L., Rosenzweig, M. R., and Lindner, B. Quantitative synaptic changes with differential experience in rat brain. *International Journal of Neuroscience,* 1971, *2,* 113–128.

Nyman, A. J. Problem solving in rats as a function of experience at different ages. *The Journal of Genetic Psychology,* 1967, *110,* 31–39.

Orbach, J. "Functions" of striate cortex and the problem of mass action. *Psychological Bulletin,* 1959, *56,* 271–292.

Peeke, H. V. S., LeBoeuf, B. J., and Herz, M. J. The effect of strychnine administration during development on adult maze learning in the rat. II. Drug administration from day 51 to 70. *Psychopharmacologia* (Berlin), 1971, *19,* 262–265.

Rabinovitch, M. S., and Rosvold, H. E. A closed-field intelligence test for rats. *Canadian Journal of Psychology*, 1951, *5*, 122–128.

Riege, W. H., and Morimoto, H. Effects of chronic stress and differential environments upon brain weights and biogenic amine levels in rats. *Journal of Comparative and Physiological Psychology*, 1970, *71*, 396–404.

Rosenzweig, M. R. Effects of environment on development of brain and behavior. In E. Tobach, L. R. Aronson, and E. Shaw (Eds.), *The biopsychology of development*. New York: Academic Press, 1971, pp. 303–342.

Rosenzweig, M. R., and Bennett, E. L. Effects of differential environments on brain weights and enzymatic activities in gerbils, rats and mice. *Developmental Psychobiology*, 1970, *2*, 87–95.

Rosenzweig, M. R., and Bennett, E. L. Cerebral changes in rats exposed individually to an enriched environment. *Journal of Comparative and Physiological Psychology*, 1972, *80*, 304–313.

Rosenzweig, M. R., and Bennett, E. L. Enriched environments: Facts, factors, and fantasies. In L. Petrinovich and J. L. McGaugh (Eds.), *Knowing, Thinking, and believing*. New York: Plenum, 1976.

Rosenzweig, M. R., Love, W., and Bennett, E. L. Effects of a few hours a day of enriched experience on brain chemistry and brain weights. *Physiology and Behavior*, 1968, *3*, 819–825.

Rosenzweig, M. R., Bennett, E. L., and Diamond, M. C. Brain changes in response to experience. *Scientific American*, 1972a, *226*, 22–30.

Rosenzweig, M. R., Bennett, E. L., and Diamond, M. C. Chemical and anatomical plasticity of the brain: Replications and extensions, 1970. In J. Gaito (Ed.), *Macromolecules and behavior*. New York: Appleton-Century-Crofts, 1972b, pp. 205–277.

Rosner, B. S. Brain functions. *Annual Review of Psychology*, 1970, *21*, 555–594.

Scheff, S. W., and Wright, D. C. Behavioral and electrophysiological evidence for cortical reorganization of function with serial lesions of the visual cortex. *Physiological Psychology*, 1977, *5*, 103–107.

Schwartz, S. Effect of neocortical lesions and early environmental factors on adult rat behavior. *Journal of Comparative and Physiological Psychology*, 1964, *57*, 72–77.

Smith, C. J. Mass action and early environment. *Journal of Comparative and Physiological Psychology*, 1959, *52*, 154–156.

Tees, R. C. Depth perception after infant and adult visual neocortical lesions in light- and dark-reared rats. *Developmental Psychobiology*, 1976, *9*, 223–235.

Thompson, W. R., and Grusec, J. E. Studies of early experience. In P. H. Mussen (Ed.), *Carmichael's manual of child psychology* (3rd Edition). New York: John Wiley and Sons, 1970, pp. 565–654.

Tryon, R. C. Genetic differences in maze learning in rats. *National society for the study of education, the thirty-ninth yearbook*. Bloomington, Ill.: Public School Publishing, 1940.

Walsh, R. N., Budtz-Olsen, O. E., Penny, J. E., and Cummins, R. A. The effects of environmental complexity on the histology of the rat hippocampus. *Journal of Comparative Neurology*, 1969, *137*, 361–366.

Weinstein, S., and Teuber, H.-L. The role of preinjury education and intelligence level in intellectual loss after brain injury. *Journal of Comparative and Physiological Psychology*, 1957, *50*, 535–539

West, R. W., and Greenough, W. T. Effect of environmental complexity on cortical synapses of rats: Preliminary results. *Behavioral Biology*, 1972, *7*, 279–284.

Will, B. E., and Rosenzweig, M. R. Effets de l'environnement sur la récupération fonctionnelle après lésions cérébrales chez les rats adultes. *Biology of Behavior*, 1976, *1*, 5–16.

Will, B. E., Rosenzweig, M. R., and Bennett, E. L. Effects of differential environments on recovery from neonatal brain lesions, measured by problem-solving scores and brain dimensions. *Physiology and Behavior,* 1976, *16,* 603–611.

Will, B. E., Rosenzweig, M. R., Bennett, E. L., Hebert, M., and Morimoto, H. Relatively brief environmental enrichment aids recovery of learning capacity and alters brain measures after postweaning brain lesions in rats. *Journal of Comparative and Physiological Psychology,* 1977, *91,* 33–50.

Wilson, M., Warren, J. M., and Abbott, L. Infantile stimulation, activity, and learning by cats. *Child Development,* 1965, *36,* 843–853.

Witkin, H. A. "Hypotheses" in rats: An experimental critique. II. The displacement of responses and behavior variability in linear situations. *Journal of Comparative Psychology,* 1941, *31,* 303–336.

Wittrig, J. J. Extravisual plasticity of posterior cortex in rats as a function of variations in proximal and distal input during development. *Perceptual and Motor Skills,* 1966, *23,* 211–219.

13

Sensory Restriction and Recovery of Function

BARRY S. LAYTON, GEORGE E. CORRICK, AND ARTHUR W. TOGA

1. INTRODUCTION

Changes in brain function having detrimental behavioral consequences may be produced by factors other than those associated with trauma or disease. In this chapter we consider recent evidence which indicates that isolation from normal sensory experience is one of these factors. Our goal is to outline some of the conditions of visual deprivation which may result in physiological and behavioral aberrations and to discuss several hypotheses concerning the mechanisms of these effects. Additionally, and in substantially greater detail, we review investigations of recovery of function following deprivation.

The deprivation literature is vast and rapidly growing, and this chapter is in no way intended to represent a complete review of the field. We restrict our discussion to studies concerning changes in cortical physiology and behavior following visual deprivation in the cat as they are relevant to recovery of function (some particularly relevant human material is also included). With this goal in mind the chapter is divided into two broad sections. The first is more general and describes some of the immediate effects of deprivation on cortical physiology and

BARRY S. LAYTON • Departments of Neurology and Psychology, St. Louis University, St. Louis, Missouri 63104   GEORGE E. CORRICK • Department of Psychology, Indiana University, Bloomington, Indiana 47402   ARTHUR W. TOGA • Departments of Neurology and Psychology, St. Louis University, St. Louis, Missouri 63104

behavior. The major interpretive problems in this field are discussed, as are some of the experimental strategies that have been developed to resolve them. The second section is concerned with functional recovery following deprivation and is organized independently of the first part in order to facilitate a finer level analysis of a more restricted subject matter. Detailed reviews of sensory deprivation in general may be found in Riesen (1975) and among the many reviews of visual deprivation experiments those of Barlow (1975) and Ganz (1975) are of particular interest. Because research involving deprivation in other modalities (cf., e.g., Reisen, 1975) has not yet evolved to the same degree as the work in vision, the question of the generality of the phenomena discussed in this chapter is open.

This chapter is primarily intended as an examination of the evidence concerned with determining the degree of functional restitution that occurs under various conditions following isolation from the normal visual environment. But the material discussed also furnishes insight into the various phenomena of functional recovery which occur following traumatic brain damage. Regarding the general problems of recovery from the tangent of visual deprivation provides a surprisingly rich perspective, and, although we do not have the space to exploit this potential fully, the reader who is familiar with the recovery literature will quickly appreciate it.

2. EFFECTS OF DEPRIVATION

2.1. Functional Attributes of the Normal Adult and Neonatal Inexperienced Visual Cortex

2.1.1. The Adult

The effects of deprivation on visual cortical function can be understood only in relation to the cortex of the normal adult, the properties of which can be analyzed from a variety of perspectives. The organization presented below reflects the focus of most of the literature reviewed in this chapter and provides a standard with which to evaluate the effects of deprivation. Except where otherwise noted, the normative data are based upon the work of Hubel and Wiesel (e.g., 1962).

2.1.1a. Binocular Connectivity. In the normal adult cat, the large majority of cells in the striate cortex receive input from both eyes. These units summate in response to simultaneous stimulation of the appropriate areas of both eyes. The degree to which a cortical cell is influenced varies from complete control by one eye to equal influence by both eyes and is termed *ocular dominance*.

   2.1.1b. Orientation Specificity.   The receptive fields of most striate cells are arranged so that they respond best to linear stimuli (e.g., bars, edges) of one orientation. Response activity of such units falls off as the orientation of the stimulus deviates from the preferred angle. Cells that are orientation-specific for stimuli of any one angle are represented about equally, and for binocular cells, the preferred orientation is identical in both eyes.

   2.1.1c. Direction Selectivity.   Most cells of the adult striate cortex are selective in their response, not only to orientation, but also to the direction of movement of stimuli across the visual field.

   2.1.1d. Disparity Specificity.   Each binocular cortical cell responds optimally to stimuli having small vertical and horizontal discrepancies between the retinae (Barlow, Blakemore, and Pettigrew, 1967; Nikara, Bishop, and Pettigrew, 1968). The disparity selectivity of binocular cells in the striate cortex has been hypothesized to be the physiological basis of binocular depth discrimination (Barlow *et al.*, 1967).

2.1.2. Visually Inexperienced Neonatal Cortex

   Do the effects of deprivation to be discussed below operate to destroy, render inefficient, or otherwise disrupt neural connections that are present prior to experience, or do they prevent environmentally guided development of an unconnected system? Obviously, this question can be resolved only by studying the pristine neonatal brain. If neonatal connectivity is identical to that of the normally experienced adult, then deprivation must produce its effects by active disruption of these connections. Passive prevention of environmentally guided development is implied if the neonatal brain is "unconnected."

   2.1.2a Binocular Connectivity.   Hubel and Wiesel (1963) recorded from two kittens without visual experience, one 8 days and the other 16 days old. The cells they encountered in the younger animal were sluggish and rapidly habituating; in the older animal, they were less so. However, the units had adult-like binocular interaction in both kittens. This finding has been reconfirmed many times (e.g., Blakemore and Van Sluyters, 1974; Pettigrew, 1974).

   2.1.2b. Orientation Specificity.   Hubel and Wiesel concluded that the cells in their kittens demonstrated orientation selectivity, although the range of preferred stimuli was somewhat broader than in the adult. Later studies (Blakemore and Van Sluyters, 1974; Imbert and Buisseret, 1975; Pettigrew, 1974) have challenged the conclusion that orientation specificity is a property of the neonatal cortex. More recently, however, Sherk and Stryker (1976) performed a series of experiments replicating Hubel and Wiesel's original results.

2.1.2c. Direction Selectivity. Investigations concerning the status of this property are also contradictory and inconclusive (Hubel and Wiesel, 1963; Imbert and Buisseret, 1975; Pettigrew, 1974; Sherk and Stryker, 1976).

2.1.2d. Disparity Specificity. Although the data are too sparse to allow any definitive conclusions concerning this property, Pettigrew (1974) found no evidence that binocularly activated cortical cells in the inexperienced neonate were selective in terms of retinal disparity.

2.1.3. Conclusions

The research cited indicates that the binocular connectivity characteristic of the adult is present in visually inexperienced brains. Apparently this propery is innate, and, therefore, any binocular aberrations following deprivation must be the result of a disruptive process.

Since data concerning the presence of orientation, direction, and disparity selectivity in the neonate are sparse or inconsistent, there is no way of telling, at this time, whether the effects of deprivation to be discussed below are to prevent environmentally guided development or to alter genetically determined connections mediating these properties. For this reason, conclusions concerning the causes of deprivation effects on these properties must await further research.

2.2. Deprivation Experiments

The studies to be reviewed use one or more of several techniques of visual deprivation. Depending on the age of the animal and the duration of deprivation, these procedures have varying effects on adult physiology and behavior.

1. *Dark-rearing* eliminates, and *lid-suture* or *black-contact-lens occlusion* effectively reduce, retinal illumination.
2. *Translucent-contact-lens occlusion* eliminates pattern vision while permitting about 3 log units more retinal illumination than the first method (Wiesel and Hubel, 1963a).
3. *Selective deprivation* refers to several different procedures, each of which permit only limited visual stimulation along one or more dimensions. The rearing of kittens in environments containing linear contours of only one orientation is an example.

of the orientation that would have been blurred when uncorrected than when triggered by orthogonal stimuli. If the evoked-potential response is assumed to correlate with quantity of neural activity, then these results indicate that there are fewer units sensitive to the orientation that is blurred when uncorrected than to other orientations.

The assumption that early uncorrected astigmatism produces a permanent neural deficit has been directly tested in kittens by fitting them with lenses that artificially created varying degrees of astigmatism resulting in the blurring of certain specific contours (Freeman and Pettigrew, 1973). A control group wore nonastigmatic lenses. Recording immediately following the period of deprivation showed that this relatively mild alteration of the early visual environment does indeed have a noticeable effect on the distribution of orientation-selective cells in the cortex. In the experimentally reared kittens, units clustered about the axis that was in focus, and few were encountered orthogonal to that angle. This effect was graded; that is, the kittens wearing lenses that produced a more severe distortion showed a greater cortical aberration. Also of interest is the fact that of the units having a preferred orientation distant from the meridian of clear focus, most had unusually broad response limits, firing less selectively than the more finely tuned cells clustered about the preferred orientation. It appears, then, that the *degree* of selectivity as well as the number of units responding to a particular orientation may be a function of exposure to angles of that orientation.

2.2.3. Movement Deprivation

It has been found that cortical direction selectivity, like binocular connectivity and orientation specificity, can be affected by environmental conditions. In one study, Cynader, Berman, and Hein (1973) reared kittens in stroboscopic illumination so that movement across the retina was prevented. Less than half of the units recorded from the strobe-reared cats were direction selective compared with more than 80% of the cells studies in a normally raised control group.

In a later study (Cynader, Berman, and Hein, 1975), kittens were reared so that the only visual input was a continuously leftward-moving series of irregularly shaped patches of luminescent paint. In the normal cat, right and left selective cells are equally represented in the striate cortex. In the experimentally reared kittens, more than half of the neurons encountered had a leftward component in their preferred direction and only about one-quarter had a rightward component. Tretter *et al.* (1975) and Daw and Wyatt (1976) have reported similar results.

2.2.4. Alteration of Disparity Relations

To test the plasticity of binocular disparity specificity in cortical cells, Schlaer (1971) raised newborn kittens in darkness except for a 1-hour/day period in the light, during which time they wore specially designed eyeglasses that introduced a large or small vertical disparity between corresponding areas of the retinae. After 4 months of this treatment, cortical recordings were made. Those kittens raised with the greater disparity showed a shift in the normal cortical disparity distribution approximately compensating for the conditions of rearing. Those raised in the less severe condition showed a similar though smaller shift.

2.2.5. Critical-Period Concept and Brief-Exposure Experiments

2.2.5a. Critical Period. In their original experiments, Wiesel and Hubel (1963*b*, 1965*b*) recognized that the physiological and behavioral effects resulting from eye-closure were more or less profound depending on age of onset and duration of deprivation. Later, a series of parametric studies was conducted to demonstrate the effects of these variables more precisely (Dews and Wiesel, 1970; Hubel and Wiesel, 1970). By systematically varying the time of eye-closure and its duration, it was concluded that, in the kitten, the period between the 4th and 12th weeks of life is one of high sensitivity to the effects of MD and BD. The sensitive or critical period starts at a peak, drops off between the 6th and 8th weeks, and seems to gradually disappear by the end of the 12th week. These studies also showed that the duration of eye-closure has a graded effect depending on the time it is initiated during this period. For example, a 6-day closure at the beginning of the critical period produced as profound an effect on cortical binocularity and visually guided behavior as closure for the entire period, whereas a closure for the same duration at any other time within the sensitive 2 months had a much less severe effect (Hubel and Wiesel, 1970). There is some evidence that the peak of the critical period for direction deprivation is not identical to that for MD and BD (Daw and Wyatt, 1976).

If there are effects of eye-closure following the critical period, they are too small to have been observed with the behavioral and physiological procedures used to demonstrate the gross effects of such treatment during the critical period. In cats form-deprived after 3 months of age for up to 14 months, there are no noticeable effects on cortical physiology (Hubel and Wiesel, 1970) or visual placing and acuity (Dews and Wiesel, 1970). There is, however, evidence from a more selective deprivation procedure indicating that at least the re-

sponse properties of visual cortical cells may be influenced by the env:-
ronment well into adulthood. Creutzfeld and Heggelund (1975) contour deprived adult cats who had had normal visual experience during
the critical period. Recording immediately following a period when
only vertical stripes could be viewed indicated that the cortex was domi-
nated by cells with preferred orientations clustering about the *horizontal.* The permanence of the effect was not investigated, but whatever its
time course, this study suggests that the critical-period concept may be
relative rather than absolute, an hypothesis that figures prominently in
some explanations of recovery of function from critical period deprivation (see Section 3).

    2.2.5b. Brief Exposure. Hubel and Wiesel (1970) investigated the
minimum period of deprivation required to show an environmental effect on the visual system and found that only 3 days of monocular
closure during the 4th week will produce extensive cortical abnormalities. The mirror image of the technique in which a short deprivation
period is maintained within a period of visual experience involves al-
lowing a "window" of visual experience within a period of deprivation.
This method has resulted in the somewhat surprising discovery that
permanent cortical adjustments having potential perceptual consequences require only a brief exposure to the environment. Blakemore
and Mitchell (1973) kept kittens in a dark room during the entire critical period except for 0, 1, 3, 6, 18, 27, or 33 hours around the 28th
day—the time of peak sensitivity to the environment. Exposure was
limited to vertical stripes. Recording at 6 weeks of age showed that the
cortex of the kitten kept in the dark room for the entire period (0
hours exposure) had no neuron with more than a very vague orientation preference and many visually unresponsive cells. The cortex of the
kitten with 1-hour exposure was quite different in that almost every
unit encountered was adult-like in terms of response latency and orientation specificity. The receptive fields of these units were clustered
within a narrow range about the vertical. Cells more sensitive to other
angles were infantile in their response characteristics. Exposure longer
than 1 hour produced only a slight further maturation of response
characteristics and selectivity about the vertical, so that the difference
between 0 and 1 hour of exposure was much more striking than that
between 1 and 33 hours.

    Peck and Blakemore (1975) found similar but less striking results
when they limited the visual experience of kittens to 1, 6, or 20 hours
in a *normal* visual environment. In this study, changes of ocular dominance and degree of orientation selectivity were the variables of interest. Exposure was on the 29th day. Six or 20 hours of monocular vision
resulted in a shift of the ocular-dominance distribution in favor of the

experienced eye. The cells activated by this eye showed distinct orientation selectivity. These changes were less evident when recording immediately following exposure than when a "consolidation" period of 2 days intervened. The fact that 1 hour of exposure to the normal environment had no noticeable effect on cortical physiology while 1 hour in an environment of vertical stripes produced profound changes suggested to Peck and Blakemore that different contours may somehow compete for domination of individual cells, thereby defeating the strong organizing influence on the cortex of a one-contour environment. As Blakemore and his colleagues have suggested, the analogy between the results of their studies summarized above and the process of learning is difficult to resist. The neural substrate of behavioral plasticity may involve neural alterations which are triggered by environmental occurrences of brief duration. The possibility that potentially analogous changes in the visual cortex can be produced in very brief periods combined with evidence that these changes are more apparent after a period of consolidation like that demonstrated to exist in behavioral studies of learning (cf. Milner, 1970, Chapter 20) suggests that one significant by-product of visual-deprivation research may prove to be a powerful methodology in the search for the engram. Also relevant to this issue are reports by Pettigrew, Olson, and Barlow (1973) and Pettigrew and Garey (1974), who induced changes of ocular dominance, orientation preference, and disparity selectivity in striate neurons of kittens without visual experience *while the units were under observation.* The procedure involved first determining the response properties of an encountered unit and then attempting to condition changes in these properties by exposing them to nonpreferred stimuli. The observed effects were more dramatic when a "consolidation" period was interpolated between conditioning and testing.

The data reviewed in Section 2 establish that visual deprivation may disrupt normal visual physiology and behavior. It is now necessary to examine the degree to which the physiological and behavioral abnormalities are permanent and if and under what conditions recovery of function can occur.

3. RECOVERY OF FUNCTION

In order to facilitate a more detailed exposition of the problem of recovery,* Section 3 is organized differently from Section 2. First the

---

* Our use of the term "recovery" in the context of deprivation research may seem to imply that any "recovered" physiological or behavioral capacity has existed at some prior time in the organism's history (whether or not its existence has actually been de-

issue of behavioral recovery is treated, followed by a discussion of recovery on the physiological level. The interesting and problematic relationship between the two is also subjected to analysis.

3.1. Behavioral Recovery

It is commonly recognized that normal visual behavior requires both visuomotor coordination and appreciation of form or pattern. These two visual functions can be experimentally dissociated (Held, 1968) and hypotheses have been advanced suggesting that they are subserved by separate neural mechanisms (e.g., Schneider, 1969). Examination of research investigating recovery following visual deprivation indicates that it is crucial to distinguish between these functions when evaluating recovery potential.

Tasks which tap the ability to appreciate form or pattern involve discrimination procedures of the type familiar to most behavioral scientists and will be more fully described when appropriate. The tasks most commonly used to assess visuomotor behavior may be less familiar. They include:

1. Obstacle avoidance: the ability to avoid obstacles while freely moving is assessed.
2. Visual following or tracking: objects are moved around the animal's head; the ability to follow the object's movement is assessed.
3. Visual startle: an object is moved rapidly toward the animal's head; the presence of an eye blink is noted.
4. Jumping: the smoothness and lack of hesitation in making jumps from elevated platforms is assessed.
5. Visually triggered extension: the animal is slowly lowered toward a smooth surface; extension of the forelimbs is noted.
6. Visually guided placing: the animal is slowly lowered toward an interrupted surface; the ability to avoid gaps in the surface with a forelimb is noted (see Hein and Held, 1967, for a discussion of the differences between #5 and #6).

---

termined). Thus, by using this term, we may appear to be embracing a nativist position concerning the origin of the neural connections in the visual system. However, our review of the evidence regarding the structure of the neonatal visual cortex makes it clear that this position is untenable. Probably at least some of the effects of deprivation act to prevent environmentally guided development of a system that is not fully determined by genetic factors. Thus, some of the phenomena discussed in this section may be more appropriately considered cases of retarded development than cases of recovery. Our use of the latter term does not imply a nativist bias, but rather reflects its (perhaps unfortunate) ubiquity in the literature.

7. Visual cliff: stepping from a platform to a glass surface covering patterned surfaces. One pattern is placed directly under the glass (i.e., shallow side) and the other pattern is placed at some distance below the glass (i.e., deep side). Stepping toward the shallow side is regarded as an indication that the animal can use depth cues.
8. Optokinetic nystagmus (OKN): the animal is placed in the center of a drum with vertical stripes inside. The drum is rotated and eye movements are elicited in the direction of rotation.

Generally, tests of visuomotor capacity are more "informal" than those which are used to assess pattern vision; they are administered on a limited number of occasions and do not employ conditioning procedures. Ability as reflected by performance on a given test is typically scored as normal, deficient, or absent. Unfortunately, criteria for scoring are not always made explicit, a fact which sometimes leads to confusion when attempting to compare the results of two or more studies.

3.1.1. Binocular Deprivation: Recovery of Visuomotor Capacity

Wiesel and Hubel (1965*b*) briefly described the recovery of visual behavior in one cat binocularly lid-sutured for the first 3 months of life and then reared with one eye open. They reported that the animal appeared completely blind immediately following deprivation but that some recovery was evident during the next 3 months. There was some evidence of visual following and of the ability to avoid large obstacles. However, visual placing and graceful jumping were never observed, and small objects frequently were not avoided. There was little further improvement over the next 18 months of testing, and it was concluded that at best only minimal behavioral recovery follows binocular deprivation during the critical period.

These results stand in marked contrast to those of Baxter (1966), who found very rapid recovery for cats dark-reared for up to 1 year. When tested immediately after deprivation for visual placing, jumping, visual startle, visual following, and obstacle avoidance, the cats appeared blind. Baxter then put two cats in standard laboratory cages and took two others to his home. The former showed recovery on the visuomotor tasks after about 30 days, and the latter within only 10 days. Baxter believed that the home environment was more stimulating than that of the laboratory and hence facilitated the rate of recovery.

It is not easy to account for the dramatic differences between the results of Baxter and of Hubel and Wiesel. The length of the deprivation period cannot be a factor, since Baxter's cats were deprived much longer. Neither paper was specific as to testing procedures or criteria for recovery. It should be noted that whereas Wiesel and Hubel's cat was allowed monocular recovery, Baxter's animals recovered with both eyes open. Indications from a third study make it doubtful, however, that this manipulation could account for the behavioral discrepancy. Chow and Stewart (1972) reared cats binocularly deprived for 16–20 months, followed by at least 6 months of monocular experience. While no specifics of visuomotor testing were reported, these cats were later described as indistinguishable from normal, except for a heightened startle response.

Sherman (1973) found limited recovery in BD cats tested for visually triggered extension, visual following, and the ability to ensnare a moving object with a forepaw. Again, initially after deprivation the BD cats appeared blind, but within a short time (5 days for one cat, 17 days for the other) responses reappeared, although they were still deficient. For example, visually triggered extension was inappropriate in that the forelegs extended well before the cat was near a visible surface. When tested with both eyes open, BD cats could follow objects moving both to the right and left; however, when tested with one eye open, following occurred only to ipsiversive movement in the ipsilateral hemifield. Finally, the accuracy of forepaw reaching was judged to be "fair," but well below that of normal. In a follow-up study, Sherman (1974) observed that after up to 26 months of experience with either one or both eyes open, BD cats showed the same visuomotor deficits. Thus, one commonality emerges from the investigations reviewed to this point: whatever visuomotor recovery does occur following BD, it appears to be limited to the period of time immediately following deprivation.

More recently van Hof-van Duin (1976a) conducted a detailed study of the development of visuomotor responses in cats dark-reared for 4 or 7 months. All animals demonstrated recovery with the rate being inversely related to deprivation time. Visual tracking, obstacle avoidance, visually triggered extension, and OKN became positive within 3 weeks for the 7-month-deprivation group and in less time for the cats deprived for 4 months. The more complex visuomotor tasks, such as visually guided placing, visual cliff, and jumping, took somewhat longer to appear, but the 4-month-deprived cats showed complete recovery within 7 weeks and the 7-month-deprived cats within 10 weeks. The sequence of development of the various visuomotor responses in BD cats was found to be identical to that of the sequence of their ontogenesis in normal kittens.

There are obvious contradictions regarding the extent of recovery of visuomotor responses subsequent to BD. Wiesel and Hubel (1965b) describe severe and long-lasting deficits while Baxter (1966) and van Hof-van Duin (1976*a*) report full recovery within short periods of time. The data that Wiesel and Hubel (1965*b*) report are based on only one animal, and the specifics of testing are not elaborated; therefore, their results should be interpreted with caution. Similar criticisms can be made of the Baxter (1966) study. Van Hof-van Duin (1967*a*), however, reports on 21 animals and is very specific about testing methods. Sherman (1973, 1974), who reported on 4 BD cats and provided a detailed description of testing procedures, obtained results which lie between the extremes of no recovery and full recovery.

Differences in testing methods could explain some of these discrepancies. For example, Sherman (1973) found that visual following recovered and appeared normal in BD cats when *tested* with both eyes open. However, when tested monocularly, a permanent deficit was revealed. The other studies reporting recovery of visual following (Baxter, 1966; van Hof-van Duin, 1976*a*) did not attempt monocular testing. Differences in experience during and after deprivation could also be important factors. The cats in the study by van Hof-van Duin (1976*a*) were housed in groups of 2–4 per cage and handled daily during the deprivation period. Following deprivation the cats were housed in group cages and were allowed up to 6 hours per day in a "playroom" furnished with toys and other manipulanda. Such "enriched" conditions may facilitate recovery from traumatic brain damage (see Finger, this volume, Chapter 12) and may also have an effect on recovery from visual deprivation. Baxter suggested this explanation for the rapid recovery shown by his two house-reared cats.

One form of visuomotor behavior not yet discussed is the ability to orient to and approach a novel stimulus. Sherman used this aspect of visually guided behavior as a test to determine visual-field deficits following deprivation. He found that cats responded only to objects in the ipsilateral hemifield immediately after BD (Sherman, 1973). BD cats allowed up to 2 years of experience with either both or only one eye open showed no recovery (Sherman, 1974).

The deficits resulting from binocular deprivation on visuomotor tasks are not specific to light deprivation. Held and Hien (1963) and Hein and Held (1967) observed visuomotor deficits in cats deprived of the normal visual feedback of motor activity. In the latter study, kittens were limited to 6 hours a day of binocular experience during which time they wore an opaque collar which prevented them from seeing their own limbs and torsos. These animals showed normal extension but abnormal placing; in addition, they had difficulty in striking objects with their paws. Thus, visual guidance of the limbs is disrupted in cats that are earlier deprived of viewing their own appendages. However, recovery from deprivation of visuomotor coordination is rapid. Hein and Held (1967) reported good coordination after only 18 hours of normal experience.

In the earlier study, Held and Hein (1963) raised pairs of kittens in the dark, except for daily binocular exposure under special conditions. During exposure one kitten was free to move while the other was carried passively in a "gondola"; thus, only the "active" kitten was allowed to correlate its movements with sensory stimulation. When tested for visually guided placing, visual following, and visual startle and on the visual cliff, the "passive" kitten was always deficient. Again, recovery was rapid. Within 2 days of normal movement the "passive" kitten showed positive responses on all tests.

Although BD is generally considered in the context of the elimination of light or pattern, it is clear from the work of Held and Hein that this procedure also deprives the animal of the opportunity for visuomotor coordination. From this perspective, the profound deficits resulting from BD and whatever recovery subsequent to eye-opening is achieved may be at least partially due to the disruption and reestablishment of sensorimotor feedback.

3.1.2. Binocular Deprivation: Recovery of Pattern Vision

There have been few studies investigating recovery of pattern discrimination following binocular deprivation in cats. In one, Ganz, *et al.* (1972) deprived kittens binocularly for up to 6 months and then tested them in a runway apparatus on flux, contour (i.e., horizontal versus vertical striations), and form (i.e., upright versus inverted triangles) discrimination problems. Training was monocular. Each BD cat eventually mastered all of the problems but required more trials than normals on some of them. The flux-discrimination was mastered at the same rate as MD cats using their experienced eye. Aarons, Halasz, and Riesen (1963) have also shown that dark-reared cats learn flux discriminations at the same rate as normal animals. However, acquisition of orientation and form discriminations by BD cats required, respectively, about 2 and 5 times as many trials as MD cats who used their nondeprived eye (Ganz *et al.*, 1972). BD cats thus seem to be able to master visual discrimination problems, but at a retarded rate for more complex tasks.

Chow and Stewart (1972) also found good recovery following binocular deprivation. They raised two cats with binocular suture for about 20 months and then allowed 12–14 months experience with only one eye open. When tested in a runway apparatus using a go–no-go procedure, the BD cats easily mastered flux- and grid-orientation problems, but only one achieved criterion on a form (i.e., disc versus cross) discrimination; the other cat, while failing to meet criterion after 975 trials, was nevertheless performing above chance when training was terminated.

Both Ganz *et al.* (1972) and Chow and Stewart (1972) demonstrated that BD cats can eventually master flux, orientation, and form discriminations. The important difference in these two studies lies in the rate of acquisition of the discriminations. Ganz *et al.* (1972) began training without a period of normal experience, and the rate of acquisition of orientation and form problems was considerably retarded compared to MD cats using their initially open eye. Chow and Stewart (1972) showed that BD cats given a long period of normal usage of one eye acquire orientation discriminations at rates similar to MD cats using the normal eye. The single BD cat that mastered the form discrimination required only about twice as many trials as MD cats with the normal eye. Chow and Stewart argue that their training and testing procedures may explain the degree of recovery which they obtained, especially in their MD cats (see below). While not conclusive, these data suggest that monocular experience following BD may facilitate the rate of acquisition of visual discrimination problems.

In summary, the deficits induced by binocular deprivation are profound immediately following deprivation, although subsequent visual experience may result in considerable recovery. Visuomotor responses recover rapidly to nearly normal levels. Visual discriminations are possible after BD, and visual experience tends to facilitate the rate at which they can be acquired. However, there are permanent deficits in the extent of the visual fields of each eye as a result of BD. Sherman (1974) pointed out that these results are not necessarily contradictory. BD cats could quite possibly learn to use their abnormal visual fields in a manner enabling successful visuomotor and discrimination performance. If BD cats do require time to adapt to visual-field deficits, this may help explain the common observation of severe initial deficits followed by good recovery. Thus, although BD cats may eventually succeed in terms of experimenter-defined ends, the means used to achieve these ends are not necessarily identical to those used by nondeprived cats (see Laurence and Stein, this volume, for a full discussion of the means–end approach to recovery studies).

3.1.3. Monocular Deprivation: Recovery of Visuomotor Capacity

Given the evidence reviewed above demonstrating that the immediate physiological and behavioral effects of MD are more severe than those of BD, it should not be surprising to find that behavioral recovery following MD is more limited. Wiesel and Hubel (1965*b*) monocularly deprived kittens for the first 3 months of life and then reverse sutured the eyes so that only the initially deprived eye received later visual experience. Only minimal behavioral recovery was observed. Some recovery of visual following was seen during the first 3 months, but little more was noted with extended experience. Large obstacles could be avoided, but not small ones, and jumping was never graceful. It was also reported that visually triggered extension never returned. The latter result has not been replicated. Ganz and Fitch (1968) found rapid recovery of visually triggered extension in cats monocularly deprived from 1 to 3 months after birth. Animals deprived for longer periods required up to 1 month for triggered extension to reappear. That recovery of visually triggered extension is rapid following MD and reverse suture was recently confirmed by van Hof-van Duin (1976b). Cats in this study were deprived for longer periods than in the Ganz and Fitch (1968) and Wiesel and Hubel (1965b) studies, but visually triggered extension was first seen as early as 8 days and no later than 24 days after reverse suture. Sherman (1973) reports recovery of visually triggered extension to be rapid (i.e., 8 days) following reverse suture in one case and delayed (i.e., 95 days) in another. However, in all cases the response topography was abnormal and remained so after 2 years of forced usage of the deprived eye (Sherman, 1974).

The other component of visual placing (Hein and Held, 1967), visually guided placing, is more resistant to recovery than visually triggered extension. Van Hof-van Duin (1976b) reported that all MD cats were deficient on this task even after 3 years of forced usage of the deprived eye. Ganz and Fitch (1968) described two cats that exhibited abnormal visually guided placing after long periods of reverse suture. Dews and Wiesel (1970) reported that recovery of visually guided placing is dependent on the duration of MD. If deprivation was confined to about 6 weeks or less (still within the critical period), recovery was good (see also Movshon, 1976b). However, if deprivation was extended for 3–4 months, recovery occurred only after prolonged reverse suture; littermates deprived for comparable times but allowed only binocular experience did not show visually guided placing.

According to van Hof-van Duin (1976b) all other visuomotor behaviors are impaired following MD and do not recover even after forced usage of the deprived eye. Obstacle avoidance was impaired, but the deficit was noted only if tested in a novel environment. Ganz and Fitch (1968) described improvement of obstacle avoidance over a 3–5 month period of recovery to a point where MD cats resembled normals, but these cats had some residual deficits. Often obstacles were avoided only after their vibrassae contacted the object. Van Hof-van Duin (1976b) pointed out that deficits of MD cats may be masked by testing in a familiar environment, an idea which may explain the recovery of obstacle avoidance observed by Ganz and Fitch (1968).

Visual cliff performance was also found to be permanently impaired by van Hof-van Duin (1976*b*), although recovery on this task was noted by Ganz and Fitch (1968). In the latter study, however, the cats were deprived for shorter periods (22 weeks as opposed to 8–10 months), so the rate of recovery on the visual cliff may be dependent on the duration of deprivation. Movshon (1976*b*) reported recovery on the visual cliff for short deprivation periods (5–7 weeks) within the critical period when the effects of deprivation are more easily reversible. Thus, the appreciation of monocular depth cues, as revealed by the visual cliff test, is impaired following long-term MD and reverse suture but may be subject to recovery when the period of deprivation is shorter. Parenthetically, it may be noted that AMD cats do not develop an ability to use binocular depth cues even after up to 2 years of normal binocular experience (Blake and Hirsch, 1975).

Some data already reviewed indicate that reverse suturing results in some advantage in recovery from MD in comparison to simple binocular experience. Additionally, Ganz and Fitch (1968) reported that reverse suturing confers an advantage to the deprived eye when tested for OKN. The initially deprived eye of MD cats given binocular experience had a deficient OKN response; however, following reverse suture the initially deprived eye showed OKN responses equivalent to the initially open eye. Van Hof-van Duin (1976*b*) also reported that OKN responses become normal with reverse suture following longer deprivation. However, the OKN was positive only if the direction of rotation of the drum was from temporal to nasal; response to movement in the opposite direction was deficient when tested immediately after deprivation and remained so for up to 2.5 years. The OKN response asymmetry was also observed in the nondeprived eye when tested during the deprivation period. Thus, the asymmetry is not due simply to light deprivation but rather results from disruption of the normal synergistic input from both eyes during development. The fact that a similar asymmetry was not described in BD cats (van Hof-van Duin 1967*a*) supports this notion.

The visual field of the deprived eye of MD cats is also abnormal (Sherman, 1973). The visual field of a normal eye extends from about 90° ipsilateral to about 45° beyond the midline into the contralateral visual field; the fields of each eye thus overlap in an area that extends to about 45° on either side of the midline. However, the binocular portion of the visual field of an MD eye is absent and only the monocular part of the deprived eye field is preserved. That is, the visual field of an MD eye extends from 90° ipsilateral to only 45° ipsilateral (Sherman, 1973).

There are no changes in the extent of the deprived eye's field following either long-term reverse suture or binocular experience (Sherman, 1974).

The data reviewed above suggest that MD severely disrupts visuomotor behavior and that little recovery is demonstrable even after forced usage of the initially deprived eye. Visually triggered extension is the only visuomotor behavior that fully recovers following long-term MD and reverse suture. Recovery is noted on other tasks but usually following only briefer deprivation periods. Reverse suturing appears to facilitate recovery in comparison to experience with both eyes open. The fact that recovery potential is greater if the period of initial deprivation is shorter is consistent with the notion that there is a period of marked physiological plasticity following birth when the visual system is most sensitive to modification by environmental factors (e.g., Blakemore and van Sluyters, 1974).

Movshon (1976b) recently provided evidence showing that the plasticity of the sensitive period applies to visuomotor responses. By monocularly depriving cats for 5, 6, or 7 weeks, and then reverse suturing them for 3–63 days, Movshon was able to track recovery of funtion over time. He showed that the ability of the two eyes to support normal visuomotor behavior reverses following reverse suture; that is, performance guided by the initially deprived eye improves while that of the initially experienced eye deteriorates. The rate of reversal between the two eyes is dependent on the duration of the initial deprivation. Following 5 weeks of deprivation, reversal takes only about 6 days while after 6 weeks of MD reversal takes 24 days. However, after 7 weeks of deprivation, reversal does not occur before 63 days. Thus, after 7 weeks of deprivation, behavioral plasticity already appears limited (see also Dews and Wiesel, 1970). If deprivation extends beyond the end of the sensitive period, behavioral plasticity as revealed by visuomotor tasks is very limited (e.g., Sherman, 1974; van Hof-van Duin, 1976b).

3.1.4. Monocular Deprivation: Recovery of Pattern Vision

Ganz and Fitch (1968) found that, immediately following monocular deprivation, cats failed to discriminate a vertical from a horizontal rectangle with their deprived eye but were successful with their experienced eye. Two cats were also given up to 5 months of forced usage of the deprived eye to facilitate recovery, but both still failed to make the original horizontal versus vertical discriminations.

Dews and Wiesel (1970) provided evidence that forced usage of the deprived eye can result in eventual recovery of some discriminative abilities. Kittens monocularly deprived for 3 months and then given up to 2 years of binocular experience failed to discriminate between continuous and interrupted lines, but kittens deprived for comparable times and then reverse sutured succeeded. However, the extent of recovery was again dependent on the duration of the initial deprivation. Cats deprived longer than 3 months failed to make the gap discrimination regardless of whether they were forced to use the deprived eye or given only binocular experience. In comparison, forced usage did aid recovery on visually guided placing. These results indicate that recovery of visual discriminative behavior is limited at best when monocular deprivation is extended beyond the sensitive period.

In contrast, Chow and Stewart (1972) found evidence for recovery of pattern discrimination when MD was extended well beyond the sensitive period. The cats in their study were deprived for 20–22 months, then reverse sutured for 7–12 months. Using the deprived eye, flux and horizontal versus vertical grid discriminations were mastered. Only one of three cats performed above criterion on a form discrimination (i.e., cross versus disc), but the other two cats performed well above chance on this problem during the later stages of training.

There are procedural differences that could account for the apparently discrepant data collected by Chow and Stewart (1972). In the experiments of Ganz and Fitch (1968) and Dews and Wiesel (1970), the behavioral apparatus was a modified Yerkes box; the animal faced the positive and negative stimulus panels from a distance and had to approach the positive stimulus. Thus, this task involved simultaneous discrimination, correct orientation, and approach to the correct side. Chow and Stewart (1972) also used a runway apparatus but employed a go–no-go procedure. Positive and negative stimuli were presented on separate trials and the task required the cat to approach the positive stimulus and to remain still to the negative stimulus. Chow and Stewart reasoned that this method avoids the spatial complexities involved in the simultaneous discrimination procedures. Thus, deficits of visuomotor coordination resulting from deprivation would be less likely to interfere with performance. In addition, these investigators were very responsive to affective variables. Their cats were handled affectionately after each trial to aid in maintaining behavior, and if a succession of errors disrupted performance, a previously mastered problem was reintroduced until normal behavior was reestablished.

Additional evidence of the importance of task variables in evaluating recovery of visual-discrimination behavior following MD has been provided by van Hof-van Duin (1976*b*). Permanent deficits were found on a number of visuomotor tasks in cats monocularly deprived for 8–10 months and then reverse sutured (see above). Pattern discrimination in these same animals was found to recover well. On a horizontal versus vertical grid discrimination, the cats performed as well with the deprived eye as with the nondeprived eye. The animals also performed well on a series of problems requiring them to discriminate vertical from oblique grids at various angles. Form discrimination was also found to be good when the figure–ground relationships of the form problems were reversed. This result implies that pattern discrimination was based on stimulus shape and not on local flux cues. Good transfer after figure–ground reversal was also found by Rizzolatti and Tradardi (1971).

The apparatus used by van Hof-van Duin (1976*b*) was unique in that the cats were not required to walk down runways. The cat sat in a box and faced the stimuli that covered two small gates in one wall. To select a stimulus and obtain reinforcement it had only to push the gate open. Thus, the demands of good visuomotor coordination were reduced or eliminated, enabling a more direct assessment of discriminative abilities. On the basis of the results obtained in this apparatus, van Hof-van Duin (1976*b*) suggested that MD produces visuomotor deficits but not deficits in sensory discrimination. This conclusion is in agreement with that of Myers and McCleary (1964).

That MD cats can perform visual discriminations again raises the question of whether they use the same cues as normal cats use in these problems. Deprived animals using the deprived eye commonly take more trials to master a problem than when using the nondeprived eye (e.g., Chow and Stewart, 1972; Dews and Wiesel, 1970; Ganz and Haffner, 1974; van Hof-van Duin, 1976*b*), and this suggests that MD animals may in fact be utilizing alternate strategies. Ganz and Haffner (1974) set out to determine how MD cats solve discrimination problems under a variety of stimulus transformations, reasoning that, in normal perception, recognition of objects can occur independently of changes in size, brightness, or orientation.

Ganz and Haffner (1974) monocularly deprived their cats for 3–5 months and then reverse sutured them for a period comparable to the length of the initial deprivation. Training and testing was in a Yerkes-type apparatus and cats were trained on flux, grid orientation, and form discriminations. MD cats using their deprived eye managed to master all three problems, but required many more trials than normal controls, MD cats using the nondeprived eye, or BD cats. The effects of reverse suturing were evident only on the form discrimination (i.e., upright versus inverted triangles): All of the reverse-sutured animals mastered this task but none of the MD animals with subsequent binocular experience did so. Forced usage thus facilitated recovery, but only on the most difficult task.

The transposition tests more clearly revealed the considerable advantage of the reverse-sutured animals. On the grid-orientation problem transpositions of the stimuli included reversing the positions of the black and white stripes and making the stripes thicker or thinner. Reverse-sutured and normal cats transposed successfully on all tests; their performance never fell below 95% correct. MD cats with no forced usage failed most of the tests: One cat transposed successfully on 3 of 10 problems and the other cat transposed on only 1 of 10. Ganz and Haffner interpreted this result to mean that the normal and reverse-sutured cats solved this problem on the basis of orientation, independently of flux cues, whereas the MD cats with later binocular experience relied on local flux cues. If the local flux distribution was disrupted by, say, narrowing the black stripes, the latter cats failed to transfer the discrimination.

Transposition tests were also run on the form problem; however, MD cats without reverse suture were not included, since they did not master the original discrimination. The transpositions of the form problem consisted of changing the size of the triangles, reversing the figure–ground relationships, and presenting only the bottom or top portion of the triangle. The normal animals transposed to all but the last test. This indicates that only the portion of the stimulus near the point where the cats pushed to obtain reinforcement was used to make the original discrimination. The deprived animals failed all but the "bottom" transposition. The results of this experiment indicate two things. First of all, discrimination of orientation in MD animals takes place independently of local flux cues. Secondly, form discriminations are acquired more slowly and transpose less readily, if at all, in reverse-sutured animals than in normal cats. Since they do not transpose to local flux alterations, the reverse-sutured animals apparently use local flux cues to master form discriminations. These results clearly demonstrate the importance of taking a means–end approach to the results of behavioral recovery experiments following visual deprivation.

It is clear that the weight of the evidence reviewed favors the proposition that MD cats can recover many discriminative abilities. But the mechanisms of such recovery are obscure. Attacking the problem using the lesion method, Spear and Ganz (1975) have investigated the role of various areas of the visual cortex in recovery of pattern discrimination after monocular deprivation. Combined lesions of areas 17, 18, and 19 produced a total loss of the preoperatively learned discriminations. Thus, visual cortex appears crucially involved in recovery.

Sherman's data (1973, 1974) showing that the visual field for the deprived eye of MD cats includes only the peripheral monocular segment suggests that recovery in MD cats may be based on some new use of the monocular field. Spear and Ganz (1975) showed that removal of the monocular segment of area 17 (a portion of the cortex containing cells which receive input from only one eye) produced no deficit in the retention of form discrimination in MD or normal cats. Therefore, recovery of pattern discrimination is not dependent on the monocular part of area 17 alone.

Finally, Spear and Ganz investigated effects of lesions that *spared* only the monocular segment of area 17. The results of such lesions were variable, but three of the four cats with lesions relearned the discriminations with savings; their performance was better than the animals with lesions of areas 17, 18, and 19. These results show that the central retinal projection zone of area 17 is not crucial to recovery from monocular deprivation, nor are areas 18 and 19 critical to recovery (see also Winans, 1971).

The work of Spear and Ganz (1975) demonstrated that recovery of function following MD may not be dependent on a single cortical locus, a finding which suggests that behavioral recovery is mediated by the small number of cortical cells that are still responsive to stimulation through the deprived eye. The investigators did not, however, consider the possibility that recovery may be mediated either peripherally (e.g., at the lateral geniculate) or centrally (e.g., at the Clare–Bishop area) to areas 17, 18 and 19.

3.2. Physiological Recovery

A fundamental aim of neurobiology is the correlation of behavioral phenomena to physiological mechanisms. Finding a correlation between behavioral recovery and recovery of the normal response properties of cortical cells following deprivation has, therefore, been the aim of many workers in the deprivation field. Unfortunately, this goal has not been achieved. The previous sections have outlined the extent of behavioral and perceptual recovery after deprivation, and it has been shown that in some situations such recovery is considerable. However, a corresponding degree of physiological recovery has not been observed.

3.2.1. Physiological Recovery Following Binocular Deprivation

We have already noted that the distribution of ocular dominance of cortical cells following BD is roughly like that of a normal animal; however, BD results in more unresponsive cells and more cells with abnormal receptive-field properties. Wiesel and Hubel (1965*b*) reported on a single cat that was binocularly deprived for 3 months and then allowed more than 1 year of experience with one eye open. Following this period, there was no obvious change in cortical ocular dominance relationships; the open eye did not show any predominance in driving cortical cells. However, there were signs of other physiological changes. For example, the number of binocularly driven cells decreased, a result similar to that seen in cats reared with artificial strabismus or alternating monocular deprivation (Hubel and Wiesel, 1965). Chow and Stewart (1972) obtained similar results. This finding implies that the lack of synergistic input during monocular recovery exerts a small but measurable effect on cortical ocular dominance. It has also been found that monocular experience following BD leads to a decrease in the proportion of unresponsive cortical neurons (Chow and Stewart,1972; Wiesel and Hubel, 1965*b*). Thus, modification of the physiological properties of cortical cells is possible well beyond the end of the critical period.

The receptive field properties of cortical neurons may also have the potential to be altered beyond the sensitive period. Wiesel and Hubel (1965*b*) found an increase in the proportion of cells which lacked orientation specificity in BD cats with later monocular experience. Twice as many of the abnormal receptive fields were in the eye opened during the recovery period. On the other hand, Chow and Stewart (1972) found that aside from sluggish and rapidly adapting responses, the receptive-field properties of cortical cells in their BD cats were normal following long monocular experience.

More recently Cynader, Berman, and Hein (1976) provided a detailed comparison of the receptive-field characteristics of cortical cells in BD cats immediately following deprivation and after prolonged binocular experience. Just after deprivation about a third of the cells were unresponsive to light stimulation and most of the responsive cells fatigued rapidly. But the most marked abnormality of the visually responsive cells was their lack of specificity: 88% had neither orientation nor direction specificity as compared to only 4% without such specificity in normal cats. Following a 6–12-month period of binocular experience, there was a marked increase in the number of cells with specific receptive fields: orientation specificity was seen in about half of the units, but there was little increase in the percentage of direction-selective cells. There was also a decrease in the number of unresponsive cells.

Taken together these studies suggest that there is a degree of plasticity in cortical cells following the sensitive period; that is, after binocular deprivation, environmental factors can still influence the response properties of cortical cells. Although monocular experience after BD may cause an increase in the proportion of abnormal receptive fields (Wiesel and Hubel, 1965b) binocular experience increases the proportion of cells with receptive-field specificity (Cynader *et al.*, 1976). This difference seems to reflect the deleterious effects of the absence of synergistic input to cortical cells and shows, furthermore, that these effects may be exerted beyond the sensitive period. Nevertheless, neither binocular nor monocular experience following BD completely establishes or reestablishes normal cortical physiology, a fact that stands in contrast to the reports of behavioral recovery subsequent to BD (e.g., van Hof-van Duin, 1976a). Although there is a variety of possible alternative explanations, this discrepancy may simply reflect a difference in the power of resolution between electrophysiological and behavioral techniques. Thus, the physiological abnormalities that remain after "recovery" from binocular deprivation either may not influence visual behavior or may not be detectable using behavioral procedures.

3.2.2. Physiological Recovery Following Monocular Deprivation

Behavioral recovery following MD is dependent on both the time when deprivation is ended and the nature of postdeprivation experience. The effects are more reversible if deprivation is ended within the first few months and the animal is forced to use the deprived eye. Physiological recovery is dependent on the same factors, but the degree of recovery is more limited.

The period of maximum susceptibility to MD begins about 4 weeks postnatally and extends until about the 12th week (Hubel and Wiesel, 1970; Blakemore and van Sluyters, 1974). During this period even very short episodes of MD can markedly alter the ocular dominance of cortical cells such that most are driven by the nondeprived eye (Hubel and Wiesel, 1970; Olson and Freeman, 1975). Under certain conditions these effects can be reversed as easily as they are produced. If cats are monocularly deprived until 5 weeks and then reverse sutured, nearly all cortical cells are then driven by the initially deprived eye. However, if reverse suturing is delayed until 14 weeks, there is little shift in cortical ocular dominance (Blakemore and van Sluyters, 1974). Thus, the effects of MD on ocular dominance are completely reversible if the deprivation conditions are reversed during the critical period.

Recovery is also dependent on the nature of the postdeprivation experience. Hubel and Wiesel (1970) monocularly deprived cats for 5 weeks during the critical period and allowed binocular experience for 12–14 months. Only small changes in ocular dominance were observed subsequent to this experience; most cells were still predominantly driven by the initially open eye. Blakemore and van Sluyters (1974) demonstrated extensive shifts in ocular dominance after equivalent deprivation periods followed by only 9 weeks of reverse suture. In this latter case, ocular dominance was shifted such that the initially deprived eye drove most cortical cells. Extending the deprivation period further into the sensitive period followed by reverse suture produced less marked shifts in ocular dominance (Blakemore and van Sluyters, 1974).

The rate of ocular dominance shifts is also dependent on the time that reverse suturing takes place. If it is done early in the sensitive period, the initially deprived eye begins to drive cortical cells within 3 days, and by 12 days the shift of ocular dominance is complete. As reverse suture is delayed, ocular dominance shifts are delayed in both onset and completion (Movshon, 1976*a*).

Movshon concluded from these and other data that cortical plasticity within the sensitive period has two phases. Initially, the ocular dominance of all cortical cells is modifiable by experience, but the rate at which changes may be effected declines with age. Thus, reverse suturing at 4 weeks shifts the ocular dominance of cortical cells faster than reverse suturing at 5 weeks. During the later stages of the sensitive period, increasing numbers of cells are "committed" to one eye and the remaining cells retain the ability to shift their ocular dominance but do so at different times; the "uncommitted" cells, however, are as plastic as they were during the early stages of the sensitive period. Movshon (1976*b*) found a good correlation between the ability of the two eyes to support visuomotor behavior and the rate of ocular dominance reversal for animals reverse sutured at 5 or 6 weeks. The correlation broke down for animals reverse-sutured at 7 weeks, in which case the deprived eye was behaviorally normal 6 days after reverse suture but physiologically could drive only about one-quarter of the cortical cells.

Receptive-field properties are also modifiable during the critical period. Following reverse suture, as the eyes are shifting in their ability to drive cortical cells, receptive-field specificity also changes. Generally, in the MD animal, when one eye provides most of the influence on a cortical cell, the receptive field of that eye is orientation specific whereas the receptive field in the nondominant eye is nonoriented (Blakemore and van Sluyters, 1974; Movshon, 1976*a*). However, following a longer period of reverse suture, some cells may have oriented fields in each eye but the preferred orientations may differ by as much as 90° (in normal cats orientation preference is identical in both eyes). Thus, reversal of the effects of MD by reverse suturing cannot establish identical receptive-field characteristics in each eye.

Although the effects of MD on ocular dominance are reversible within the critical period, deprivation continued throughout the critical

5. REFERENCES

Aarons, L., Halasz, H. K., and Riesen, A. H. Interocular transfer of visual intensity discrimination after ablation of striate cortex in dark reared kittens. *Journal of Comparative and Physiological Psychology*, 1963, *56*, 196–199.

Barlow, H. B. Visual experience and cortical development. *Nature*, 1975, *258*, 199–204.

Barlow, H. B.,, Blakemore, C., and Pettigrew, J. D. The neural mechanism of binocular depth discrimination. *Journal of Physiology*, 1967, *193*, 327–342.

Baxter, B. L. Effect of visual deprivation during postnatal maturation of the electroencephalogram of the cat. *Experimental Neurology*, 1966, *14*, 224–237.

Blake, R., and Hirsch, H. V. B. Deficits in binocular depth perception in cats after alternating monocular deprivation. *Science*, 1975, *190*, 1114–1116.

Blakemore, C., and Cooper, G. F. Development of the brain depends on the visual environment. *Nature*, 1970, *228*, 477–478.

Blakemore, C., and Mitchell, D. E. Environmental modification of the visual cortex and the neural basis of learning and memory. *Nature*, 1973, *241*, 467–468.

Blakemore, C., and Papaiannou, J. Does the vestibular apparatus play a role in the development of the visual system? *Journal of Physiology*, 1974, *236*, 373–385.

Blakemore, C., and van Sluyters, R. C. Reversal of the physiological effects of monocular deprivation in kittens: Further evidence for a sensitive period. *Journal of Physiology*, 1974, *237*, 195–216.

Blakemore, C., and van Sluyters, R. C. Innate and environmental factors in the development of the kitten's visual cortex. *Journal of Physiology*, 1975, *248*, 663–716.

Chow, K. L., and Stewart, D. L. Reversal of structural and functional effects of long-term visual deprivation in cats. *Experimental Neurology*, 1972, *34*, 409–433.

Cool, S. J., and Crawford, M. L. J. Absence of binocular coding in striate cortex units of Siamese cats. *Vision Research*, 1972, *12*, 1809–1814.

Creutzfeldt, O. D., and Heggelund, P. Neural plasticity in visual cortex of adult cats after exposure to visual patterns. *Science*, 1975, *188*, 1025–1027.

Cynader, M., Berman, N., and Hein, A. Cats reared in stroboscopic illumination: Effects on receptive fields in visual cortex. *Proceedings of the National Academy of Science*, 1973, *70*, 1353–1354.

Cynader, M., Berman, N., and Hein, A. Cats raised in a one-directional world: Effects on receptive fields in visual cortex and superior colliculus. *Experimental Brain Research*, 1975, *22*, 267–280.

Cynader, M., Berman, N., and Hein, A. Recovery of function in cat visual cortex following prolonged deprivation. *Experimental Brain Research*, 1976, *25*, 139–156.

Daw, N. W., and Wyatt, H. J. Kittens reared in a unidirectional environment: Evidence for a critical period. *Journal of Physiology*, 1976, *257*, 155–170.

Dews, P. B., and Wiesel, T. N. Consequences of monocular deprivation on visual behavior in kittens. *Journal of Physiology*, 1970, *206*, 437–455.

Duffy, F. H., Burchfiel, J. L., and Snodgrass, S. R. Ammonium acetate reversal of experimental amblyopia. Paper presented at the Society for Neuroscience, 6th Annual Meeting, Toronto, Canada, 1976.

Duffy, F. H., Snodgrass, S. R., Burchfiel, J. L., and Conway, J. L. Bicuculline reversal of deprivation amblyopia. *Nature*, 1976, *260*, 256–257.

Freeman, R. D., Mitchell, D. E., and Millodot, M. A neural effect of partial visual deprivation in humans. *Science*, 1972, *175*, 1384–1386.

Freeman, R. D., and Pettigrew, J. D. Alteration of visual cortex from environmental asymmetries. *Nature*, 1973, *246*, 359–360.

Freeman, R. D., and Thibos, L. N. Electrophysiological evidence that abnormal early visual experience can modify the human brain. *Science,* 1973, *180,* 876–878.

Ganz, L. Orientation in visual space by neonates and its modification by visual deprivation. In A. H. Riesen (Ed.), *The developmental neuropsychology of sensory deprivation.* New York: Academic Press, 1975.

Ganz, L., and Fitch, M. The effect of visual deprivation on perceptual behavior. *Experimental Neurology,* 1968, *22,* 638–660.

Ganz, L., and Haffner, M. E. Permanent perceptual and neurophysiological effects of visual deprivation in the cat. *Experimental Brain Research,* 1974, *20,* 67–87.

Ganz, L., Hirsch, H. V. B., and Tieman, S. B. The nature of perceptual deficits in visually deprived cats. *Brain Research,* 1972, *44,* 547–568.

Hein, A., and Held, R. Dissociation of the visual placing response into elicited and guided components. *Science,* 1967, *158,* 390–392.

Held, R. Dissociation of visual functions by deprivation and rearrangement. *Psychologische Forshung,* 1968, *31,* 338–348.

Held, R., and Hein, A. Movement-produced stimulation in the development of visually guided behavior. *Journal of Comparative and Physiological Psychology,* 1963, *56,* 872–876.

Hirsch, H. V. B. Visual perception in cats after environmental surgery. *Experimental Brain Research,* 1972, *15,* 405–423.

Hirsch, H. V. B., and Spinelli, D. N. Visual experience modifies distribution of horizontally and vertically oriented receptive fields in cats. *Science,* 1970, *168,* 869–871.

Hirsch, H. V. B., and Spinelli, D. N. Modification of the distribution of receptive field orientation in cats by selective visual exposure during development. *Experimental Brain Research,* 1971, *13,* 509–527.

Hubel, D. H., and Wiesel, T. N. Receptive fields, binocular interaction and functional architecture in the cat's visual cortex. *Journal of Physiology,* 1962, *160,* 106–154.

Hubel, D. H., and Wiesel, T. N. Receptive fields of cells in striate cortex of very young, visually inexperienced kittens. *Journal of Neurophysiology,* 1963, *26,* 994–1002.

Hubel, D. H., and Wiesel, T. N. Binocular interaction in striate cortex of kittens reared with artificial squint. *Journal of Neurophysiology,* 1965, *28,* 1041–1059.

Hubel, D. H., and Wiesel, T. N. The period of susceptibility to the physiological effects of unilateral eye closure in kittens. *Journal of Physiology,* 1970, *206,* 419–436.

Imbert, M., and Buisseret, P. Receptive field characteristics and plastic properties of visual cortical cells in kittens reared with or without visual experience. *Experimental Brain Research,* 1975, *22,* 25–36.

Kratz, K. E., Spear, P. D., and Smith, D. C. Postcritical period reversal of effects of monocular deprivation on striate cortex cells in the cat. *Journal of Neurophysiology,* 1976, *39,* 501–511.

LeVere, T. E. Neural stability, sparing, and behavioral recovery following brain damage. *Psychological Review,* 1975, *82,* 344–358.

Meyers, B., and McCleary, R. A. Interocular transfer of a pattern discrimination in pattern deprived cats. *Journal of Comparative and Physiological Psychology,* 1964, *57,* 16–21.

Milner, P. *Physiological psychology.* New York: Holt, Rinehart and Winston, Inc., 1970.

Movshon, J. A. Reversal of the physiological effects of monocular deprivation in the kitten's visual cortex. *Journal of Physiology,* 1976a, *261,* 125–174.

Movshon, J. A. Reversal of the behavioral effects of monocular deprivation in the kitten. *Journal of Physiology,* 1976b, *261,* 175–187.

Muir, D. R., and Mitchell, D. E. Visual resolution and experience: Acuity deficits in cats following early selective visual deprivation. *Science,* 1973, *180,* 420–422.

Nikara, T., Bishop, P. O., and Pettigrew, J. D. Analysis of retinal correspondence by studying receptive fields of binocular single units in cat striate cortex. *Experimental Brain Research*, 1968, *6*, 353–372.

Olson, C. R., and Freeman, R. D. Progressive changes in kitten striate cortex during monocular vision. *Journal of Neurophysiology*, 1975, *38*, 26–33.

Packwood, J., and Gordon, B. Stereopsis in normal domestic cat, Siamese cat and cat raised with alternating monocular occlusion. *Journal of Neurophysiology*, 1975, *38*, 1485–1500.

Peck, C. K., and Blakemore, C. Modification of single neurons in the kitten's visual cortex after brief periods of monocular visual experience. *Experimental Brain Research*, 1975, *22*, 57–68.

Pettigrew, J. D. The effect of visual experience on the development of stimulus specificity by kitten cortical neurons. *Journal of Physiology*, 1974, *237*, 49–74.

Pettigrew, J. D., and Garey, L. J. Selective modification of single neuron properties in the visual cortex of kittens. *Brain Research*, 1974, *66*, 160–164.

Pettigrew, J. D., Olson, C., and Barlow, H. B. Kitten visual cortex: Short-term, stimulus-induced changes in connectivity. *Science*, 1973, *180*, 1202–1203.

Pettigrew, J. D., Olson, C., and Hirsch, H. V. B. Cortical effect of selective visual experience: Degeneration or reorganisation? *Brain Research*, 1973, *51*, 345–351.

Riesen, A. H. (Ed.). *The developmental neuropsychology of sensory deprivation.* New York: Academic Press, 1975.

Rizzolatti, G., and Tradardi, V. Pattern discrimination in monocularly reared cats. *Experimental Neurology*, 1971, *33*, 181–194.

Schneider, G. E. Two visual systems. *Science*, 1969, *163*, 895–902.

Sherk, H., and Stryker, M. P. Quantitative study of cortical orientation selectivity in visually inexperienced kittens. *Journal of Neurophysiology*, 1976, *39*, 63–70.

Sherman, S. M. Visual field defects in monocularly and binocularly deprived cats. *Brain Research*, 1973, *49*, 25–45.

Sherman, S. M. Permanence of visual perimetry deficits in monocularly and binocularly deprived cats. *Brain Research*, 1974, *73*, 491–501.

Sherman, S. M., Guillery, R. W., Kaas, J. H., and Sanderson, K. J. Behavioral, electrophysiological and morphological studies of binocular competition in the development of the geniculo-cortical pathways of cats. *Journal of Comparative Neurology*, 1974, *158*, 1–18.

Shlaer, R. Shift in binocular disparity causes compensatory change in the cortical structure of kittens. *Science*, 1971, *173*, 638–641.

Spear, P. D., and Ganz, L. Effects of visual cortex lesions following recovery from monocular deprivation in the cat. *Experimental Brain Research*, 1975, *23*, 181–201.

Spinelli, D. N., Hirsch, H. V. B., Phelps, R. W., and Metzler, J. Visual experience as a determinant of response characteristics of cortical receptive fields in cats. *Experimental Brain Research*, 1972, *15*, 289–304.

Stryker, M. P., and Sherk, H. Modification of cortical orientation selectivity in the cat by restricted visual experience: A reexamination. *Science*, 1975, *190*, 904–906.

Tretter, F., Cynader, M., and Singer, W. Modification of direction selectivity of neurons in the visual cortex of kittens. *Brain Research*, 1975, *84*, 143–149.

van Hof-van Duin, J. Development of visuomotor behavior in normal and dark-reared cats. *Brain Research*, 1976*a*, *104*, 233–241.

van Hof-van Duin, J. Early and permanent effects of monocular deprivation on pattern discrimination and visuomotor behavior in cats. *Brain Research*, 1976*b*, *111*, 261–276.

Wiesel, T. N., and Hubel, D. H. Effects of visual deprivation on morphology and physiology of cells in the cat's lateral geniculate body. *Journal of Neurophysiology*, 1963*a*, *26*, 978–993.

Wiesel, T. N., and Hubel, D. H. Single-cell responses in striate cortex of kittens deprived of vision in one eye. *Journal of Neurophysiology,* 1963*b*, *26,* 1003–1017.

Wiesel, T. N., and Hubel, D. H. Comparison of the effects of unilateral and bilateral eye closure on cortical unit responses in kittens. *Journal of Neurophysiology,* 1965*a*, *28,* 1029–1040.

Wiesel, T. N., and Hubel, D. H. Extent of recovery from the effects of visual deprivation in kittens. *Journal of Neurophysiology,* 1965*b*, *28,* 1060–1072.

Winans, S. S. Visual cues used by normal and visual-decorticate cats to discriminate figures of equal luminous flux. *Journal of Comparative and Physiological Psychology,* 1971, *74,* 167–178.

PART **V**

ACCOUNTING FOR SPARING AND RESTITUTION

14

Recovery after Brain Damage and the Concept of Localization of Function

SCOTT LAURENCE AND DONALD G. STEIN

1. INTRODUCTION

Although damage to the central nervous system often results in permanent disruption or loss of behavioral function, a remarkable degree of recovery or restitution may occur under certain circumstances. In some cases, there is a return to normal or near-normal levels of performance even after extensive loss of nervous tissue. However, there is considerable disagreement over the nature of, and reasons for, such recovery and consequently over its meaning for our understanding of nervous system organization and activity in the intact organism. There seem to be at least two principal reasons for the lack of a unitary approach to recovery of function. First, varying methodologies and the large number of complex and interdependent factors which influence recovery of function often prevent any one specialist from making meaningful generalization of findings to areas removed from his or her immediate area of inquiry. Second is the confusion generated by the ambiguous and sometimes meaningless nature of the terms and concepts used to describe and interpret the operations of the nervous system and the mechanisms thought to subserve restitution of function after damage. In this chapter we hope to provide some clarification of

SCOTT LAURENCE AND DONALD G. STEIN • Department of Psychology, Clark University, Worcester, Massachusetts 01610

various explanatory constructs used to interpret or explain recovery, and we will discuss some of the underlying assumptions concerning the relationships between central nervous system structure and function that are evident within these various approaches to the problem.

1.1. Problems of Definition

Given the rather recent and substantial interdisciplinary interest in the area of central nervous system plasticity, it is not surprising to find considerable heterogeneity in the way of the concepts of recovery and neural plasticity have been used and defined. This confusion has apparently contributed to misunderstandings over the implications of the recovery process for our knowledge of "normal" brain structure and function.

For our purposes, recovery of function can be generally defined as a return to normal or near-normal levels of performance, following the initially disruptive effects of injury to the nervous system. In animal studies, the extent of recovery can be operationally defined and empirically determined and usually involves a direct comparison of selected pre- and posttraumatic behaviors. In clinical cases, recovery is often judged against normal performance on various neurological and neuropsychological tests; information concerning the patients' premorbid history is also used. Despite the fact that these procedures allow for explicit and consistent measurement of "recovered" behavior, there is considerable room for disagreement over whether the behavior represents "true" restitution of function or whether the subject simply learns to substitute a new set of strategies for those lost as a result of injury (Gentile, Schmelzer, Green, Neiburgs, and Stein, in press; Goldberger, 1974). This disagreement has implications for the problem of the relationship between recovery and localization of function and appears to center in part on ambiguity in the meaning and usage of the term "function."

Essentially, we may conceive a function in terms of goals (the accomplishment of an experimenter-defined end) or in terms of means (an emphasis upon the specific behaviors used to attain those ends). We usually think of recovery in terms of a renewed ability to achieve certain ends, but a failure to analyze the specific means used by brain-damaged organisms can result in a failure to detect a true deficit (see Isaacson, 1975, for example). A combination of means and ends analyses is crucial if recovery is to be used either as a method of studying nervous organization or as part of any debate concerning localization of function. Clearly, recovery need not imply plasticity, reorganization, or any other term intended to indicate changes in the neural topography of localized functions if the "recovered," brain-damaged organism is able to achieve goals through the employment of novel tactics or unusual behaviors (e.g., Goldberger, 1974; Lashley, 1960).

The ability to use novel tactics when familiar means of achieving ends have been blocked is one of the fundamental characteristics of biological activity, and it must always be considered when analyzing a particular instance of recovery. Sometimes the use of novel tactics is obvious, but often highly similar behaviors mask unique compensatory devices, and subtle techniques may be required to clarify "real" differences (e.g., Gentile *et al.*, 1974; Goldberger, 1974).

In the following discussion we will interpret as "recovered" any behavior or set of behaviors which allow an organism to attain a goal, given that the organism was capable of accomplishing that goal prior to, but not immediately following, neural injury. The assertion that a specific function has or has not "recovered" should represent a clear definition of what constitutes the normal or preoperative range of activities and how the postoperative functions differ from and/or are similar to them. To be complete, studies of recovery should include a clear description of the goal (if a goal analysis is being employed) and the means being used to accomplish that goal (e.g., Gentile *et al.*, in press).

Recovery can be used to describe many different processes taking place in the CNS, and means–ends analyses can help to avoid some of the confusion generated by this ambiguity of meaning.

1.2. Recovery and Sparing

A good example of recovery of function from our point of view has been provided by Teitelbaum (1971) and Teitelbaum and Epstein (1962), who studied the effects of lateral hypothalamic lesions on eating in rats. While it is generally accepted that rats with bilateral lesions of the lateral hypothalamic (LH) area display both adipsia and aphagia, these authors demonstrated that there is a specific and invariant sequence of recovery in rats with LH lesions that closely parallels the ontogenesis of eating in the normal rat. Although the "recovered" LH rats eventually appear "normal," a study by Teitelbaum and Cytawa (1965) underscores how different the recovered animals can be from intact rats. They showed that recovered rats with LH lesions once again became adipsic and aphagic after potassium chloride was applied to the overlying cortex to induce spreading depression. This temporary loss of cortical functioning reintroduced the full lateral hypothalamic syndrome, and artificial support and forced feedings were required to keep the animals alive.

Differences in the behavior of "normal" and "recovered" animals have been demonstrated in a number of studies. For example, Gentile and her colleagues (in press) created one- or two-stage lesions of medial parietal (motor) cortex in adult rats and then tested the animals on an elevated runway. There was initial impairment in both groups of brain-damaged rats, although those with serial lesions recovered more rapidly. All of the animals eventually recovered to preoperative criterion, but high-speed cinematographic analysis revealed that the two groups used different strategies to navigate the runway. Thus, "normal" behavior in these two lesion groups may have been mediated by different patterns of reorganization in the CNS.

As differentiated from the concept or definition of recovery, *sparing* of function refers to a failure to detect any loss of behavioral efficiency even immediately after neural damage. In an experimental paradigm, this usually means that the spared animals are compared to other subjects that exhibit a deficit. Stein, Rosen, Graziadei, Mishkin, and Brink (1969), for example, have shown that rats suffering hippocampal damage in two unilateral stages, spaced 1 month apart, are significantly less impaired in tests of passive avoidance and visual-spatial discrimination than are one-stage animals who have received the same damage in a single session. In fact, two-stage animals were similar in performance to sham-operated controls. Strictly speaking then, the rats of Stein *et al.* did not reveal a gradual return to normal function but rather an absence of deficit on the tasks they studied. It is worth noting, however, that some aspects of recovery may be inferred from observations of sparing. Thus, it should be realized that sparing and recovery of function can be two logically separable issues which *may* require different types of explanation and may involve separable physiological mechanisms (see Teuber, 1974, for example). Reference will be made to both phenomena throughout this section.

Many studies are designed and/or described in a manner which makes it very difficult to determine whether sparing, recovery, or a combination of the two has occurred (e.g., Bekoff, Lockwood, and Meikle, 1972). Often, animal studies employ cumulative scores (such as errors or trials to criterion) to study differences between pre- and post-traumatic behavior or between, say, the effects of a single versus a two-stage lesion. In such instances, sparing which may be noticeable only in the first few days following injury may be obscured. A learning paradigm may actually involve retraining, and other more "natural" or "spontaneous" processes of recovery or sparing may be overlooked. Here the human clinical literature, with its emphasis upon an intensive if often qualitative analysis of a single subject over a long period of time, provides very useful information (e.g., see Geschwind, 1974). It must be remembered that the type of testing situation employed, the definition of the goal or criterion, and the type of data analysis used can individually and in combination affect the interpretation of the recovery process. As we discuss below, these factors may also play a role in developing the constructs used to explain sparing or recovery.

2. STRUCTURAL EXPLANATIONS OF RECOVERY

Structural explanations of recovery are based on conceptions relating to the anatomical organization of the intact brain. They are *static* constructs in the sense that no special, particular process is alluded to; rather, recovery is seen as a necessary consequence of the way the brain is organized. However, these static explanations are actually applicable only to sparing, and not to recovery, a fact which is often overlooked (Rosner, 1970). Of course, they may be used in combination with more dynamic constructs to account for recovery as well. This naturally implies that however good these constructs may be, they are directly applicable to only a restricted range of phenomena. Under structural explanations we include *redundancy* and *multiple control*.

2.1. Redundancy

Redundancy, or redundant representation (Rosner, 1970), refers to the possibility that a part of a neural system may adequately mediate the function normally subserved by the system as a whole. That is, when some, or even most, of a particular area is destroyed, there may still be enough tissue remaining to carry out a goal-directed behavior in a manner apparently indistinguishable from the normal.

Before elaborating on the notion of redundancy itself, it may be worthwhile to discuss its affiliation with Lashley's (1929) concept of *equipotentiality*. Lashley argued that within a given region of the brain, function was mediated equally by all of the tissue *within* that region. Thus, if a particular structure (such as the temporal area) were partially damaged, the remaining intact tissue would continue to mediate the behavior. Such "equipotentiality" would mean the effects of a lesion would depend more on the amount of tissue destroyed within a structure than upon the specific portion of substructure destroyed.

It is clear that *redundancy* and *equipotentiality* are closely related terms. However, Lashley used *equipotentiality* in reference to the homogeneity of structure and function he presumed to exist within particular areas of the rat cortex, consisting of relatively undifferentiated and unspecialized substructures in which the exact emplacement of a lesion seemed to be unrelated to the degree and type of behavioral disruption measured. Chow (1967) has discussed how such a notion is less applicable to the primate cortex, with its greater degree of "lateralization" and "specialization." For Rosner, redundancy seems to signify a relationship between two anatomically distinct but functionally related substructures. To quote Rosner:

> . . . a local region of sensory surface such as skin or retina projects to many neurons at any particular stage of the relevant afferent pathway. Loss of some of these neurons leaves others at the same level that can still process signals from the local peripheral region (p. 555).

This difference may be of little more than scholarly importance.* While the two terms seem to refer to different physiological mechanisms, it is clear that they each refer to similar types of phenomena and the same types of empirical evidence apply to each. For this reason, we will use the term *redundancy* to encompass both equipotentiality and redundant representation.

Wall (unpublished report) points out that redundancy has also been envisaged as a series of hierarchically ordered systems in which more recently evolved areas (such as the cerebral cortex) inhibit the functions of lower, less-evolved centers. After damage to so-called higher centers, the more primitive areas (presumably subcortical) would be released from inhibition, thus permitting some aspects of the previous behavior to unfold. As Wall points out, however, the partial or inefficient recovery observed might be due, not to the release of "lower control centers," but to a "disordered function of a single, integrated nervous system."

The chief difficulty with studies that fail to find deficits (e.g., Beach, *et al.* 1960), and hence provide some support for redundancy, is that there always remains the possibility that the analysis was not refined enough to detect a significant loss in quality of performance (Dawson, 1973; Isaacson, 1975). Another way of looking at the problem is to assume that redundancy may not be a structural feature of the brain but rather a consequence of surplus information in the testing situation (or test–organism system). Destruction of a particular part of the brain may in fact completely and/or irrevocably eliminate the perception of certain cues for example, but the testing situation may still contain other cues (or, alternatively, a small but sufficient quantity of the same class of cue that has been destroyed) sufficient for the discrimination to be made. The inability of the experimenter to detect a deficit may be a reflection of the animal's capacity to rely on a reduced amount of information (assuming that in the normal situation sufficient or surplus in-

---

* It is interesting to note that Lashley used such notions as equipotentiality and mass action in support of a holistic and relational conception of neural organization, while for Rosner redundant representation helps explain apparently anomalous results from the localizationist position.

formation was available) or to develop totally new or compensatory strategies for solving a problem (Rosen and Stein, 1969). One way in which testing for a deficit situation is refined, then, is to fully eliminate this surplus information. As Zeki (1969) has shown, sometimes differences in performance can be revealed by simply taking a closer look at the actual data collected and by not relying too heavily on measures of global performance.

While the elimination of multiple-model cues (such as the confounding of position with visual cues) is common practice, the elimination of intramodal cues may be very difficult. For example, Winans (1967) had cats learn to discriminate between upright and inverted triangles, then made lesions in areas 17, 18, and 19 in a single stage, and retrained them on the task. All the animals were able to relearn this discrimination. One could conclude from these data that either small remaining areas of the striate cortex were able to mediate this kind of complex perception (equipotentiality) or that pattern perception was not "localized" in the striate area and could be accomplished in other areas as well. Such conclusions might be unwarranted because consistent local luminous flux cues (at either the apex or bottom border of the figures) were not controlled. All that the cats would need to discriminate between such figures is the ability to detect brightness differences in a very restricted part of their visual field.

Other studies with cats (e.g., Spear and Braun, 1969) have tried to eliminate consistent local luminous flux cues by requiring animals to discriminate between vertical and horizontal stripes, and by randomly alternating the bottom-most or right-most stripe as either black or white. Even in these studies, however, it is possible for the animals to discriminate the figures by moving their eyes and detecting differential rates of brightness change, (see Galambos, Norton, and Frommer, 1967; Pasik, Pasik, and Schilder, 1969). It is important to note that in those studies where most of the surplus information has been reduced (e.g., Spear and Braun, 1969), the number of trials required for relearning is very large (see for example Spear and Barbas, 1975). Zeki's (1969) analysis of studies on the secondary visual system of the monkey reveal how performance similar to control animals' (Meyer, Harlow, and Ades, 1951) may be a function of subtotal lesions, overtraining, and/or setting a criterion of "deficit" which is too high.

From the viewpoint of common sense, it is difficult to contend that the destruction of any particular substructure cannot have some behavioral effects. Certainly, such effects may only be noticeable under certain conditions, since organisms can perform some goal-directed activities through a number of means (which allows for considerable compensation in the face of loss) and since all testing situations involve a certain degree of surplus information.

2.2. Multiple Control

The concept of multiple control has been discussed by Rosner (1970). As an explanation for *sparing* of function, it is both simple and comprehensive. Briefly stated, multiple control relies upon the notion of multiple localization; a specific function is conceived as being controlled by more than one center. Hence, destroying one governing substructure still leaves another intact. This differs from "redundancy" since, in the latter, sparing is conceived as being due to the ability of a single governing substrate to mediate a function, despite damage.

Insofar as recovery of function is concerned, multiple control, like redundancy, is a "static" concept, and cannot by itself account for the process of initial deficit followed by a gradual return to normal; the concept implies no mechanism that would account for such a change. If the concept is to account for both sparing and recovery, it must be understood how in some cases no deficit is apparent, while in others there is a temporary deficit.

Another problem for the concept of multiple control, at least in its simple and strictly localizationist form, is that it is an untestable and therefore unfalsifiable hypothesis. This makes it weak from the theoretical point of view. This difficulty is evidenced in an example of multiple control used by Rosner (1970). Cytawa and Teitelbaum (1967) studied the effects of cortical spreading depression on rats who had recovered from the effects of bilateral septal destruction. Usually, rats suffering such lesions demonstrate heightened sensitivity to stimuli, or hyperreactivity. This "emotional" reaction gradually subsides or recovers, usually within 3–10 days.

After applying potassium chloride to the overlying cortex of such recovered rats, Cytawa and Teitelbaum noted a complete return of this hyperreactivity, lasting for about 10 days. The conclusion, proposed by Rosner, that both the cortex and septum represent control centers for emotion can be tested only by depressing the activity of both areas. If recovery of hyperreactivity were still found after such lesions, however, one could simply postulate yet another control center. In fact, Clark, Meyer, Meyer, and Yutzey (1967) have found that septal emotionality does disappear with combined septal and cortical lesions, although such recovery is slower than it is with a septal lesion alone. To propose the existence of a third control center for emotionality is consistent, but it indicates an infinite regress.

Insofar as "emotionality" is concerned, other difficulties with multiple control emerge. First of all, it is apparent that if such dual or multiple centers exist, then they do not share the same "status"; cortical destruction alone, for example, does not lead to hyperreactivity (Clark *et al.*, 1967). Further, the "cortical center" cannot be really specified in more detail, a fact which leads one to suspect that the effects of cortical dysfunction are more the results of distributed and mass-action effects. Clark *et al.* have demonstrated that 80–90 percent removal of the cortex (following septal damage) had the same effects as did bilateral ablation of either anterior or posterior cortex. Further difficulties come from studies of combined septal and amygdaloid lesions. Since such destruction, when performed simultaneously, leads to greater emotional reactivity (Kleiner, Meyer, and Meyer, 1967), one should conclude that the amygdala also constitutes another control center for emotion. Such a conclusion is complicated by the results of Schwartzbaum and Gray (1966). These authors found that amygdaloid lesions made subsequent to septal destruction actually reduced the amount of reactivity. A simple notion of multiple control, then, can neither predict nor account for differential effects with simultaneous and sequential lesions of different structures. The differential effects of simultaneous and sequential lesions of the hippocampus (Stein *et al.*, 1969), caudate nucleus (Schultze and Stein, 1975), reticular formation (Adametz, 1959), feline visual cortex (Bekoff *et al.*, 1972), or sulcus principalis in the monkey (Rosen, Stein, and Butters, 1971) cannot be explained by multiple control, for example, since the same tissue is destroyed under both the simultaneous and sequential conditions.

3. PROCESS APPROACHES TO RECOVERY

It is obvious that recovery of function takes place over time. Hence, constructs which emphasize events and mechanisms which occur after the lesion offer an inherent advantage over structural or static explanations. Unlike redundancy and multiple control, which are best applicable to the phenomenon of sparing, process approaches are more directly concerned with recovery of function.

3.1. Functional Substitution

One alternative to multiple control is the closely related notion of functional substitution. This construct refers to the possibility that one subsystem can take over the "functions" of another in the event of neural damage to the latter. Here "function," of course, must be understood in its teleogical sense; we may say that one subsystem has taken over the "role" or "purpose" of another. Further, one should not require that the replacement subsystem perform the function in a manner identical to the "normal" subsystem; it must, however, be performing the same duties. That is, if there exists a "brightness discrimination" subsystem which can be selectively destroyed, one can be certain that this operation has been taken over functionally only if the new subsystem also performs brightness discrimination (even if it does so in a different way) and does not merely compensate for the loss by changing eye-scanning patterns, head movements, etc.

Functional substitution is quite clearly a direct extension of localization of function. However, it admits of a certain plasticity of function as well; we might characterize this position as asserting that particular areas of the brain are specialized for performing particular (teleological) functions, but that the "assignments" of function to structure within this system may change depending upon circumstance (especially early or infant lesions; Fass, Jordan, Rubman, Seibel, and Stein, 1975; Goldman, 1972; 1974).

Functional substitution may operate in two distinguishable ways. One can conceive of a subsystem undergoing some kind of reorganization in order to perform different goals. This process may be akin to learning, but how it might occur is a complete mystery. This view of functional substitution was postulated by Kennard (1938) to explain the recovery of motoric functions. Alternatively, we may conceive of a whole new subsystem emerging in the brain, a unique organization set in motion by injury. This possibility has been put forward by Horel, Bettinger, Royce, and Meyer (1966) and by Meyer (1973). Note that both of these views concentrate on the events which take place after a lesion and postulate that the intact areas of the damaged brain undergo some special process. Since one may suppose that such processes can be manipulated, functional substitution is in principle a testable concept, a fact which gives us great advantage over multiple control. The first alternative, however, posits no special mechanisms (although they may exist), while the second alternative requires that there in fact be some unique process. While no hard experimental evidence (or proposed mechanisms exists) for or against the first alternative, we can examine some support for the second.

Horel *et al.* (1966) invoked this latter form of functional substitution in explanation of their experimental findings. These authors demonstrated that rats with posterior neocortical lesions could acquire a black–white discrimination in approximately the same number of trials as do normal rats. Further, rats trained on the discrimination task and then given a lesion reacquired the discrimination in about the same number of trials as did the other two groups. This similarity in overall performance, however, concealed a difference in learning rates. The success of the groups with striate lesions in the early part of training or retraining was related to the fact that these animals, unlike normal rats, did not consistently avoid the white stimulus card. This difference led the authors, and later Meyer (1973), to conclude that ". . . at least two different mechanisms are available for black/white discrimination" (p. 117). While this may be interpreted as an example of multiple control, Meyer goes on to say that ". . . some other part of the brain vicariously took over the function after the visual cortex was removed" (p. 118). This sounds like the "reorganizational" hypothesis of Kennard (1938), but Meyer cites a study by Goodman and Horel (1966) as evidence that this "substitution" is an indication of a unique system which may emerge in response to a lesion.

It should be noted, however, that one need not hypothesize the existence of such a system in order to explain the results of Horel *et al.*; it is quite enough to say that visual cortex lesions lead to a decreased amount of visual input, which in turn leads to less aversiveness to bright stimuli. The results of Goodman and Horel (1966) need further explaining *only* if it is assumed that brightness discrimination is localized within a particular system and, further, that this system was completely destroyed by the lesions. It is also possible that the overall similarity in performance concealed differential strategies (in eye-scanning, use of local luminous flux cues, etc.) between the different groups; differences which are not so much representative of new and different systems for black–white discrimination *per se,* but which represent different "parts" of a more general system which allows for brightness discrimination through a number of alternative means. A lesion may eliminate the possibility for using some of these strategies but not others.

Another experiment which bears on the question of functional reorganization was recently performed by Fass *et al.* (1975). These investigators studied the effects of one-or two-stage lesions of the lateral hypothalamic area (LH) on food intake and weight regulation in rats. The animals with one-stage lesions developed the classical symptoms of aphagia and adipsia. After the first (unilateral) lesion in the two-stage group, there was also a postoperative inability to regulate body weight, but this deficit gradually disappeared. After the second operation destroyed the contralateral LH, no changes in food intake or weight regulation were observed. This finding could be interpreted to indicate that some sort of reorganization of hypothalamic (or larger neural subsystem) function had occurred since the same lesion in contralateral, homologous tissue did not have the same behavioral or metabolic consequences. It is unlikely that, in this context, different response strategies were used "to attain the goal" of weight regulation for Ss with two-stage lesions. Here it may well be the case that functional reorganization of CNS tissue was involved in the disappearance of the deficit.

It should be pointed out in this section that if one is determined to accept the concepts of both localization and substitution of function by another structure after the "critical locus" for a given behavior is destroyed, some caution is necessary. A substitution theory would have to explain how the "substituted" area can mediate its own functions and "take over" new responsibilities without some change in its capacity or efficiency. Milner's (1974) theory of the development of language disorders after brain damage in children may serve as a good example of what might be happening when a secondary area substitutes for the primary, damaged area. In very young children, it appears that both hemispheres are involved in the development of language. Milner claims that as development continues, the left hemisphere suppresses the right and becomes more important in mediating linguistic functions. While early lesions often "spare" language ability, there is a price to be paid in the form of reduction of overall intellectual capacity (retardation). Milner hypothesizes that such retardation "may be the result of 'crowding,' that is, the mediation of additional functions by the nondominant right hemisphere as it compensates for damage to the dominant left hemisphere" (p. 215).

3.2. Plasticity, Radical Reorganization, and Reorganizational Compensation

The terms *plasticity* (Stein *et al.*, 1969) *radical reorganization* (Luria, 1948), and *reorganizational compensation* (Rosner, 1970) have been used to indicate that at least some instances of recovery and/or sparing are the result of global changes in neural organization which take place in response to injury. Luria has been most insistent in concluding that perhaps all instances of recovery involve "radical" change, while Rosner sees reorganizational compensation as just one possible explanation applicable to a restricted range of recovery phenomena.

Plasticity seems to connote a kind of morphological flexibility, and the term is often used to describe such anatomical changes as axonal sprouting and regeneration, "pruning" effects, etc. (see Bernstein and Goodman, 1973). Another definition of plasticity can be seen as more radical. One can assume that each substructure does have a consistent and identifiable role to play within the brain, but that such specialized functions may "shift" in response to injury or other factors. This should be considered as a shift in *subsystem specialization*. The existence of this form of plasticity receives some support from the work of Goldman (1972), and has been discussed (from an entirely different perspective) by Hecaen (1969).

Shifts in function of CNS structures need not occur only in response to brain injury, but may also be the natural consequence of development processes that continue throughout life (Goldman, 1974). Recently, Stein and Firl (1976) removed the frontal cortex of aged rats in either one or two stages and studied the effects of these lesions on the performance of spatial and avoidance tasks. In young rats one-stage lesions result in permanent deficits (Stein, 1974), while two-stage lesions of the same area result in sparing of function. In the old rats there were no significant deficits on spatial performance when the animals with one- or two-stage lesions were compared to age-matched, nonoperated controls. Cell counts in the thalamus showed that there were no significant differences in number of intact neurons between aged, intact rats, old rats with lesions, and young, brain-damaged counterparts. Stein and Firl proposed that the brain damage inflicted upon the old rats had no effect on spatial behavior because the frontal cortex or the rest of the brain had changed its function; thus, removing an area that was partially nonfunctional would not be expected to have much effect.

A third and most radical view of plasticity would hold that recovery of function after brain damage is indicative of a continual transformation in global and specialized operations—that one cannot localize functions (however conceived) and that the operations of the brain's constituent neural subsystems may change according to ontogenetic history, injury, and a host of environmental variables. The discovery that a particular substructure undergoes anatomical change, however, may mean one of three quite different things, and this ambiguity in meaning points to the major difficulty with any vaguely conceived reorganizational or plasticity hypothesis.

First of all, it is clear that a change in substructure, even a "radical" one, does not necessarily indicate that a structure's role or teleological "function" has changed. That is, a change in structure may occur in response to injury, but the system may still accomplish the same ends. For example, Glassman (1970) created lesions in motor cortex of cats and observed a deficit in reaching behavior that was required to obtain morsels of food placed in a small tube. As the behavior recovered, Glassman noted a return of potentials in the motor cortex surrounding the damaged area. During the period in which the deficit was manifest, recordings from the same electrodes were flat or abnormal. Thus, even though the structure (in this case motor cortex) was damaged, it still appeared to play some role in the mediation of the motor response. Here one may also speak of relearning or compensation such as discussed by Rosner (1970) and demonstrated by Gazzaniga (1969a, b) in his investigations of cross-cuing strategies in split-brained monkeys and humans (also see Geschwind, 1974).

It might be thought that such processes as axonal sprouting represent "functional" plasticity uniquely related to injury and perhaps the construction of a new substructure which is intimately related to recov-

ery. However, such growth may be representative of normal growth
processes as well and is merely an indication of a general and ongoing
reorganization which alters the ability of the organism to meet ends in
the face of continually changing environmental exigencies, while not
representing any fundamental change in the "ground rules" by which
the brain operates. This first meaning of plasticity is therefore related
to the ability of an organism to act under diverse sets of circumstances,
including those which are due to brain damage. Here, plasticity or
reorganization in response to injury should not be considered as any
more "radical" or fundamental than changes which occur in any learning situation. Although we will discuss physiological hypotheses of recovery in a later section, it is important to note here that it would be exceedingly difficult to demonstrate that the generation of new synaptic
contacts is responsible for the recovery of function; not only would it
be necessary to demonstrate that no sparing of function has occurred
(either because not enough of a particular structure was destroyed or
because other areas may also be involved in its control), but it would be
necessary to ensure that no alternative or compensatory strategies were
being used by the animals and that no other processes were responsible. Further, merely correlating the emergence of new synaptic connections with behavior would not be sufficient to demonstrate their role
in recovery; such growth may only be indicative of a dynamic synaptogenesis which is always occurring under normal conditions (Chambers, Liu, and McCouch, 1973; Pribam, 1971; Rose, Malis, Kruger, and
Baker, 1959; Rose, Malis, and Baker, 1961; Sotelo and Palay, 1971).
Such widespread synaptic changes may be the underlying physiological
mechanism for a general relearning or compensatory process which is
actually responsible for recovery. It would be particularly difficult to
control this possibility, since the same manipulation may affect both the
"normal" and "unique " synaptic formations equally and the time factors involved in both processes may be very similar.

The same types of distinctions as discussed in the preceding paragraphs apply, *mutatis mutandis,* to the notions of radical reorganization
and reorganizational compensation. There is an obvious ambiguity in
any reorganizational hypothesis; it may indicate that the types of operations of the whole or a part of the brain have been fundamentally altered, or that the brain simply performs old operations in different
ways.* It is often assumed that any morphological change must be

---

* Among compensation explanations involving an ambiguous degree of reorganization
we count Goldberger's (1972, 1974) superb investigations into "restitution" of pathologic grasp in monkeys after area 6 ablations. He interprets this recovery as due to an
"enhancement of its opposite reflex, that of tactile evasion" (p. 79). Although one can
disagree with his assertion that such an enhancement is separable from a reorganiza-

"basic," while any changes at other levels (electrophysiological, behavioral) are less radical, but it would seem that such an assumption rests upon a false dichotomy between structural and functional change.

However radically one wishes to conceive of reorganization or plasticity, it is quite clear that Luria (1948) and especially Rosner (1970) see reorganization on the level of substructure specialization. Of course, for Luria this position represents a simple extension of his theory of dynamic localization, wherein the brain is seen as organized on the basis of widely distributed functional systems, while for Rosner reorganizational compensation represents one way in which specialized substructures may learn to interact with themselves and with the environment to perform old acts in new ways. In fact, the notion of compensation implies that recovery has not "really" taken place, but rather that the organism has simply "adjusted" to damage and now performs many tasks in a different and less efficient manner, or perhaps has altered its environment (or has had it altered by others) in such a way as to lessen the demands placed upon it.

There is a great deal of attraction for any theory which proposes a global reorganization change behind recovery, for, if nothing else, it obviates many of the logical and empirical difficulties inherent within any attempt to specify more exactly the subsystems "responsible" for recovery. However, it is quite clear that plasticity, reorganizational compensation, and radical reorganization possess an inherent ambiguity in meaning which makes it very difficult to generate specific hypotheses. This difficulty seems related to the fact that the level of extent of "fundamental" change remains ambiguous. This, in turn, may represent the specious assumption that structural changes are more basic than are those changes which occur at the level of behavior.

4. PHYSIOLOGICAL PROCESSES AND RECOVERY

Throughout the foregoing discussions we have emphasized a theoretical approach to recovery at the expense of analyzing empirical data which might appear relevant to a physiological explanation or orientation. There are a number of reasons why physiological processes have been more or less ignored. Primarily, it seems that a great deal of the confusion and contradiction within the scientific community dealing with recovery of function is more a result of conceptual ambiguity than

tional hypothesis (such a belief seems to rest upon a notion of reflex akin to an automatic mechanism reducible to localizable pathways of inhibition and excitation), a notion which is unsupported (Bizzi and Evarts, 1971; Burke, 1971), Goldberger's work does show that compensation can involve highly specifiable behavioral strategies.

of a lack of empirically gathered fact. Second, there seems to be no necessary relationship between any particular physiological approach and any particular theoretical one; we have already discussed how physiological changes such as axonal sprouting may be taken as support for widely differing positions, and we will expand upon this point below. Finally, a presentation or review of the various physiological approaches to recovery would be rather redundant in the face of the numerous in-depth and comprehensive summaries which have recently appeared in the literature. Very extensive reviews and analyses of axonal sprouting and regeneration within the mammalian CNS have been presented by Stenevi, Björklund, and Moore (1973 and by Moore (1974). Bernstein and Bernstein (1973) have similarly reviewed sprouting and regeneration in the spinal cord. Schneider (1973) and Schneider and Jhavari (1974) have discussed empirical and theoretical issues relevant to various aspects of neuromorphological plasticity, including developmental effects and the "pruning" phenomenon (the increase in axonal elaboration after transection of its terminal process). Recent symposia (Bernstein and Goodman, 1973; Stein *et al.*, 1974) have presented a comprehensive overview of the area and a detailed examination of some specialized topics. Consequently, we will attempt to present only an analysis of how these various explanations may be interpreted within the context of the conceptual approaches discussed earlier.

4.1. Diaschisis and Restitution of Function

Of the various physiological approaches to recovery, diaschisis is perhaps the oldest and best known. It is actually a much better and certainly more specific explanation for certain types of loss resulting from a lesion than it is an explanation for recovery from that loss. In 1914, von Monakow defined diaschisis as

> . . . an "interruption of function" appearing in most cases quite suddenly . . . and concerning widely ramified fields of function, which originates from a local lesion but has its points of impact not in the whole cortex (corona radiata, etc.) like apoplectic shock but only at points where fibers coming from the injured area enter into primarily intact grey matter of the whole central nervous system. . . . Speaking quite generally, the process of diaschisis may be regarded as being caused by abolition of excitability (functional standstill) due to local disruption of the brain substance within one neuron group, which is transmitted to neuron groups closely adjacent to and directly related with the affected part of the brain . . . (pp. 28, 29).

Diaschisis, then, represents a type of "secondary" or distributed effect dependent upon the tightly coupled or interconnected nature of the nervous system. It is not entirely clear how von Monakow conceived of this "functional shock," and the term has been rather loosely applied to a wide range of phenomena. Luria, Naydin, Tsvetkova, and Vinarskaya (1969) seem to interpret diaschisis as a kind of general, inertial trauma which temporarily suppresses activity in areas far from the site of the lesion because of the widespread effects of such processes as edema and extracellular blood flow. This interpretation is consonant with von Monakow's statement that diaschisis is transmitted to "closely adjacent" parts of the brain; such disruptions as are due to edema and interruptions in vascular flow would seem to be dependent upon the proximity of a particular area with the substructure which has been damaged. Conceived as such, recovery from diaschisis is identical to the notion of *restitution of function* hypothesized by Rosner (1970). Whatever von Monakow's original intent, we do not think that diaschisis is best understood in this way (as a part of "vegetative" disruption). Von Monakow certainly wished to stress functional loss in areas sometimes far removed from the site of the lesion. Not all such losses, however, can be reduced to edema, vascular interruption, or changes in biochemical milieu (Luria *et al.*, 1969). For example, since Nauta (1971) has shown extensive parietal-occipital efferents to the frontal lobes in man, one would expect that an occipital lesion would have some effect on frontal lobe function due to the loss of regulative input from the occipital area. Wickelgren and Sterling (1969) have found direct evidence for this form of distributive loss after cooling or damaging the feline visual cortex. These authors noticed a loss of inhibitory input into the superior colliculus, and hence an alteration in the latter structure's response to input from the contralateral eye. In short, a functional loss could be related to proximity as well as to the amount of input from the damaged area into another.

While it must be remembered that such "vegetative" changes as edema may contribute to an initial deficit and that the recovery from such effects may be an important correlate to recovery of function,* there is heuristic merit in distinguishing "vegetative" and "functional" disruption. In some cases this may be a practical impossibility. For example, as mentioned earlier, Glassman (1970) was able to correlate disruption and recovery of a sensorimotor task with the disappearance and return to electrophysiological activity in the areas immediately surrounding the lesion. In such cases the areas which have been destroyed have both vascular and functional relations with the areas that immediately surround it, and any attempt to ferret out the type(s) of secondary

---

* Isaacson (1975) has discussed 16 variables which could temporally suppress CNS activity after traumatic injury but which gradually diminish in their effects.

disturbance(s) which is active here would be very difficult. In contrast, the superior colliculus and visual cortex are easily separable substructures with no direct vascular linkages, and it is quite likely that the effects found by Wickelgren and Sterling are due to the loss of regulative input *per se*. This is strongly supported by the fact that cooling and destroying the cortex gave identical results.

Distinguishing diaschisis as understood in this purely functional sense from other secondary processes has important bearing on the notion of recovery of function. There is little difficulty in conceiving how such processes as edema and vascular interruption may occur and diminish (since such changes are not unique to the nervous system and seem to be a general feature of reparative, metabolic activity), but how is one to describe the recovery following loss of regulative input? Surely von Monakow's assertions that recovery from diaschisis is due to a "regression" of shock due to "a struggle for the preservation of the disrupted nervous function" (p. 32)—"The diaschisis which is spreading as a form of passive inhibition is met by a movement of reparative character, originating from the primarily intact parts of the nervous system representing the most vital function" (p. 32)—are vague and speculative and, more important, offer no mechanisms through which such recovery might occur.

If the spatiotemporal relations between various substructures have any functional significance at all, then the loss of such regulative input cannot be recovered spontaneously. If only some of the inputs of a substructure have been destroyed, then it is possible to imagine some kind of reorganizational process taking place—an adaptation of sorts to a decreased amount of input which would allow the downstream structure to function normally. As indicated below, both axonal sprouting and degeneration supersensitivity may be related to such reorganization. Such an hypothesis requires the interposition of some special process(es) unlike reparative recovery, however, and even this hypothesis cannot account for those instances in which all input has been severed. In any case, it is clear that diaschisis itself, although applicable to an understanding of distributive *loss, cannot,* if understood in a strictly functional sense, account for recovery of function.

4.2. Regenerative and Collateral Sprouting

Stenevi *et al.* (1973) have identified two forms of neural sprouting within the CNS as a response to injury. *Regenerative sprouting* refers to proximal regeneration of the axon after it has been transected and the distal portion degenerates. The newly generated axon may or may not reinnervate the denervated areas. In contrast, *collateral sprouting* refers to sprouting from intact cells to a denervated region after some or all of its normal input has been destroyed.

Very little is known about regenerative sprouting, but its relevance to mammalian recovery of function, except in an indirect way, is probably minimal. (Regenerative sprouting does reinforce the view that a continual dynamic synaptogenesis occurs in the intact brain; Sotelo and Palay, 1971.) A number of studies (see Moore, 1974, for a review) have demonstrated regenerative sprouting in central adrenergic neurons, and recently Björklund, Johansson, Stenevi, and Svengaard (1975) have shown that regenerated CNS pathways can be physiologically functional. This sprouting seems to be very similar to the sprouting earlier discovered in the peripheral nervous system (Stenevi *et al.*, 1973). As Bernstein and Bernstein (1973) have pointed out, such sprouting is of doubtful functional importance in the CNS, since the marked complexity of the central nervous pathways and the glial and connective tissue scars which form after neural damage probably prevent many regenerated axons from innervating any sites. Once the conditions necessary to promote point-to-point connections within CNS are known (and this would seem to result from a better understanding of neural ontogenesis), regenerative sprouting may come under the control of scientific manipulation, and this may represent a significant advance in our ability to direct and increase recovery of function.

Collateral sprouting from intact central axons in response to denervation of nearby areas has been investigated by a number of authors (Goodman and Horel, 1966; Lund and Lund, 1971; Lynch, Matthews, Mosko, Parks, and Cotman, 1972; Moore, Björklund, and Stenevi, 1971; Raisman, 1969), but the conditions contributing or causal to collateral sprouting are poorly understood, and it is not well known how frequently and within what areas of the brain it can occur. Adrenergic areas, because they can be easily studied using the histochemical method of Falck and Hillarp (Falck, 1962), have received the major focus of investigation. Stenevi *et al.* (1973), however, believe that collateral sprouting is not restricted to adrenergic areas only.

Collateral sprouting has been demonstrated to some degree in the septal nucleus and anteroventral thalamic nucleus after damage to the hippocampus afferents (Raisman, 1969; Moore *et al.*, 1971; Stenevi *et al.*, 1973), in the dorsal lateral geniculate nucleus after visual cortex lesions (Stenevi *et al.*, 1973), in the olfactory tubercle after olfactory bulb destruction, and in the cerebeller cortex after superior cerebeller penduncle lesion (Stenevi *et al.*, 1973). Stenevi et al. also report that no collateral sprouting has been observed in the lateral preoptic area and lateral mammillary nucleus of the hypothalamus after hippocampal destruction, in the dorsal lateral geniculate nucleus after optic nerve transection, in the superior colliculus after optic nerve and/or visual cortex lesions, in the hypothalamus after amygdaloid lesions, in the suprachiasmatic nucleus after raphé and optic nerve lesions, and/or in the lumbar gray of the spinal cord after spinal and subthoracic hemisection. An analysis of those substructures in which central adrenergic collateral sprouting does and does not occur have led Stenevi *et al.* (1973) to conclude that at least three general conditions are necessary before such sprouting can be easily observed. "First," they indicate,

> . . . there must be a minimal density of the adrenergic innervation within the denervated area for reinnervation to be demonstrable. . . . Second, the denervation of nonadrenergic elements must be substantial. Third, the adrenergic axons should be distributed within the denervated areas in sufficient proximity to vacated synaptic sites to promote collateral sprouting. It is not now possible to quantify these statements but they should serve as general guidelines (p. 128).

One factor that may influence the extent and time course of collateral sprouting is the rate at which axonal debris resulting from a lesion is removed from the damaged area. Raisman and Field (1973) have recently demonstrated that until the products degeneration are removed, collateral sprouting cannot occur. It is possible that collateral sprouting occurs in some areas but not others and that it reflects the degree to which lesion debris remains and the rate at which the products of degeneration can be removed from the injured area.

An interpretation of what either regenerative or collateral sprouting may mean, especially insofar as recovery of function is concerned, depends upon an understanding of what triggers this type of reaction and whether or not it is a specialized response to injury or merely representative of other more important and essentially normal synaptogenetic processes. We have discussed this point earlier in relation to the notion of functional substitution, where we emphasized the great difficulty inherent in any experimental attempt to determine if sprouting is the "cause" of recovery. There are two mechanisms through which sufficient neural "vacancies" may open in the normal brain to allow sprouting to occur. Pribram (1971) and Rakic (1975) have shown that the division of glia in response to neural stimulation may allow a growing axon to find its way through the cellular cleavage and innervate another cell. Another possibility is that neuraxonal death, which appears to be a part of normal, regulative processes during embryogenesis (Cowan, 1973), may serve a similar function in the mature nervous system. Cells may die, leaving a number of vacated sites which can be filled by intact cells. In this way, the mature brain may differ from the immature one by virtue of the greater number and complexity of its interneural connections and the elaboration made at the expense of absolute cell numbers. Whatever the stimulus for normal sprouting may be, it is certainly possible that it is a frequently occurring process. The parallels between normal ontogenetic growth and that seen in sprouting have been described by Goodman and Horel (1966), Goodman *et al.* (1973), Raisman (1969), Rose *et al.* (1959; 1961), and Sotelo and Palay (1971).*

One way in which the importance of sprouting for recovery might be investigated would be to study the degree of dendritic and axonal elaboration (or contraction) in areas far removed from the side of the lesion. It is possible that the entire brain might respond to the destruction of its substructures by increasing connectivity in intact areas. Such an investigation is necessary, in any case, if the causal role of regenerative or collateral sprouting in recovery of function is to be known.

Finally, a very important problem that still remains to be solved is the determination of whether or not the presence of collateral sprouts or anomalous projections (which may be physiologically "functional"; see West, Deadwyler, Cotman, and Lynch, 1975) are functionally adaptive for the organism. In a recent series of elegant experiments, Schneider (1973) has shown that if the superficial layer of the superior colliculus is damaged in the neonatal hamster, fibers coming from the retina will be redirected and will grow into the deeper layers of the stratum profondum. If extensive unilateral damage to the superior colliculus in newborns is sustained, retinal fibers will cross the midline and invade appropriate (homologous) layers of the colliculus contralateral to the damaged side. In these two cases anomalous sprouts would be "competing" for the same synaptic space normally occupied by the appropriate contacts arriving from the retina. Given the crowding and competition for synaptic space, it is unlikely that the anomalous sprouts would mediate recovery. In fact, Schneider's animals showed abnormal orientation behavior to visual stimuli which led him to propose that recovery of visual orientation might be enhanced by the destruction of the anomalous sprouts.

Schneider also described a rather curious phenomenon which he called the "pruning effect." He noted that after axons are cut, there is a tendency to preserve, as much as possible, their terminal arborizations. Thus, removal of the distal portion of the axon would engender sprouting closer to the cell body. Such sprouts would be likely to make synaptic contacts (if at all functional) in areas not directly associated

---

* One reason why a more generalized interpretation of sprouting would be more helpful for and understanding of recovery is that localized sprouting, as discussed by Stenevi *et al.* (1973), seems to occur under such restrictive conditions that its relevance for many instances of neural destruction would seem to be minimal. Sprouting in intact areas may be more important and is probably not subject to such restrictions.

with the initial projections. These new terminals might then introduce considerable "noise" into an area that may have previously functioned normally. In this case, as well as in the one mentioned above, sprouting could have maladaptive consequences for the organism.

4.3. "Relatively Inefficient" Synapses

Although the possibility that collateral sprouting can enhance or mediate recovery is still an intriguing one, there are, as we pointed out in an earlier section, a number of serious limitations in using observed samples of anomalous connections to explain functional restitution. To avoid some of the difficulties that are inherent to explaining recovery in the CNS by growth of new terminals, Wall and his associates (1976) have recently proposed that already existing, but "relatively ineffective," pathways might be able to mediate neural function when primary sensory afferentation is eliminated.

In one experiment, Wall and Egger (1971) removed the nucleus gracilis in rats and thereby eliminated hindlimb sensory representation to the nucleus ventralis lateralis of the thalamus. After removal of the gracilis, the medial part of the VPL will not respond to skin stimulation of the hindlimb but will respond to skin stimulation of the forelimbs. When the rats were allowed to survive, it appeared that the area responding to forelimb stimulation expanded "in an orderly fashion" into the area which had previously responded to the hindlimb. Although these findings could be interpreted in terms of sprouting of forelimb afferents into the denervated hindlimb area, Wall proposed that there might have been "silent cells already connected to the area which do not function in the intact animal" but which can become active when primary afferents are removed.

To test this hypothesis, Merrill and Wall (1972) studied the receptive field properties of afferents into lamina 4 of the cat spinal cord. Neurons in this area have very restricted receptive fields which do not vary and have a very definite edge. By sectioning the dorsal roots or blocking them, Merrill and Wall were able to show that all of the afferents into the lamina are limited to a very small "micro bundle" consisting of a few fibers. When the fibers were blocked, the receptive field disappeared. Merrill and Wall then stimulated neighboring dorsal roots electrically (instead of with tactile stimulation, which was ineffective) and the same cell again responded. The authors claim that the electrical stimulation was able to trigger a volley in masked, ineffective terminals that fed into the same cell from neighboring afferents. Natural stimulation failed to produce effective excitation of the cell. Wall suggests that the response of these "relatively ineffective afferents" occurs almost immediately after deafferentation of the primary roots and that therefore the reappearance of the unit response is not likely to be due to anomalous sprouts replacing the normal afferents that were damaged in the adult animals.

To support his position further, Wall provides other evidence which was derived from experiments using acute and reversible techniques of deafferentation. First, Wall (unpublished) mapped the receptive-field properties of the dorsal column nuclei of the cat and selected cells which responded to the stimulation of the foot. He then blocked the spinal cord in the L4 segment with ice technique. Wall found that most of the cells "lost their response to peripheral stimulation" but were capable of ongoing activity. Some of the cells, however, "lost their receptive fields on the foot and gained one on the abdomen. When the cold block was removed, the receptive fields reverted to the foot." Wall interpreted his data to indicate that at least some of the cells in the spinal cord have alternative inputs which can become effective (unmasked) as soon as normal input is removed. Similar findings and interpretations have recently been made by Eidelberg, Kreinick, and Langescheid (1975).

In essence Wall and his associates have provided physiological evidence for a type of redundant mechanism in the CNS, but much more research will need to be done to determine whether the presence of "relatively ineffective synapses" can mediate functional restitution after brain damage. Wall's findings and interpretations, however, do demand further thought and examination. If the existence of parallel pathways can be understood in terms of the role they may play in reorganizing the activity of the CNS after damage, Wall's findings may have very important practical and theoretical consequences.

4.4. Denervation Supersensitivity

One of the most intriguing explanatory models for recovery of function is that of denervation supersensitivity. The term refers to the phenomenon of increased postsynaptic responsiveness (sensitivity) to neurotransmitter substances or their agonists after input to an area has been denervated. Such denervation may be accomplished surgically (Trendelenburg, 1963), by trauma, by chemical means (through the use of 6-hydroxydopamine, Trendelenburg, 1972), or "functionally" by using such drugs as alpha-methyl-para-tyrosine (^{a}m^{p}t) which inhibit adrenergic synthesis and therefore neurotransmission (Glick, 1974). Glick (1974) has described a series of studies interpreted within the context of the supersensitivity model of recovery and has postulated that loss of inputs into a particular area can be compensated for by increased sensitivity of the postsynaptic membrane to a decreased amount of transmitter substance.

The usefulness of this model is indicated by the fact that a relatively simple physiological change can explain a wide variety of complicated and apparently discrepant phenomena. Glick (1974) has applied it to the anorexic effect of amphetamine and has resolved previously discrepant data related to this phenomenon. This model is also consistent with the reactions of frontally ablated monkeys and rats to a wide range of agonistic and antagonistic drugs, including pretreatment with ^{a}m^{p}t, and it affords a simple explanation of initial deficits and recovery from nigro-striatal lesions (Glick, 1974). The specificity of the model is well illustrated by a study by Glick and Greenstein (1973a,b), the results of which also afford an attractive explanation for some types of serial-lesion effects. Glick and Greenstein hypothesized that since the catecholamines had been implicated both in feeding behavior (Grossman, 1962; Margules, Lewis, Dragovich, and Margules, 1972) and in recovery following lateral hypothalamic lesions (Berger, Wise, and Stein, 1971; Zigmond and Stricker, 1973), recovery following LH lesions might be due to supersensitivity of intact neurons involved in feeding to remaining catecholaminergic inputs. They also interpreted the transient aphagia followed by recovery and changes in sensitivity to D-amphetamine after frontal lesions in mice to the loss of catecholaminergic efferents from the frontal lobe. They argued that if frontal lobe lesions were performed 30 days prior to LH lesions (a time period which gives supersensitivity more than sufficient time to develop), then remaining LH neurons might already be supersensitive, and hence recovery from LH lesions might occur at a faster rate. Their experimental findings supported this argument, and this was further strengthened by the fact that simultaneous frontal and LH lesions did not facilitate recovery. This represents support for the denervation supersensitivity model and, perhaps of even greater interest, it affords a good physiological explanation for some serial-lesion effects (see Glick and Zimmerberg, 1972). It may be that many instances of savings or recovery correlated with multiple, spaced lesions (as opposed to single-stage destruction) are related to the supersensitivity of downstream neurons induced by the first lesion. Of course, there are only a few lesion paradigms which satisfy the necessary restraints of the denervation supersensitivity model, and hence not all serial-lesion effects can be so easily explained.

Despite its elegance, the denervation supersensitivity model of recovery of function faces a number of obstacles. None of these problems are insurmountable, but they should prevent an all-encompassing acceptance of this particular model.

In comparisons between normal and brain-damaged animals regarding their reactions to various drugs, specificity of drug action and a homogeneity between the intact areas of the normal and damaged brain should not be assumed to exist. Claims of specificity may be unwarranted if it is assumed that such drugs as $^amp^t$ act only on denervated areas; norepinephrine-containing neurons are extensively located throughout the brain (Skolnick and Daly, 1974) and we should expect that they too are affected by such injections. Lack of homogeneity between intact and damaged brains contributes to difficulties in assuming drug-action specificity; after a frontal ablation it should not be assumed that the remaining areas of the brain react normally to chemical stimulation. For example, there is no reason to assume that a 5 mg/kg injection of D-amphetamine given to brain-damaged animals is comparable (in its effects on CNS activity) to an identical dose given to a normal subject. There are other important problems of interpretation as well. Ungerstedt, Ljungberg, Hoffer, and Siggins (1975) point out that when neurotransmitter analogues are used to test for supersensitivity, there is little specificity of drug action and effect. There are also marked differences in the time course of supersensitivity observed after peripheral and central deafferentation (e.g., only 24 hours after interruption of dopamine transmission). Because of this, Ungerstedt *et al.* pose the question of whether the "supersensitivity" observed after CNS lesions is due to a real increase on sensitivity of dopamine receptors or a possible compensatory decrease in transmission of dopamine antagonists.

From the perspective of those interested in a broad range of recovery phenomena, perhaps the most disappointing attribute of the supersensitivity model is its applicability to only a special combination of neuroanatomical locus and lesion parameters. First of all, it is quite clear that the model is applicable to only those situations involving the destruction of inputs into a particular area, leaving the receptive neurons intact. Recovery from damage to such structures as the visual or motor cortex, for example, does not conform to this requirement because *both* afferents and their receptive fields are destroyed. If all inputs into an area are destroyed, of course, then supersensitivity of the postoperative membrane would be useless. Further, in those instances involving destruction of large numbers of heterotype inputs, it is highly unlikely that supersensitivity could bring about a full recovery of information flow. Generally speaking, it is curious that the effects of input destruction should be exactly counterbalanced by an increase in post synaptic sensitivity, unless one is prepared to accept the remote possibility that supersensitivity evolved specifically as a mechanism of recovery. Studies are needed which would determine the precise relationships between the amount of input destruction, the degree of supersensitivity, and the extent of recovery. There are probably interesting differences between the behavior of such "recovered" animals and unoperated animals, and these differences also require further study.

5. LOCALIZATION AND RECOVERY OF FUNCTION

It is evident that the various concepts used to interpret or explain recovery or sparing, whatever their individual merits and deficiencies, represent a set of assumptions concerning the way the "normal" or uninjured brain is organized. In part, this may be due to the fact that recovery of function has only rarely received attention as a phenomenon worthy of study in its own right and that virtually all investigations have studied only a single factor thought to influence the process of recovery, although the available evidence indicates that recovery results from the interactive effect of many processes (Isaacson, 1975).

Theories of recovery reflect theories about normal brain organization because recovery cannot be divorced, either conceptually or physiologically, from a consideration of these "normal" processes. Granted, the possibility that new neural circuits or subsystems occur within the brain as a result of damage leaves us with the possibility that the "normal" and "recovered" brains do not operate in exactly the same way, but this difference is obviously not a fundamental one. Further, there is no firm evidence that such localized alterations in subsystem circuitry are solely or even partly responsible for instances of recovery. As we have stressed previously, the physiological theories or events should not be seen as competitive with more "conceptual" approaches to recovery and physiological events which occur prior to, or concomitantly with, recovery are in accord with virtually all of the conceptual (structural and process) theories. The underlying physiology of recovery, in other words, has the same relationship to such processes as learning, attention, behavior, and the myriad other vaguely defined and "normal" activities of organisms as does the more "usual" physiology of the nervous system.

Many of the approaches to recovery discussed in this chapter reflect a localizationist interpretation of CNS function. However, there exists considerable disagreement over the implications of recovery of function for theories of localization. Some see the fact of both sparing and recovery as a direct challenge to the principle of localization (Stein, 1974), while others see recovery as consistent with, and explainable by, localization doctrine (Geschwind, 1974; LeVere, 1975; Rosner, 1970).

Localization of function is a pervasive concept within the neurosciences. It is a notion both ambiguous and broad in meaning, and its various forms constitute the paradigmatic base to most biochemical, electrophysiological, and ablation studies of the mammalian central nervous system. Even so, localization of function has been subject to remarkably little conceptual analysis, and even the most cursory glance at current theoretical and empirical literature reveals tremendous variation in the way in which the notion is used.

There are many "types" of localization of function, some of which have opposable meanings; these various types differ along a number of dimensions. Some of the dimensions of lesser importance include (1) the size of the "localizable area" (ranging from a discussion of the functions of an entire hemisphere, for example, to the functions of certain subcellular organelles); (2) whether or not a function is attributed to a "regionalized" area of the brain (a relatively well-circumscribed chunk of tissue such as the hypothalamus, for example) or to a distributed system (such as the "cholinergic system"); a particular localization scheme may fall in an intermediary position between the highly regionalized and the highly ramified or distributed forms; (3) the type of category system used to investigate and/or explain a particular phenomenon (that is, the terminology may be couched within electrophysiological, biochemical, behavioral, or psychological terms, and localization of function statements may refer to any one of the various relationships between these and other categories). The categories used by a particular author may be self-consistent and nonoverlapping, or they may be mixed (such as using behavioral terms in describing the localizable electrophysiological responses of a single cell), and different terms may be used to refer to similar phenomena.

The single most important distinction regarding localization of function, however, and the dimension most relevant to the relationship between recovery and localization of function is that of "means" versus "ends." It is the failure of many authors to be explicit concerning their use of "function" within one of these two contexts which has led to a great deal of conceptual confusion.

As discussed earlier, when discussing ends, we refer to a process or function in reference to the *goal* it has accomplished, the *result* or *effects* it has within a particular context, or the *role* it has within a larger system. Conversely, an emphasis upon means disregards the final product of a particular process and emphasizes instead the *way* in which that goal was accomplished; the actual behavior of an organism, for example (or the biochemical changes, etc.), is therefore described. It should be clear that there are no rigid or necessary relationships between means and ends; that is, a particular goal may be accomplished through a number of means, and identical means may, in different contexts, accomplish entirely different ends.

This distinction between means and ends is central to an understanding of localization, for if we understand function to imply the accomplishment of certain ends, it is very difficult and oftentimes meaningless to talk of localization of function, while if we imply by *function* the "pure" description of a particular process, then localization of function is simply tautological.

It is often meaningless to talk of a teleologically construed function as localized within a particular substructure of the brain since virtually all goals can be accomplished in widely diverse ways and because each goal usually requires the simultaneous and sequential orchestration of many separate processes. Clearly, since there are differences among goals according to their generality, complexity, abstractness, or simply in the time over which they occur, some localization statements are more troublesome than are others; the greater the generality, the less likely it is that it is a highly localizable function. No one would seriously argue that such a highly general and complex function as house-building, for example, is a localizable function, and it is possible that were there agreement on which functions are highly synthetic, goal-oriented activities and which are elementary operations of the nervous system, we would then have no argument about whether or not a particular function is a localizable one. In fact, localization schemes are in constant flux and often change in accordance with our changing notions about what a particular function (such as memory, movement, or language) really is. As a single function comes under greater scrutiny, it becomes less and less possible to view it as an elementary and simple process, and it begins to assume the shadowy outline of a widely ramified *system* (in this case a unified collection of even smaller functions, inseparable from all of the other, formerly distinct functions). The scientific goal, here, of course, is the widely accepted practice of searching for the basic *units* or building blocks of the nervous system; it is assumed that it is these units which are truly localized, and that our present language, as cumbersome and incorrect as it is, reflects a true philosophy of the nervous system.

If the concept of function is thought of in its means or operational connotation, localization of function becomes a tautological rather than a meaningless notion. In this case, we are asserting nothing more than that a particular biochemical or electrophysiological process *exists,* and that it is an identifiable or knowable process. (This means that it has a certain *invariant* quality to it, or that it is not undergoing complete and constant flux. We usually identify "the" operations of a particular substructure or subsystem with this invariant quality, a fact which requires us to adopt ever-increasingly abstract or formalized forms of description.) Employing localization of function in this way contributes little to our understanding of the relationships between such processes as neural and behavioral events, but it is conceptually harmless unless improper categories are used to describe neural events. A common example of such "category confusion" is the use of behavioral terminology in description of neural processes (such that single cells within the cortex act as brightness or contour "analyzers"). Such terminology too often gives the impression that a psychological or behavioral act is accomplished within the brain; it is important to realize that the only processes accomplished by the nervous system *per se* are *neural* processes.

The assumption that one can relate specific behavioral processes within specific subregions of the brain is in large part based upon the assumption that deficits resulting from extirpation or damage to a specific neural area adequately and accurately reflect the behavioral functions mediated by the area under investigation. Even before the turn of the century, Jackson warned that localization of symptoms following CNS injury is not the same as localization of function in normal, healthy tissue. In 1910, Morton Prince, then President of the American Neurological Association wrote that:

> The present doctrine of cerebral localization regarded as a mapping of the brain into areas within which lesions give rise to particular groups of symptoms is one of the triumphs of neurology which cannot be valued too highly. Regarded as a localization of the psychophysiological functions represented by these symptoms within narrowly circumscribed areas, it is in large part naive to a degree which will excite the smiles of future neurologists (p. 340).

Even a brief scan of today's contemporary journals in the field of neuroscience would demonstrate that no one is smiling. Indeed, there are those who have written of the development of a "new phrenology" emphasizing that localization of function can be carried out with greater precision than ever before (see the recent symposium text edited by Zülch, Creutzfeldt, and Galbraith as an example of this trend, 1975).

Prince (1910) was well aware of how these two different conceptions of function could bedevil one's thinking about localization:

> The doctrine of cerebral localization acquires a very different significance according to whether it means that the brain can be mapped out into a number of circumscribed areas in each of which can be located a definite psychophysiological faculty . . . or whether it means only that these areas contain anatomical elements which are made use of for the physiological expression of a function; or that a given area is such an integral element of

a functioning mechanism widely distributed in the cortex, that an injury to
the "center" not only destroys the element but throws the whole of this
function out of commission by dynamic influences upon other areas and
thus produces a group of symptoms (p. 338).

Prince, in fact, was echoing Claude Bernard (1865) who wrote years
earlier that, "It does not suffice to destroy an organ to understand what
functions it serves" (p. 239).

While it would be foolhardy to deny that lesions produce highly
consistent behavioral and physiological effects, this does not mean that
the effects produced represent the functioning of the structure prior to
damage. In fact, the results of lesions may tell us more about how such
damage alters the operations of those areas remaining intact. Seen in
this light, recovery of function poses no challenge to localization if that
doctrine is conceived in terms of specifiable neural operation or if we
think in terms of the localization of symptoms rather than of
psychological or behavioral functions.

In spite of anatomical and morphological boundaries (even natural
cleavages) between structures, there is no a priori reason to assume that
the influence of any one part of the CNS over any other part remains
constant. It is likely that there is a constant interplay of influence, and
the outcome of a lesion may very much depend on the time at which
the lesion is made (Goldman, 1974, 1975; Stein and Firl, 1976), the
genetic endowment (Isaacson, 1975), past experience (Will and Rosenzweig, 1976), motivation of the subject (see Gazzaniga, 1974), or structural alteration of the part or any of the other parts of the system
before or after the lesion is created (Isseroff, Leveton, Freeman, Lewis,
and Stein, 1976).

It has been known for a long time that both the immediate and
long-term effects of brain damage (or other kinds of CNS manipulation) are not limited just to the site of the lesion. Recent studies in
which degeneration stains are employed (see for example Hicks and
d'Amato, 1975) have shown that even small, well "localized" lesions can
alter projection pathways from the structure to distant regions in the
brain. In addition, lesions occurring as a result of accident or those
created in the laboratory often sever fibers of passage from one region
to another that may not be conducting afferent or efferent information
to or from the area in question (Isaacson, 1975). As a result of such un-
controlled artifact, there are dramatic and widespread anatomical
changes throughout the brain which could certainly serve to alter many
aspects of the subject's behavior. If such degeneration then results in
anomalous sprouting or denervation supersensitivity in structures far
removed from the site of the lesion, one could certainly predict widespread changes in function as well. One example taken from the recent

literature might suffice to demonstrate our point. Hicks and d'Amato (1975) created unilateral lesions of motor sensory cortex in rats and then used Fink–Heimer stains to trace the extent of postoperative degeneration in the mature (as well as in developing) rats. They reported that:

> There was a fairly abundant outflow of fine fibers into the caudate-putamen
> . . . from cortico-fugal fibers. Numerous degenerated fibers extended to
> the posterior cortex dorsally and into the cingulum, and they crossed in
> corpus callosum to the opposite cortex. There was abundant projection to
> many parts of the thalamus, pretectal and subthalamic regions. . . . The
> midbrain colliculi, tegmentum and the substantia nigra received fibers. The
> pons received an abundant component and few fibers entered the midline
> and regional reticular formation at this level (p. 17).

This represents only a partial description of the widespread changes produced by a relatively well-defined, unilateral cortical lesion. Clearly, changes in any and all of these areas might contribute the observed symptomatology.

Further, "distributed" effects of lesions are certainly more complex than is suggested even by such widespread anatomical changes. For example, Goldberger (1974, p. 276) notes that ". . . part of the impairment which follows corticospinal lesions in the Macaque results from the discouragement experienced by the animal at the initial post-operative failure of its affected limbs to execute movement in a rewarding manner." Naturally, such psychological variables are especially important in understanding the effects of and recovery from brain damage in humans.

If consensual validation is to serve as our only guide for defining structure–function relationships in the brain, then the pathology observed after damage to specific anatomical areas can serve to define these relationships. However, it is also possible to view brain-behavior pathology as not just representing a remnant of normal behavior, but rather as a totally new type of behavior resulting from a more or less efficient reorganization of the tissue remaining. Thus, as Head would have suggested (see Reise, 1950), the remaining tissue becomes a new whole in itself. Seen in this light, symptomatology is not due only to what is taken out, but also to the reaction of the remaining CNS to the insult inflicted upon it.

Research on recovery of function taken in this context then becomes, a question of whether it is a threat to schemas of localization, but an attempt to determine the conditions under which restitution after brain damage can or cannot occur. In other words, "what are the limits to plasticity?" Reise suggests that certain types of behaviors are more vulnerable to brain lesions than others (see, for example, Butters,

Butter, Rosen, and Stein, 1973), and in such cases one might expect to find less efficient recovery. It should be noted, however, that "vulnerability" may change with age, sex (see Goldman, 1975), or preoperative experience (Greenough, Fass, and deVoogd, 1976). Many of these variables have received little if any attention in the experimental literature, so that even where failure to find recovery has been reported, most of the variables that might influence the outcome (and amelioration) of CNS trauma have not been explored.

Thus, instead of having to defend the position that a given "function" is localized in a particular area (or system), one might be concerned, for example, with whether the type of lesion, in addition to area of destruction, plays a role in the development of symptomatology. For example, are irritative lesions more likely to produce severe symptoms than destructive lesions? As Reitan (1966) has pointed out, the functional condition of the brain at the time of damage is a very important variable (see Goldman, 1974, 1975; Isaacson, 1975; Stein and Firl, 1976), especially in humans. The functional condition of the brain, aside from the damaged area may, as Reitan indicates, vary according to the nature of the focal lesion (space-occupying, traumatic, vascular, etc.), and the functional adequacy of the remaining tissue may be more important for localization (and relocalization) than the lesion itself.

Finally, the question of localization versus nonlocalization in the CNS may be seen by future neuroscientists as a pseudo-issue resulting from our ignorance and inability to penetrate the complexities of the brain with the techniques available to us. The localization doctrine does provide a handy tool for attacking the brain and reducing it to its most "elemental" parts. Such a reductionistic attitude is entirely consistent with the empiricist approach to inquiry, but this model may not adequately reflect the complexity of the nervous system. Jackson (1888) once said:

> What all of us dislike is the complex. We may easily err in taking the subjective confusion produced in us to be the objective thing contemplated, which is really only very complex.

Since Jackson's time many of the elemental operations of the nervous system have been more or less explained. This has been possible, in part, by ignoring this great complexity of which he spoke and by concentrating instead upon those operations amenable to the theoretical and technical tools at hand. However, a full understanding of brain–behavior relationships and such phenomena as recovery of function cannot be gained by reference to highly specifiable mechanisms within isolated areas of the brain. In dealing with recovery of function, we encounter properties of the brain at their highest levels of complexity, and little is to be gained by ignoring this fact.

Of course, it is not adequate simply to assert that such processes are highly "complex," or "global" or that they involve considerable and active "reorganization" or "plasticity." In general, recovery requires a more holistic approach, but the level of organization or complexity chosen must be appropriate for the type of question being asked. In any event, an explicit and consistent use of terminology and an appropriate and unambiguously interpretable methodology are essential.

6. CONCLUDING REMARKS

In this paper we hoped to clarify some of the issues related to the problem of recovery of function by discussing the nature of the relationships between the categories of neural and behavioral events. Some of the problems associated with interpreting certain methodological approaches to recovery were also discussed. In so doing, we cannot claim to have "solved" the riddle of recovery, any more than we have "solved" the riddle of the brain. In fact, our knowledge of recovery will only parallel our knowledge of the normal operations of the brain, and in our opinion most of the ambiguity, confusion, and apparent conflict within the field of recovery is due to a lack of comprehensive, explicit, and consistent approach to the entire range of nervous system operations and effects. Ultimately, such an approach must seek explanation in terms of elementary neural operations, but in the case of such processes as recovery, the full complexity and dynamic interaction of the nervous system cannot be ignored.

We do hope that a sufficient understanding has been gained of the many logical and practical difficulties associated with interpreting recovery and that at least some of the conceptual ambiguity relevant to describing and interpreting the effects of nervous system operations and their disruption has been dispelled.

Acknowledgment

This manuscript was prepared with support of a grant from the National Institute on Aging (1 R01 AG00295-01) and a Research Career Development Award (Type II) from the National Institute of Mental Health to the second author (5 K02 MH 70177-04). We would also like to express our sincere thanks to Ms. A. Bassett for her patience in typing the many revisions of this paper.

7. REFERENCES

Adametz, J. H. Rate of recovery of functioning in cats with rostral reticular lesions. *Journal of Neurosurgery*, 1959, *16*, 85–98.

Beach, F., Hebb, D., Morgan, C., and Nissen, H. (Eds.) *The neuropsychology of Lashley: selected papers.* New York: McGraw-Hill, 1960.

Bekoff, M., Lockwood, A., and Meikle, T. H., Jr. Effects of serial lesions in cat visual cortex on a brightness discrimination. *Brain Research*, 1972, *48*, 219–220.

Berger, B. D., Wise, C. D., and Stein, L. Norepinephrine: Reversal of anorexia in rats with lateral hypothalamic damage. *Science*, 1971, *172*, 281–284.

Bernard, C. Introduction à l'étude de la médécine expérimentale, 1865, Paris. Reissued Paris: Garnier–Flammarion, 1966.

Bernstein, J. J., and Bernstein, M. E. Neuronal alteration and reinnervation following axonal regeneration and sprouting in mammalian spinal cord. In J. J. Bernstein and D. C. Goodman (Eds.), *Neuromorphological plasticity.* Basel: S. Karger, 1973, pp. 135–161.

Bernstein, J. J., and Goodman, D. C. Overview. *Brain, Behavior and Evolution*, 1973, *8*, 162–164.

Bizzi, E., and Evarts, E. V. Translational mechanisms between input and output. *Neurosciences Research Program Bulletin*, 1971, *9*, 31–59.

Björklund, A., Johansson, B., Stenevi, U., and Svengaard, N. Re-establishment of functional connections by regenerating central adrenergic and cholinergic axons. *Nature*, 1975, *253*, 446–448.

Burke, R. E. Control systems operating on spinal reflex mechanisms. *Neurosciences Research Program Bulletin*, 1971, *9*, 60–85.

Butters, N., Butter, C., Rosen, J., and Stein, D. G. Behavioral effects of sequential and one-stage ablations of orbital prefrontal cortex in the monkey. *Experimental Neurology*, 1973, *39*, 204–214.

Chambers, W. E., Liu, C. N., and McCouch, G. P. Anatomical and physiological correlates of plasticity in the central nervous system. *Brain, Behavior and Evolution*, 1973, *8*, 5–26.

Chow, K. L. Effects of ablation. In G. C. Quarton, M. Melnechuk, and F. O. Schmitt, (Eds.), *The neurosciences, first study program.* New York: Rockefeller University Press, 1967, pp. 705–713.

Clark, S. M., Meyer, P. M., Meyer, D. R., and Yutzey, D. A. Emotionality changes following septal and neocortical ablations in the albino rat. *Psychon. Science*, 1967, *8*, 125–126.

Cowan, W. M. Neuronal death as a regulative mechanism in the control of cell number in the nervous system. In M. Rockstein (Ed.), *Development and aging in the nervous system.* New York: Academic Press, 1973, pp. 19–42.

Cytawa, J., and Teitelbaum, P. Spreading depression and recovery of subcortical functions. *Acta Biologica Experimentalis*, 1967, *27*, 345–353.

Dawson, R. G. Recovery of function: Implications for theories of brain function. *Behavioral Biology*, 1973, *8*, 439–460.

Eidelberg, E., Kreinick, C., J., and Langescheid, C. On the possible functional role of afferent pathways in skin sensation. *Experimental Neurology*, 1975, *47*, 419–432.

Falck, B. Observations on the possibilities of the cellular localization of monoamines by a flourescence method. *ACTA Physiologica Scandanavica*, 1962, *56:Suppl. 197*, 1–25.

Fass, B., Jordan, H., Rubman, A., Seibel, S., and Stein, D. G. Recovery of function after serial or one-stage lesions of the lateral hypothalamic area in rats. *Behavioral Biology*, 1975, *14*, 283–294.

Galambos, R., Norton, T. T., and Frommer, C. P. Optic tract lesions sparing pattern vision in cats. *Experimental Neurology*, 1967, *18*, 8–25.

Gazzaniga, M. S. Eye position and visual motor coordination. *Neuropsychologia*, 1969a, *7*, 379–382.

Gazzaniga, M. S. Cross-cuing mechanisms and ipsilateral eye-hand control in split brain monkeys. *Experimental Neurology*, 1969b, *23*, 11–17.

Gazzaniga, M. Determinants of cerebral recovery. In D. G. Stein, J. J. Rosen, and N. Butters (Eds.), *Plasticity and recovery of function in the central nervous system*. New York: Academic Press, 1974, pp. 203–216.

Gentile, A., Schmelzer, W., Green, S., Nieburgs, A., and Stein, D. G. Disruption and recovery of locomotion and manipulation following cortical lesions in rats. *Behavioral Biology*, in press.

Geschwind, N. Late changes in the nervous system: An overview. In D. G. Stein, J. J. Rosen, and N. Butters (Eds.), *Plasticity and recovery of function in the central nervous system*. New York: Academic Press, 1974, pp. 467–508.

Glassman, R. B. Contralateral and ipsilateral transfer of a cutaneous discrimination in normal and callosum-sectioned cats. *Journal of Comparative and Physiological Psychology*, 1970, *70*, 470–475.

Glick, S. D. Changes in drug sensitivity and mechanisms of functional recovery following brain damage. In D. G. Stein, J. J. Rosen, and N. Butters (Eds.), *Plasticity and recovery of function in the central nervous system*. New York: Academic Press, 1974, pp. 339–374.

Glick, S. D., and Greenstein, S. Possible modulating influence of frontal cortex on nigro-striatal function. *British Journal of Pharmacology*, 1973a, *49*, 316–321.

Glick, S. D., and Greenstein, S. Recovery of weight regulation following ablation of frontal cortex in rats. *Physiology and Behavior*, 1973b, *10*, 491–496.

Glick, S. D., and Zimmerberg, B. Comparative recovery following simultaneous and successive-stage frontal brain damage in mice. *Journal of Comparative and Physiological Psychology*, 1972, *79*, 481–487.

Goldberger, M. E. Restitution of function in the CNS: The pathologic grasp in *macaca mulatta*. *Experimental Brain Research*, 1972, *15*, 79–96.

Goldberger, M. E. Recovery of movement after CNS lesions in monkeys. In D. G. Stein, J. J. Rosen, and N. Butters (Eds.), *Plasticity and recovery of function in the central nervous system*. New York: Academic Press, 1974, pp. 265–337.

Goldman, P. S. Developmental determinants of cortical plasticity. *ACTA Neurobiologiae Experimentalis*, 1972, *32*, 495–511.

Goldman, P. An alternative to developmental plasticity: Heterology of CNS structures in infants and adults. In D. G. Stein, J. J. Rosen, and N. Butters (Eds.), *Plasticity and recovery of function in the central nervous system*. New York: Academic Press, 1974, pp. 149–174.

Goldman, P. Age, sex, and experience as related to the neural basis of cognitive development. In N. A. Buchwald and M. A. B. Brazier (Eds.), *Brain mechanisms in mental retardation*. New York: Academic Press, 1975, pp. 379–389.

Goodman, D. C., and Horel, J. A. Sprouting of optic tract projections in the brain stem of the rat. *Journal of Comparative Neurology*, 1966, *127*, 71–88.

Goodman, D. C., Bogdasarian, R. S., and Horel, J. A. Axonal sprouting of ipsilateral optic tract following opposite eye removal. *Brain, Behavior and Evolution*, 1973, *8*, 27–50.

Greenough, W. T., Fass, B., and deVoogd, T. The influence of experience on recovery following brain damage in rodents: Hypotheses based on development research. In R. N. Walsh and W. T. Greenough (Eds.), *Environments as therapy for brain dysfunction*. New York: Plenum Press, 1976.

Grossman, S. P. Direct adrenergic and cholinergic stimulation of hypothalamic mechanisms. *American Journal of Physiology,* 1962, *202,* 872–882.

Hecaen, H. Aphasic, apraxic and agnosic syndromes in right and left hemisphere lesions. In P. J. Vinken and G. W. Bruyn (Eds.), *Handbook of clinical neurology.* Vol. 4. Amsterdam: North Holland Publishing Company, 1969, pp. 176–179, 391–411.

Hicks, S. P., and d' Amato, C. J. Motor-sensory cortex-corticospinal system and developing locomotion and placing in rats. *American Journal of Anatomy,* 1975, *143,* 1–42.

Horel, J. A., Bettinger, L. A., Royce, G. J., and Meyer, D. R. Role of neo-cortex in the learning and re-learning of two visual habits by the rat. *Journal of Comparative and Physiological Psychology,* 1966, *61,* 66–78.

Isaacson, R. L. The myth of recovery from early brain damage. In N. R. Ellis, (Ed.) *Aberrant development in infancy.* Potomac, Md.: Lawrence Erlbaum, 1975.

Isseroff, A., Leveton, L., Freeman, G., Lewis, M., and Stein, D. G. The limits of behavioral recovery from serial lesions of the hippocampus. *Experimental Neurology,* 1976, *53,* 339–354.

Jackson, J. H. Remarks on the diagnosis and treatment of diseases of the brain. *British Medical Journal,* 1888, *2,* 59–63.

Kennard, M. A. Reorganization of motor function in the cerebral cortex of monkeys deprived of motor and premotor areas in infancy. *Journal of Neurophysiology,* 1938, *1,* 477–496.

Kleiner, F. B., Meyer, P. M., and Meyer, D. R. Effects of simultaneous septal and amygdaloid lesions upon emotionality and retention of a black-white discrimination. *British Research,* 1967, *5,* 459–468.

Lashley, K. S. Brain mechanisms and intelligence. Chicago: *University of Chicago Press,* 1929.

LeVere, T. E. Neural stability, sparing and behavioral recovery following brain damage. *Psychological Review,* 1975, *82,* 344–358.

Lund, R. D., and Lund, J. S. Synaptic adjustment after deafferentation of the superior colliculus of the rat. *Science,* 1971, *171,* 804–807.

Luria, A. R. *Restoration of brain function after war injuries.* Izd. Acad. Med. Nauk. *SSSR* (Moscow), 1948.

Luria, A. R., Naydin, V. L., Tsvetkova, L. S., and Vinarskaya, E. N. *Handbook of clinical neurology: disorders of the higher nervous system.* Vol. III. North Holland, American Elsevier, 1969, pp. 368–433.

Lynch, G., Matthews, D. A., Mosko, S., Parks, T., and Cotman, C. Induced acetylcholinesterase-rich layer in rat dentate gyrus following entorhinal lesions. *Brain Research,* 1972, *42,* 311–318.

Margules, D. L., Lewis, M. J., Dragovich, J. A., and Margules, A. S. Hypothalamic norepinephrine: circadian rhythms and the control of feeding behavior. *Science,* 1972, *178,* 640–642.

Merrill, E. G., and Wall, P. D. Factors forming the edge of a receptive field: The presence of relatively ineffective afferent terminals. *Journal of Physiology* (London), 1972, *226,* 825–846.

Meyer, D. R., Harlow, H. F., and Ades, H. W. Retention of delayed responses and proficiency in oddity problems by monkeys with preoccipital ablations. *American Journal of Psychology,* 1951, *64,* 391–396.

Meyer, P. M. Recovery from neo-cortical damage. In G. French (Ed.), *Cortical functioning in behavior.* Glenview, Ill.: Scott, Foresman, 1973, pp. 115–138.

Milner, B. Sparing of language functions after early unilateral brain damage. In E. Eidelberg and D. G. Stein, Functional recovery after lesions of the nervous system. *Neurosciences Research Program Bulletin,* 1974, *12,* 213–216.

Moore, R. Y. Central regeneration and recovery of function: The problem of collateral reinnervation. In D. G. Stein, J. J. Rosen, and N. Butters (Eds.), *Plasticity and recovery of function in the central nervous system.* New York: Academic Press, 1974, pp. 111–128.

Moore, R. Y., Björklund, A., and Stenevi, U. Plastic changes in the adrenergic innervation of the rat septal area in response to denervation. *Brain Research,* 1971, *33,* 13–35.

Nauta, W. H. J. M. The problem of the frontal lobe: A reinterpretation. *Journal of Psychiatric Research,* 1971, *8,* 167–187.

Pasik, P., Pasik, T., and Schilder, P. Extrageniculostriate vision in the monkey: discrimination of luminous flux-equated figures. *Experimental Neurology,* 1969, *24,* 421–437.

Pribram, K. H. *Languages of the brain: Experimental paradoxes and principles in neuropsychology.* Englewood Cliffs, N. J.: Prentice-Hall, 1971.

Prince, M. Cerebral localization from the point of view of function and symptoms. *Journal of Nervous and Mental Diseases,* 1910, *37,* 337–354.

Raisman, G. Neuronal plasticity in the septal nuclei of the adult brain. *Brain Research,* 1969, *14,* 25–48.

Raisman, G., and Field, P. M. A quantitative investigation of the development of collateral reinnervation after partial deafferentation of the septal nuclei. *Brain Research,* 1973, *50,* 241–264.

Rakic, R. Timing of major ontogenetic events in the visual cortex of the rhesus monkey. In N. A. Buchwald and M. A. B. Brazier (Eds.), *Brain mechanisms in mental retardation.* New York: Academic Press, 1975, pp. 3–37.

Reitan, R. M. Problems and prospects in studying the psychological correlates of brain lesions. *Cortex,* 1966, *2,* 127–154.

Riese, W. Principles of neurology. *Nervous and Mental Disease Monographs,* 1950, *80,* 1–168.

Rose, J. E., Malis, L. I., Kruger, L., and Baker, C. P. Effects of heavy ionizing monoenergetic particles on the cerebral cortex. II. Histological appearance of laminar lesions and growth of nerve fibers after laminar destruction. *Journal of Comparative Neurology,* 1959, *115,* 243–297.

Rose, J. E., Malis, L. I., and Baker, C. P. Neural growth in the cerebral cortex after lesions produced by monoenergetic deuterons. In W. A. Rosenblith (Ed.), *Sensory Communication.* Cambridge: M.I.T. Press, 1961.

Rosen, J. J., and Stein, D. G. Spontaneous alternation behavior in the rat. *Journal of Comparative and Physiological Psychology,* 1969, *68,* 420–426.

Rosen, J. J., Stein, D. G., and Butters, N. Recovery of function after serial ablation of prefrontal cortex in the rhesus monkey. *Science,* 1971, *173,* 353–356.

Rosner, B. S. Brain functions. *Annual Review of Psychology,* 1970, *21,* 555–594.

Rosner, G. Recovery of function and localization of function in historical perspective. In D. G. Stein, J. J. Rosen, and N. Butters (Eds.), *Plasticity and recovery of function in the central nervous system.* New York: Academic Press, 1974, pp. 1–30.

Schneider, G. E. Early lesions of superior colliculus: factors affecting the formation of abnormal retinal projections. *Brain, Behavior and Evolution,* 1973, *8,* 73–109.

Schneider, G. E., and Jhavari, S. R. Neuroanatomical correlates of spared or altered function after brain lesions in the newborn hamster. In D. G. Stein, J. J. Rosen, and N. Butters (Eds.), *Plasticity and recovery of function in the central nervous system.* New York: Academic Press, 1974, pp. 65–110.

Schultze, M., and Stein, D. G. Recovery of function in the albino rat following either simultaneous or seriatum lesions of the caudate nucleus. *Experimental Neurology,* 1975, *46,* 291–301.

Schwartzbaum, J. S., and Gray, P. E. Interacting behavioral effects of septal and amygdaloid lesions in the rat. *Journal of Comparative and Physiological Psychology,* 1966, *61,* 59–65.

Skolnick, P., and Daly, J. W. Norepinephrine-sensitive adenylate cyclases in rat brain: Relation to behavior and tyrosine hydroxylase. *Science,* 1974, *184,* 175–177.

Sotelo, C., and Palay, S. L. Altered axons and axon terminals in the lateral vestibular nucleus of the rat: Possible example of neuronal remodeling. *Laboratory Investigation,* 1971, *25,* 653–671.

Spear, P. D., and Braun, J. J. Pattern discrimination following removal of visual neocortex in the cat. *Experimental Neurology,* 1969, *25,* 331–348.

Spear, P. S., and Barbas, H. Recovery of pattern discrimination ability in rats receiving serial or one-stage visual cortex lesions. *Brain Research,* 1975, *94,* 337–346.

Stein, D. G., Rosen, J. J., Graziadei, J., Mishkin, D., and Brink, J. Central nervous system: Recovery of function. *Science,* 1969, *166,* 528–530.

Stein, D. G. Some variables influencing recovery of function after CNS lesions in the rat. In D. G. Stein, J. J. Rosen, and N. Butters (Eds.), *Plasticity and recovery of function in the central nervous system.* New York: Academic Press, 1974, pp. 373–427.

Stein, D. G., Rosen, J. J., Butters, N. (Eds.), *Plasticity and recovery of function in the central nervous system.* New York: Academic Press, 1974.

Stein, D. G., and Firl, A. Brain damage and reorganization of function in old age. *Experimental Neurology,* 1976, *52,* 157–167.

Stenevi, U., Björklund, A., and Moore, R. Y. Growth of intact central adrenergic axons in the denervated lateral geniculate body. *Experimental Neurology,* 1972, *35,* 290–299.

Stenevi, U., Björklund, A., and Moore, R. Y. Morphological plasticity of central adrenergic neurons. *Brain, Behavior and Evolution,* 1973, *8,* 110–134.

Teitelbaum, P. The encephalization of hunger. In E. Steller and J. M. Sprague (Eds.), *Progress in Physiological Psychology.* Vol. 4. New York: Academic Press, 1971, pp. 319–346.

Teitelbaum, P., and Cytawa, J. Spreading depression and recovery from lateral hypothalamic damage. *Science,* 1965, *147,* 61–63.

Teitelbaum, P. and Epstein, A. The lateral hypothalamic syndrome: Recovery of feeding and drinking after lateral hypothalamic lesions. *Psychological Review,* 1962, *69,* 74–90.

Teuber, H. L. Recovery of function after lesions of the central nervous system: History and prospects. In E. Eidelberg and D. G. Stein, *Functional recovery after lesions of the nervous system.* Vol. 12. Neurosciences Research Program Bulletin, 1974, pp. 197–211.

Trendelenburg, U. Supersensitivity and subsensitivity to sympathamimetic amines. *Pharmacological Review,* 1963, *15,* 225–277.

Trendelenburg, U. Factors influencing the concentration of catecholamines at the receptors. In H. Blaschko and E. Muscholl (Eds.), *Catecholamines: Handbuch der Experimentellen Pharmakologie, XXXIII,* Berlin: Springer-Verlag, 1972.

Ungerstedt, U., Ljungberg, T., Hoffer, B., and Siggins, G. Dopaminergic supersensitivity in the striatum. In D. B. Calne, T. N. Chase, and A. Barbeau (Eds.), *Advances in neurology,* Vol. 9. *Dopaminergic Mechanisms.* New York: Raven Press, 1975, pp. 57–66.

von Monakow, C. Diaschisis. (1914). Excerpted in K. H. Pribram (Ed.), *Mood, States, and Mind.* London: Penguin Books, 1969, pp. 27–37.

Wall, P. D., and Egger, M. D. Formation of new connections in adult rat brains after partial deafferentation. *Nature,* 1971, *232,* 542–545.

Wall, P. D. Plasticity in the adult mammalian central nervous system. Unpublished manuscript, 1976.

West, J. R., Deadwyler, S., Cotman, C. W., and Lynch, G. Time-dependent changes in commissural field potentials in the dentate gyrus following lesions of the entorhinal cortex in adult rats. *Brain Research,* 1975, *97,* 215–233.

Wickelgren, B. G., and Sterling, P. Influence of visual on receptive fields in cat superior colliculus. *Journal of Neurophysiology*, 1969, *32*, 16–23.

Will, B. E., and Rosenzweig, M. Effets de l'environnement sur la recuperation fonctionnelle après lesions cerebrales chez les rats adultes. *Biology of Behaviour*, 1976, *1*, 5– 16.

Winans, S. S. Visual form discrimination after removal of the visual cortex in cats. *Science*, 1967, *158*, 944.

Zeki, S. M. The secondary visual areas of the monkey. *Brain Research*, 1969, *13*, 197–226.

Zigmond, J. J., and Stricker, E. M. Recovery of feeding after 6-hydroxydopamine (6-HDA) or lateral hypothalamic lesions: The role of catecholamines. *Federation Proceedings of American Society for Experimental Biology*, 1973, *32*, 754.

Zülch, K. J., Creutzfeldt, O., and Galbraith, G. C. *Cerebral localization.* Berlin: Springer-Verlag, 1975.

15

Is Seeing Believing: Notes on Clinical Recovery

MICHAEL S. GAZZANIGA

A persistent phenomenon in the neurological clinic is that patients who experience mild to severe cerebral damage and who show at the onset serious behavioral deficits usually recover some, if not all, of the lost function. While this is an enormous benefit to the patient, for which all are thankful, it is downright disconcerting to the neuropsychologist, who is trying to identify steady-state changes in behavior that are traceable to specific neurological lesions.

There have been several attempts at trying to understand this recovery process. The easiest and clearly the least controversial is the recovery seen as a consequence of reduced cerebral edema, when the function lost was simply a by-product of a state of transient swelling. This, of course, is a common event and holds little mystery. What is more perplexing is the recovery of function seen following cases of real tissue damage, loss, or disconnection. Our first observations on the phenomenon were from the last category and out of that came insights into the mechanisms active in the first two. In general, it is our belief that recovery almost invariably is the product of an alternate behavioral strategy being brought into play, with a patient in a sense solving a behavioral task by taking a different "road to Rome."

MICHAEL S. GAZZANIGA • Department of Psychology, State University of New York, Stony Brook, New York 11794, and Department of Neurology, Cornell Medical College, New York, New York 10021

1. CROSS-CUING IN THE SPLIT BRAIN

1.1. Somesthesia

One of the earliest observations of ours that suggested the importance of changing behavioral strategies to cover for an actual and persistent neurological deficit came from the way split-brain patients learned how to identify objects from a limited set held in the left hand. Immediately after commissurotomy, the patients were unable to identify objects of any kind in the left hand. In time, however, they became adept at identifying the objects if they were told that it was one of two items. Thus, if a ball and a square were given to the left hand and the patient had to say which was which, good performance was soon seen in the commissure-sectioned cases. This meant that somehow somatosensory information from the left hand was getting to the left speech hemisphere.

On the surface, one interpretation was that stereognostic information from the left hand was somehow making its way to the left hemisphere either through subcallosal pathways or perhaps through ipsilateral routes. It turned out, however, that neither of these possibilities was the case. Instead, the ipsilateral tracks coursing up to the left hemisphere could carry quantitative information (Gazzaniga, 1970), and the patients learned to deduce by presence or absence of stimulation, by duration of feeling an edge, and the like what one of the two objects it might be. If these same objects, however, were placed in a larger set and there was no limit on what the objects might be, their performance quickly fell to chance. In other words, when the left hemisphere knew what the objects were, it could deduce from quantitative cues available to it from the ipsilateral pathways which of the two was being presented on a given trial. It did not know them because of a stereognostic sense of what the objects were.

Working with the somatosensory system, then, we find a clinical–surgical case in which there seems to be recovery of function for the recognition of objects. Yet, by careful behavioral analysis, it turns out that the knowledge of the object comes from quite a different behavioral and neurological base than is normally used by the patient.

1.2. Visual Functions

Perhaps a more dramatic example of apparent recovery came from our results (Gazzaniga and Hillyard, 1971) on visual testing of the right hemisphere. In visual testing of patient L.B., we noticed in a particular training session that he was able to name one of two numerals flashed to the right hemisphere from the speech center on the left. At first we felt that perhaps the subcallosal pathways were opening up and able to transfer simple perceptual information. This proved not to be the case, however, and a careful behavioral analysis revealed that what appeared as recovery was instead the appearance of a sophisticated behavioral strategy.

In presenting the simple numerals, we suddenly flashed L.B. a new numeral, the number 2. After the trial, he winced, looked at me, and said, "That's not a zero or a one," and I replied that he was correct, and told him that from here on in, we were going to present a series of numerals. To our great surprise, after a few trials, L.B. was beginning to name not only the zero and the one, but any numeral up to eight.

Again, at first glance, this was a remarkable shift in behavior, and we concluded that either the right hemisphere was capable of some simple speech or the left hemisphere was now a recipient of subcallosal information. Both hypotheses, however, proved to be grossly incorrect. Careful analysis of the reaction time to each of the numerals showed that L.B. took more time to respond to one than to zero, two than one, four than three, five than six, and so on. What we discovered he was doing was using a very sophisticated cross-cuing strategy (Gazzaniga and Hillyard, 1971). The left hemisphere commenced a count, and with that process there was a slight head movement. When the number flashed coresponded to the counted number, the right hemisphere signaled the left hemisphere by stopping the head. The left hemisphere observed this and said to the experimenter "four" or "three," or whatever the number might be on a particular trial. This was evident because when the subject was not allowed an indeterminate time to respond, scores on the presented information dropped to chance.

Again, what looked like a major change in behavior, with neurological implications for recovery, turned out to be a sophisticated behavioral strategy.

2. THE NEUROLOGICAL PATIENT

2.1. Disorder in Manipulo-Spatial Skills

It is my opinion that the same kind of process of what is essentially self-cuing goes on in more traditional cases of brain damage. For example, in a recent analysis of a patient with a large right parietal infarct, it became clear that the kind of recovery one sees in much of that syndrome was a function of switching behavioral strategies. In particular, in the first weeks after the infarct, the ability of the patient to construct blocks, perform the Milner wire-figure test, and carry out other tasks usually thought to require proper right parietal lobe functioning was extremely poor, at best. Approximately 5 weeks after the infarct, however, the patient began to recover some ability to perform the block-design tasks, even though the performance was tedious and painfully slow, and in no way natural. The patient, who had a 139 verbal IQ, seemed to be putting the blocks together, not because of a return of the manipulo-spatial skills required (Le Doux, Wilson, and Gazzaniga, 1977), but by a verbal strategy and deduction, a skill that was clearly remaining to him. However, when the wire-figure test was used at the same point in time when he was performing better on the block design, his score immediately dropped to chance again. This task, which did not lend itself to easy verbal description, proved to be continuing to manifesting his deficit.

Our interpretation of these observations is that the actual deficit in manipulo-spatial activities produced by the right hemisphere lesion is persistent. The apparent return of abilities on the more verbalizable block test is a product of the verbal processor coming into play and assisting in solution of the task (Le Doux, Wilson, and Gazzaniga, 1978).

2.2. Disorders in Language

A frequent yet little-considered phenomenon in the neurologic clinic is that patients with dominant hemisphere disease frequently suffer from an anomia or dysnomia. This inability to find nouns is in marked contrast to the ability to use verbs. What is remarkable about this language disorder, as with many others, is that the deficit appears to recede. Recent experimentation of ours on a new split-brain patient offers us a clue on one of several possible underlying mechanisms that allows for this.

Verbal commands were presented to the right hemisphere of a split-brain patient (Gazzaniga, Le Doux, and Wilson, 1977) with a high language ability. The patient was able to carry them out. Thus, if the word "point" was flashed to the right hemisphere, the patient would point with the left hand. Under more routine conditions, words flashed to the right hemisphere that involve no discrete graphic motor response go undescribed because the speech center in the left hemisphere is disconnected from the right half-brain. In test situations like this, however, the patient, when asked what he saw, says "Oh, 'point.' " When the word "rub" was flashed, the patient rubbed the back of his head, and when asked what the command has been, he said, "Uh, 'itch.' "

What the patient is doing is this: The left hemisphere, watching the movement being produced and under the control of the right half-brain, then simply describes the action much as he would describe the action of another person. When the response is unequivocal, like pointing, his description is accurate. When it could easily be the result of a number of commands, such as words like "rub," he works at a chance level.

One can immediately see a possible parallel with the clinical problem of anomia. It is common experience to see that such a patient will be unable to name an object like a comb. Yet when the patient picks it up and starts to use it, and is asked "What are you doing?" he typically says "Combing—oh, it is a comb." When a paper clip is placed in front of the patient, he says he is unable to name it. When he is asked what he is doing, when he is using it, he says typically "Clipping papers—oh, a clip."

It would appear that the ability to name is a function of a stragegy. The item must be considered by its use, which then allows the object to become a verb, and verbs can still be accessed in these patients. The clever patient need not go through the actual action, but merely has to be asked how it is used.

3. SUMMARY

In example after example from the clinic, one can point to alternative behavioral strategies that seem to be active in covering for a neurological deficit. These clinical examples serve up fair warning that the improvement in function following neurological insult may not reflect recovery of function in neurological sense. They may reflect the ingenious ability of the organisms to maintain a behavioral status quo by using other mental and behavioral resources.

ACKNOWLEDGMENT

This work was aided by USPHS Grant No. 25643.

4. REFERENCES

Gazzaniga, M. S. *The bisected brain.* New York: Appleton-Century-Crofts, 1970.
Gazzaniga, M. S., and Hillyard, S. A. Language and speech capacity of the right hemisphere. *Neuropsychologia,* 1971, *9,* 273–280.

Gazzaniga, M. S., Le Doux, J. E., and Wilson, D. H. Language praxis and the right hemi-
    sphere: Clues to some mechanisms of consciousness. *Neurology,* in press. (1977)
Le Doux, J. E., Wilson, D. H., and Gazzaniga, M. S. Manipulo-spatial aspects of cerebral
    lateralization: Clues to the origin of lateralization. *Neuropsychologia,* in press. (1977)
Le Doux, J. E., Wilson, D. H., and Gazzaniga, M. S. Block design performance following
    callosal sectioning: observations in functional recovery. *Arch. Neurol.,* in press.
    (1978)

Index

Ablation, *see* Brain lesion studies
Acetylcholine, in septal-rage syndrome, 288
Age, serial lesions and, 150
Age—brain damage relationship, 115-132
  age factor in, 116-119
  delayed effects in, 121-122
  future research in, 130-132
  recovery mechanisms in, 119-120
  regional brain differences in, 120-121
Age factor, in lesion experiments, 82-83
Agnosia, visual, *see* Visual agnosia
Alpha-methyl-para-tyrosine, 391
Alternating monocular deprivation, 336-337
AMD, *see* Alternating monocular deprivation
6-Aminodopamine, 95
Amphetamine, ipsilateral rotation and, 285
Amphetamine-induced hyperactivity, 289
Amphetamine injection, behavior recovery and, 176-177
Amphetamine sensitivity, functional recovery and, 290-291
Amygdalectomy, in kittens and monkeys, 125-126
Anatomical considerations, in lesion experiments, 71-85
Anatomical models, in brain-lesion studies, 322-323
Animal models, in lesion-momentum studies, 137-141
Aphagia, from hypothalamic lesions, 171
Aphasia
  left hemispheric damage and, 135-136
  visual agnosia and, 60
Army General Classification Test, 318

Audition
  frequency discrimination in, 260-262
  subtotal lesions and, 260-265
Auditory cortex, ablation of, 40-41
Auditory cortical evoked potentials, 261-262
Auditory localization, subtotal lesions and, 263-265
Auditory system, tonotopic organization of, 265
Axon
  changes in, 77
  transection of, 77

BD, *see* Binocular deprivation
Behavior, *see also* Behavioral recovery
  anatomical structure and, 24
  associations and dissociations in, 4
  class-common, 36-38
  hypothalamic control of, 44-45
  lesion momentum and, 135-160
  lesions and, 24
  training level and, 201
Behavioral capacity
  brain damage and, 131
  sparing and, 178
Behavioral change, vs. behavioral recovery, 168-169
Behavioral data
  brain function and, 16-18
  stimulus-response events in, 199-200
  testing procedures and interpretation of, 199-215
Behavioral deficiency, 178
  cause of, 201
  defined, 193-194
  delayed, 121-122
  training level and, 211-212

415